DRUG INTERACTIONS

MONOGRAPHS OF THE MARIO NEGRI INSTITUTE FOR PHARMACOLOGICAL RESEARCH, MILAN

SERIES EDITOR: SILVIO GARATTINI

Amphetamines and Related Compounds
Edited by E. Costa and S. Garattini

The Benzodiazepines
Edited by S. Garattini, E. Mussini, and L. O. Randall

Chemotherapy of Cancer Dissemination and Metastasis
Edited by S. Garattini and G. Franchi

Isolated Liver Perfusion and Its Applications
Edited by I. Bartosek, A. Guaitani, and L. L. Miller

Drug Interactions
Edited by P. L. Morselli, S. Garattini, and S. N. Cohen

Insolubilized Enzymes
Edited by M. Salmona, C. Saronio, and S. Garattini

Mass Spectrometry in Biochemistry and Medicine
Edited by A. Frigerio and N. Castagnoli, Jr.

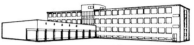

MONOGRAPHS OF THE MARIO NEGRI INSTITUTE FOR PHARMACOLOGICAL RESEARCH, MILAN

Drug Interactions

Editors

P. L. Morselli, M.D.
Head, Clinical Pharmacology
  Department
Mario Negri Institute for
  Pharmacological Research
Milan, Italy

S. Garattini, M.D.
Director, Mario Negri Institute
  for Pharmacological Research
Milan, Italy

S. N. Cohen, M.D.
Division of Clinical Pharmacology
Stanford University School of Medicine
Stanford, California

Raven Press ■ New York

Distributed in the Eastern Hemisphere by
North-Holland Publishing Company ■ Amsterdam

Made in the United States of America

International Standard Book Number
0-911216-59-6
Library of Congress Catalog Card Number
74-77802.

ISBN outside North and South America only:
0-7204-7522-8

Preface

It has been known for quite some time that the combination of two or more drugs often produces therapeutic or toxic results which may be quite different than what would be expected knowing the pharmacological action of each of the single compounds involved. Thus, it has been recognized that certain drugs may interact with others in the organism, either enhancing or abolishing their beneficial or adverse effects. Only recently, however, have some of the mechanisms of such interactions become more clearly understood.

The purpose of the international and interdisciplinary symposium upon which this volume is based is not only to present all the information available on the most important types of drug interactions reported so far, but also to discuss the various basic molecular events underlying these processes.

While in the past, pharmacologists tended to consider drug interactions as phenomena taking place only at certain receptor sites, the current feeling is that there may be many other factors involved. This is based on recent findings that a number of drug interactions may occur outside the receptor sites and take place at the level of absorption, excretion, metabolism, tissue distribution, protein binding, and subcellular localization. Thus it is of crucial importance to consider all these alternative possibilities when trying to determine the chemical and biochemical mechanism, and the actual site of drug action or interaction. Also, the role of pharmacogenetic differences and exogenous factors, which may modify the human response to drugs, must be considered.

Although, at present, most of the attention is being focused on the adverse reactions and drug antagonism resulting from drug combinations, it is evident that beneficial therapeutic effects could also be obtained by combining certain carefully selected compounds, and using them in appropriate doses, modes, and schedules of administration.

It is hoped that this volume will help in placing drug therapy on a more rational basis and thus facilitate the task of clinicians, pharmacologists, and other scientists who are concerned with drug combinations and interactions. Although they may approach this problem at different levels, depending on their particular discipline, all their efforts are directed toward the same goal —attaining a better understanding of the many different factors involved in drug therapy, so that it may be individually tailored to suit the particular needs of each individual patient.

S. Garattini
*Director, Mario
Negri Institute of
Pharmacological Research*

Contents

IMPORTANCE OF MEASURING DRUG LEVELS IN THERAPY

DESIGN OF PROTOCOL FOR EVALUATING DRUG INTERACTIONS

DRUG INTERACTION INFORMATION SYSTEMS

Drug Interactions, edited by P. L. Morselli,
S. Garattini, and S. N. Cohen. Raven Press,
New York © 1974

Drug Interactions: Historical Aspects and Perspectives

J. J. Burns and A. H. Conney

Roche Research Center, Nutley, New Jersey 07110

INTRODUCTION

The need for an international symposium on drug interactions is obvious in view of the great interest in this subject today. Literally an explosion of information has occurred since the first major conference on drug interactions held at the Royal Society of Medicine in London in 1965 (1). The organizing committee should be congratulated for putting together a comprehensive and well-balanced program. The clinical relevance of observations in animals is appropriately stressed, and proper emphasis is also given to the importance of new methodology for the measurement of extremely small amounts of drugs and their metabolites during the investigation of drug interactions. The need for a proper perspective in this field is paramount, since compilations are appearing that list an enormous number of drug interactions, many of which are based solely on animal experiments or poorly documented clinical reports (2–4). This volume should do much to establish a scientific basis for considering drug interactions and to facilitate an understanding of their importance in drug therapy. In order to gain some perspective, two types of drug interactions are discussed in this presentation. The first, enzyme induction, has attracted considerable attention, whereas the other, ascorbic-acid interactions, is less well known.

ENZYME INDUCTION

The activities of drug-metabolizing enzymes in liver microsomes are markedly increased when animals are treated for several days with drugs, insecticides, carcinogens, hormones, or other endogenous or foreign chemicals (5–10). A great many enzymes are affected, including those that catalyze N-, S-, and O-dealkylation, hydroxylation deamination, sulfoxidation, azo-link reduction, and glucuronidation. This increase in enzyme activity appears to represent an increased concentration of enzyme protein and is referred to as "enzyme induction."

Two important points become obvious when one considers enzyme induction. First is the question of whether a change in enzyme activity *in vitro* is reflected by a corresponding change in the metabolism and action of a drug *in vivo*. The magnitude of the change in the action of a drug that may occur after enzyme induction in animals is illustrated by data obtained from rats treated with the muscle relaxant zoxazolamine (11). A high dose of this drug paralyzed rats for more than 11 hr, but after pretreatment with phenobarbital for 4 days, rats were paralyzed for only 102 min. After pretreatment with 3,4-benzpyrene for 1 day, the same dose of zoxazolamine paralyzed the rats for only 17 min. The biological half-life of zoxazolamine is 9 hr in control rats, 48 min in phenobarbital-treated rats, and 10 min in 3,4-benzpyrene-treated animals.

The second point is the extrapolation from an *in vitro* effect in animals to significance in therapy. This is illustrated by the observation that phenobarbital stimulates the activity of enzymes that metabolize bishydroxycoumarin and warfarin in the rat (12, 13), and that administration of phenobarbital decreases the blood level and anticoagulant activity of these coumarin anticoagulants in man (12, 14). Hundreds of examples of enzyme induction have been reported (1–10), but their actual relevance in human drug therapy has only been established for a few. An interesting new drug interaction has recently been reported by Brooks et al. (15). These investigators showed that the administration of phenobarbital decreased the plasma half-life of dexamethasone and decreased the effectiveness of a glucocorticoid during therapy of the asthmatic patient.

There are a number of future needs for research on enzyme induction, and some of these are given below.

(a) Many environmental chemicals, including chlorinated hydrocarbon insecticides, carcinogenic hydrocarbons, food additives, and cigarette smoke, cause enzyme induction (10). Increased metabolism of phenylbutazone and antipyrine in workers occupationally exposed to lindane and DDT is reported by B. Kolmodin-Hedman in this volume. Decreased plasma levels of phenacetin were observed in cigarette smokers (Table 1) (16). Al-

TABLE 1. *Plasma levels of phenacetin in cigarette smokers and nonsmokers at various intervals after the oral administration of 900 mg of phenacetin*

| | Hours after phenacetin administration | | | |
	1	2	$3\frac{1}{2}$	5
Subjects	Phenacetin in plasma (μg/ml)			
Nonsmokers	0.81 ± 0.20	2.24 ± 0.73	0.39 ± 0.13	0.12 ± 0.04
Smokers	0.33 ± 0.23	0.48 ± 0.28	0.09 ± 0.04	0.02 ± 0.01

Each value represents the mean $\pm$SE for nine subjects (16).

though all of the nonsmokers studied had appreciable blood levels of phenacetin, several of the smokers had no detectable levels of this drug. Increased activity of benzpyrene hydroxylase was observed in the placentas of pregnant females who smoked cigarettes (17). Although we are all exposed to many environmental chemicals during our daily life, the effects of this exposure on the safety and efficacy of drugs needs to be determined.

(b) Administration of a variety of drugs and other foreign chemicals stimulates their own metabolism in animals. The importance of enzyme induction in the interpretation of chronic toxicity studies is illustrated by two examples. After the first day of administration of a high dose of phenylbutazone to rats, the animals developed gastrointestinal lesions and had high plasma levels of the drug, but after daily administration of phenylbutazone for 2 weeks, the lesions disappeared, and the plasma levels were low (18). After a single dose of citrus red no. 2 (2,5-dimethoxyphenyl-azo-2-naphthol), a high concentration of this dye occurred in the fat of rats, but when the dye was given daily for 5 days, the concentration of dye in fat was reduced by a factor of 15 (19). After this chemical was given for 7 days, no dye could be detected in the fat. There is a need to establish the importance of enzyme induction in the safety evaluation of new drugs and environmental chemicals (20). The consequences of long-term exposure to low doses of enzyme inducers should be further investigated.

(c) Recent studies have shown that minor pathways of metabolism (i.e., N-hydroxylation or epoxide formation) may explain certain toxic reactions (21–24). Since some of these metabolites are highly reactive and combine with tissue proteins and nucleic acids, the metabolites can cause tissue lesions resulting in allergic reactions, cancer, and teratological effects. The role of enzyme inducers in altering the amounts of these minor metabolites, and thereby altering the drug's toxicity, needs to be clarified.

(d) Nutritional factors, i.e., starvation and protein or vitamin deficiency, have been shown to influence the activity of drug-metabolizing enzymes in liver microsomes. It is of interest that there are substances present in food that can cause enzyme induction. Animals on a chow diet have higher levels of microsomal enzyme activity than animals on a synthetic diet (25). In addition, it was recently shown that Brussel sprouts and other vegetables markedly stimulate the activity of hydroxylating enzymes in the intestinal mucosa of the rat (26). The significance of dietary factors in human drug therapy needs further investigation.

(e) Phenobarbital has found use in the treatment of certain diseases of hyperbilirubinemia. Chronic administration of phenobarbital lowers the serum bilirubin level in patients with chronic intrahepatic cholestasis (27), Gilbert's syndrome (28), hemolytic jaundice (29), and in some, but not all, infants with congenital nonhemolytic jaundice (30–34). The possible role of enzyme induction in treating other diseases should be explored.

ASCORBIC ACID-DRUG INTERACTIONS

There are three types of ascorbic acid-drug interactions which will be considered here:

(a) About 15 years ago, we found that compounds that cause enzyme induction also increase markedly the synthesis of ascorbic acid in the rat (35). These studies suggested, for the first time, that a wide variety of chemicals of markedly different structures and pharmacological activities could stimulate the activity of drug-metabolizing enzymes in liver microsomes. Examples of these stimulators include drugs (phenobarbital, Chloretone, phenylbutazone), polycyclic hydrocarbons (3-methylcholanthrene and 3,4-benzpyrene), and insecticides (DDT and chlordane). The marked effect of a single dose of Chloretone and 3-methylcholanthrene on ascorbic acid excretion in the rat is shown in Fig. 1. Turnover rate studies with ^{14}C-labeled ascorbic acid documented the overall stimulatory effect of these chemicals on ascorbic acid synthesis (Table 2) (36–38). Further studies showed that, in rats, drugs stimulate increased synthesis of ascorbic acid via the glucuronic acid pathway of glucose metabolism (Fig. 2). Since humans lack the enzyme system required for the conversion of L-gulonolactone to L-ascorbic acid (39), increased excretion of L-ascorbic acid does not occur following drug administration in man. However, increased excretion of D-glucaric acid (a metabolite of glucuronic acid) is observed. Interestingly enough, D-glucaric acid excretion has been used as a measure of the ability

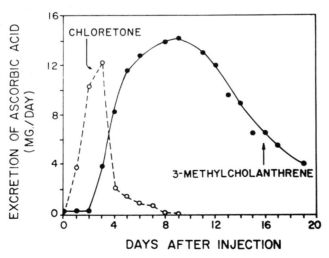

FIG. 1. Stimulation of L-ascorbic acid excretion by 3-methylcholanthrene and Chloretone. A rat was injected intraperitoneally with a 10-mg dose of 3-methylcholanthrene, and another rat was injected with a 40-mg dose of Chloretone (36).

TABLE 2. *Effect of chemicals on ascorbic acid metabolism in the rat*

Pretreatment	Body pool of AA	Turnover rate of AA	Excretion of AA	Metabolism of AA
None	10.7	2.6	0.40	2.2
Chloretone	19.2	21.5	10.2	11.3
3-Methylcholanthrene	22.5	19.0	7.1	11.9

Chloretone (45 mg) was administered orally for 4 to 7 days prior to the administration of L-ascorbic acid-1-^{14}C. 3-Methylcholanthrene (10 mg) was injected i.p. daily for 4 days, and the L-ascorbic acid-1-^{14}C was administered 5 days later. All values are given on a milligram-per-100-gram body weight basis (38).

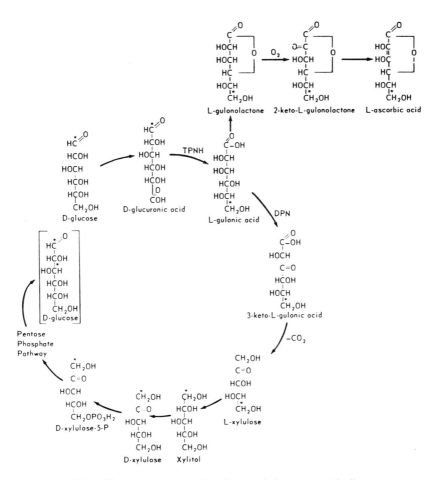

FIG. 2. The glucuronic acid pathway of glucose metabolism.

of drugs to cause enzyme induction in man (40). Similarly, increased excretion of ascorbic acid has been used to test whether compounds cause enzyme induction in rats. The mechanism by which drugs stimulate the synthesis of ascorbic acid via the glucuronic acid pathway is not known, and further research is required to determine why the same chemicals stimulate both the synthesis of ascorbic acid and the activity of drug-metabolizing enzymes.

(b) Decreased activity of drug-metabolizing enzymes occurs in guinea pigs fed an ascorbic acid-deficient diet (38). Zoxazolamine had a prolonged duration of action in vitamin C–deficient guinea pigs with no obvious sign of scurvy (Table 3). In addition, the increased duration of this drug *in vivo* can be explained by a decrease in its oxidation *in vitro* in liver microsomes prepared from vitamin C-deficient guinea pigs. Zannoni and Lynch (41) and Avenia (42) showed that levels of microsomal electron transport components, such as cytochrome P-450 and NADPH cytochrome P-450 reductase, are decreased significantly in ascorbic acid–deficient guinea pigs. Impaired activity of drug-metabolizing enzymes, and the lowered levels of electron transport components, can be restored to normal when the animals receive an adequate intake of vitamin C. The possibility that humans who have an insufficient intake of vitamin C could show increased sensitivity, and possible toxicity, to drugs should be investigated.

(c) Ascorbic acid has been reported recently to prevent the formation of nitrosamines, which come from the interaction of nitrites with secondary and tertiary amines. In studies carried out with J. Kamm, oral administration of sodium nitrite, together with aminopyrine, causes severe hepatic necrosis in the rat (43). The hepatotoxicity is presumably due to formation of nitrosodimethylamine resulting from the cleavage of aminopyrine by nitrous acid formed from sodium nitrite in the acidic environment of the rat stomach. Ascorbate prevents the rise in SGPT when coadministered with sodium nitrite and aminopyrine (Table 4), and ascorbate also prevents the microscopic changes in the liver observed when sodium nitrite and aminopyrine

TABLE 3. *Effect of ascorbic acid deficiency on drug action in guinea pigs*

Diet	Duration of zoxazolamine paralysis (min)	In vitro metabolism (μg zoxazolamine metabolized)
Ascorbic acid-supplemented	156 ± 41	36 ± 12
Ascorbic acid-deficient	309 ± 27	$12 \pm\ 8$

Guinea pigs were maintained on a scorbutogenic diet with or without the oral administration of 10 mg of ascorbic acid daily. The duration of zoxazolamine paralysis was determined after the i.p. injection of 100 mg/kg of zoxazolamine. The *in vitro* enzyme assays were carried out by incubating liver microsomes from 375 mg of liver with 100 μg of zoxazolamine for 15 min in the presence of an NADPH-generating system (38).

TABLE 4. *Effect of ascorbic acid on elevation of serum alanine aminotransferase (SGPT) activity in rats caused by sodium nitrite plus aminopyrine*

Treatment	Enzyme level (international units/liter)
Saline	16.1 ± 3.3 (N = 10)
Sodium nitrite + aminopyrine	86.2 ± 49.2 (N = 10)
Sodium nitrite + aminopyrine + ascorbic acid	16.1 ± 5.4 (N = 10)

Male rats were treated orally once a day for 2 days with saline (1.0 ml/kg), sodium nitrite (110 mg/kg), aminopyrine (130 mg/kg), and ascorbic acid (75 mg/kg). SGPT was assayed 48 hr after the last dose (43).

are administered alone. Other workers have recently found that ascorbic acid can block other toxicities caused by the interaction of amines and nitrite. Ivankovic and his associates (44) have reported that ascorbate prevents the development of hydrocephali in the offspring of rats administered ethylurea and sodium nitrite on days 10 and 11 of pregnancy. They suggest that ascorbate acts by inhibiting the formation of nitroso-ethylurea. Mirvish and his associates (45) have recently demonstrated that sodium ascorbate markedly decreases the incidence of lung adenomas in mice fed chronically either piperazine or morpholine in food in combination with sodium nitrite in their drinking water. Recently, Lijinsky and his associates (46) have shown that the chronic feeding of sodium nitrite plus aminopyrine in drinking water leads to an almost 100% incidence of liver tumors in rats. Work currently under way in our laboratory is designed to test the effect of ascorbate in this model system for aminopyrine-nitrite carcinogenicity. It is of considerable interest that nitrosopyrrolidine, a potent carcinogen in animals, is formed during the cooking of bacon and that this effect is blocked by ascorbate, which is added during the curing process (47). It is possible that the addition of high levels of ascorbate to other nitrite-containing foods will inhibit the formation of potentially toxic nitrosamines.

CONCLUSION

Many approaches are being pursued in research on drug interactions. In this presentation, some of these were illustrated from examples of investigations on enzyme induction and ascorbic acid drug interactions. In research on drug interactions, there is an urgent need to determine whether the interactions observed at the enzyme level or in laboratory animals have relevance in human drug therapy. The clinical pharmacologist plays a key role in the extrapolation of such animal data to man, and also in the proper education of the physician as to the clinical significance of drug interactions. This volume should do much to establish perspectives in the area of drug interactions. The importance of this field is evident from the activities of a number of scientific groups in the World Health Organization and the National Academy of Sciences. Research programs on drug interactions have been given a high priority by the Pharmacology-Toxicology Program of the National Institute of General Medical Sciences and by other organizations throughout the world.

REFERENCES

1. Burns, J. J., and Conney, A. H. (1965): *Proc. Royal Soc. Med. Symposium No. 7,* Clinical Effects of Interaction Between Drugs *58,* 955.
2. *The Medical Letter on Drugs and Therapeutics, 15,* 77 (1973).
3. Avery, G. S. (1973): *Drugs 5,* 187.
4. Sher, S. P. (1971): *Toxicol. Appl. Pharmacol. 18,* 780.
5. Remmer, H. (1962): *Proc. First International Pharmacology Mtg.,* Stockholm, Vol. 6, p. 235, MacMillan, New York.
6. Conney, A. H., and Burns, J. J. (1962): *Adv. Pharmacol. 1,* 31.
7. Conney, A. H. (1967): *Pharmacol. Rev. 19,* 317.
8. Gelboin, H. V. (1967): *Adv. Cancer Res. 10,* 1.
9. Selye, H. (1971): *Hormones and Resistance,* Vols. 1 and 2, Springer-Verlag, New York.
10. Conney, A. H., and Burns, J. J. (1972): *Science 178,* 576.
11. Conney, A. H., Davison, C., Gastel, R., and Burns, J. J. (1960): *J. Pharmacol. Exp. Therap. 130,* 1.
12. Cucinell, S. A., Conney, A. H., Sansur, M., and Burns, J. J. (1965): *Clin. Pharmacol. Therap. 6,* 420.
13. Ikeda, M., Conney, A. H., and Burns, J. J. (1968): *J. Pharmacol. Exp. Therap. 162,* 338.
14. MacDonald, M. G., Robinson, D. S., Sylwester, D., and Jaffe, J. J. (1969): *Clin. Pharmacol. Therap. 10,* 80.
15. Brooks, S. M., Werk, E., Ackerman, S. J., Sullivan, I., and Thrasher, K. (1972): *New England J. Med. 286,* 1125.
16. Pantuck, E. J., Kuntzman, R., and Conney, A. H. (1972): *Science 175,* 1248.
17. Welch, R. M., Harrison, Y. E., Gommi, B. W., Poppers, P. J., Finster, M., and Conney, A. H. (1969): *Clin. Pharmacol. Therap. 10,* 100.
18. Welch, R. M., Harrison, Y. E., and Burns, J. J. (1967): *Toxicol. Appl. Pharmacol. 10,* 340.
19. Radomski, J. L. (1961): *J. Pharmacol. Exp. Therap. 134,* 100.
20. Committee on Problems of Drug Safety of the Drug Research Board, National Academy of Sciences–National Research Council (1969): *Clin. Pharmacol. Therap. 10,* 607.
21. Miller, J. A. (1970): *Cancer Res. 30,* 559.
22. Reid, W. D., Christie, B., Krishna, G., Mitchell, J. R., Moskowitz, J., and Brodie, B. B. (1971): *Pharmacology 6,* 41.
23. Gillette, J. G. (1973): *Proc. Fifth International Congress on Pharmacology,* San Francisco, Vol. 2, p. 187, Karger, Basel.
24. Brodie, B. B. (1973): *Proc. Fifth International Congress on Pharmacology,* San Francisco, Vol. 2, p. 48, Karger, Basel.
25. Brown, R. R., Miller, J. A., and Miller, E. C. (1954): *J. Biol. Chem. 209,* 211.
26. Wattenberg, L. W. (1971): *Cancer 28,* 99.
27. Thompson, R. P. H., and Williams, R. (1967): *Lancet 2,* 646.
28. Black, M., and Sherlock, S. (1970): *Lancet 1,* 1359.
29. Matsuda, I., and Takase, A. (1969): *Lancet 2,* 1006.
30. Crigler, J. R., Jr., and Gold, N. I. (1966): *J. Clin. Invest. 45,* 988.
31. Crigler, J. R., Jr., and Gold, N. I. (1969): *J. Clin. Invest. 48,* 42.

32. DeLeon, A., Gartner, L. M., and Arias, I. M. (1967): *J. Lab. Clin. Med. 70,* 273.
33. Yaffee, S. J., Levy, G., Matsuzawa, T., and Baliah, T. (1966): *New Eng. J. Med. 275,* 1461.
34. Arias, I. M., Gartner, L. M., Cohen, M., BenEzzer, J., and Levi, A. J. (1969): *Amer. J. Med. 47,* 395.
35. Conney, A. H., and Burns, J. J. (1959): *Nature 184,* 363.
36. Burns, J. J., Conney, A. H., Dayton, P. G., Evans, C., Martin, G. R., and Taller, D. (1960): *J. Pharmacol. Exp. Therap. 129,* 132.
37. Burns, J. J., Mosbach, E. H., and Schulenberg, S. (1954): *J. Biol. Chem. 207,* 679.
38. Conney, A. H., Bray, G. A., Evans, C., and Burns, J. J. (1961): *Ann. N.Y. Acad. Sci. 92,* 115.
39. Burns, J. J. (1957): *Nature 180,* 553.
40. Aarts, E. M. (1965): *Biochem. Pharmacol. 14,* 359.
41. Zannoni, V. G., and Lynch, M. M. (1973): *Drug Metab. Rev. 2,* 57.
42. Avenia, R. W. (1972): Ph.D. Thesis, Cornell University, New York.
43. Kamm, J. J., Dashman, T., Conney, A. H., and Burns, J. J. (1973): *Proc. Nat. Acad. Sci. 70,* 747.
44. Ivankovic, S., Preussmann, R., Schmahl, D., and Zeller, J. (1973): *Z. Krebsforsch. 79,* 145.
45. Mirvish, S. S., Cardesa, A., Wallcave, L., and Shubik, P. (1973): *Proc. Amer. Assn. Cancer Res. 14,* 102.
46. Lijinsky, W., Taylor, H. W., Snyder, C., and Nettesheim, P. (1973): *Nature 244,* 176.
47. Herring, H. K. (1973): *Proc. Meat Indust. Res. Conf.,* pp. 47–60.

Drug Interactions, edited by P. L. Morselli,
S. Garattini, and S. N. Cohen. Raven Press,
New York © 1974

Drug Absorption Interactions — Gastric Emptying

L. F. Prescott

*Department of Clinical Pharmacology, The University Department of Therapeutics, The
Royal Infirmary, Edinburgh, Scotland*

INTRODUCTION

Many drugs influence gastrointestinal function, but absorption interactions have received relatively little attention and are rarely considered to be of clinical importance. The usual result of absorption interactions is a reduction in the rate of absorption or in the total amount of drug absorbed so that drug effects are reduced or abolished. Interactions that cause therapeutic failure are obviously important but they are unlikely to be recognized unless specifically looked for. On the other hand, the risk of drug toxicity may be increased if absorption is enhanced. From a practical point of view, it is important to differentiate between interactions that alter the *rate* of drug absorption and those that increase or decrease the *total amount* of drug absorbed, since the consequences may be quite different. A change in the rate of absorption of a long-acting drug such as warfarin would probably have little or no effect, whereas a change in the total amount absorbed may be disastrous. In contrast, if the absorption of a drug with a short biological half-life such as procaineamide is slowed down, therapeutic plasma concentrations may never be reached.

The absorption of drugs from the gastrointestinal tract is a complex process that depends on many physiological and physicochemical factors (Levine, 1970). Since the mechanisms of many drug absorption interactions are poorly understood, interactions cannot be predicted with any confidence.

I propose first to review briefly some mechanisms of absorption interactions and then to discuss in more detail interactions involving changes in the rate of gastric emptying.

MECHANISMS OF DRUG ABSORPTION INTERACTIONS

Some possible mechanisms of drug absorption interactions are listed in Table 1. Drug-induced changes in the pH of gastrointestinal fluids may have complex and unpredictable effects on the absorption of other drugs taken at the same time. According to the pH-partition theory, weak organic acids are largely absorbed from the stomach, whereas weak bases are absorbed

TABLE 1. *Possible mechanisms of drug absorption inter-actions*

pH Effects on dissolution and ionization
Changes in gastric emptying and G.I. motility
Formation of complexes, ion pairs, and chelates
Interference with active transport
Disruption of lipid micelles
Changes in portal blood flow
Toxic effects on G.I. mucosa
Changes in volume, composition, and viscosity of secretions
Effects on mucosal and bacterial drug metabolism
Changes in membrane permeability
Unknown

best from the more alkaline contents of the upper small intestine (Brodie, 1964; Binns, 1971). It is sometimes stated that the absorption of weak acids is reduced if they are given with alkali since less drug would be present in the un-ionized lipid-soluble diffusible state. However, an opposite effect may be observed. Aspirin, for example, is absorbed more rapidly from buffered alkaline solutions than from unbuffered solutions at pH 2.8 (Cooke and Hunt, 1970). This is probably due to the greater dissolution rate and aqueous solubility of aspirin in alkaline solution and rapid gastric emptying caused by an increase in the pH of the stomach contents. Contrary to the pH-partition theory, aspirin is absorbed much more slowly from the stomach than from the small intestine (Siurala et al., 1969). The stimulatory effect of alkali on gastric emptying may explain the apparent increase in propantheline absorption caused by sodium bicarbonate (Chaput de Saintonge and Herxheimer, 1973). However, alkalis and antacids may decrease the rate of absorption of other basic drugs through effects on solubility, and the inhibitory effect of sodium bicarbonate on the absorption of tetracycline may be cited as an example (Barr et al., 1971).

Drugs may interact in the gastrointestinal tract to form complexes, ion pairs, and chelates, which may be absorbed more rapidly or more slowly than the parent drugs. The absorption of tetracyclines is inhibited by the formation of insoluble chelates with metals such as calcium and iron (Neuvonen et al., 1970), dicoumarol absorption is increased by the formation of a more soluble chelate with magnesium hydroxide (Ambre and Fischer, 1973), and the absorption of a quaternary ammonium antiarrhythmic agent is enhanced by ion-pair formation with salicylate or trichloroacetate (Gibaldi and Grundhofer, 1973). Many other examples are known (Levine, 1970). The absorption of drugs may also be reduced by adsorption onto kaolin or charcoal (Binnion and McDermot, 1972) or binding to ionic exchange resins (Robinson et al., 1970).

Drugs that are analogues of naturally occurring purines, pyrimidines, sugars, and amino acids may be absorbed by small intestinal active transport, and it has been suggested that absorption may be reduced by competition between substrates such as L-DOPA and phenylalanine derived from dietary sources (Bianchine et al., 1971). It is also possible for one drug to inhibit enzymes involved in the active transport of another drug, and such an interaction has been postulated between chlorpromazine and L-DOPA (Rivera-Calimlim, 1972).

Interference with micelle formation may limit the solubility of lipids, and inhibition of absorption of cholesterol, bile acids, and vitamin A by neomycin has been attributed to this mechanism (Barrowman et al., 1973). The splanchnic blood flow may occasionally be a rate-limiting factor in drug absorption (Haass et al., 1972) and this may be of clinical significance because many drugs could have direct effects on local gastrointestinal blood flow (Curwain and Holton, 1971).

Neomycin, p-aminosalicylic acid, and colchicine have a toxic effect on the intestinal mucosa and may cause a malabsorption syndrome with impaired absorption of other drugs. Thus colchicine may cause megaloblastic anemia through interference with vitamin-B_{12} absorption (Webb et al., 1968). Drugs can also influence the volume and composition of gastrointestinal secretions (including bile), and changes in viscosity may modify drug absorption (Levy and Rao, 1972). It is now recognized that many drugs are extensively metabolized by the gastrointestinal mucosa and the gut bacterial flora, and this process might be influenced by the concurrent administration of other drugs (e.g., antibiotics).

During oral therapy, the gastrointestinal mucosa is exposed intermittently to very high drug concentrations that may alter the permeability of the gastrointestinal epithelium. In this context, it is interesting to note that insulin and many polypeptides greatly enhance the membrane transport of pethidine, isoniazid, salicylate, and chlorpromazine—drugs normally considered to cross cell membranes by passive diffusion. Thus the intestinal uptake of isoniazid is enhanced by insulin, and this effect is antagonized by ouabain (Danysz and Wisniewski, 1970). The clinical significance of such interactions is unknown. Finally, we must admit to virtually complete ignorance of the mechanisms of many drug absorption interactions.

GASTRIC EMPTYING AND GASTROINTESTINAL MOTILITY

The stomach is not an important site of drug absorption. Basic drugs and compounds absorbed by active transport are not absorbed from the stomach to any extent, and even weakly acid drugs such as aspirin, warfarin, and barbiturates and low molecular weight neutral compounds such as ethanol are absorbed much more slowly from the stomach than from the small intestine (Siurala et al., 1969; Kekki et al., 1971; Magnussen, 1968). Drugs are probably absorbed more rapidly from the upper small intestine than from the stomach because of the much greater surface area of the intestine (Levine, 1970). The rate of gastric emptying may therefore limit the rate of

TABLE 2. *Drugs that might influence gastric emptying*

Atropine and anticholinergics
Antihistamines
Tricyclic antidepressants
Phenothiazines
Sympathomimetics
Anti-Parkinson drugs
Narcotic analgesics
Nitrites
Iproniazid
Chloroquine
Metoclopramide
Anticholinesterases
Caffeine
Prostaglandins
Antacids
Antihypertensives

drug absorption and is particularly important in the context of interactions since it can be influenced by many drugs (Table 2).

Many drugs are absorbed more slowly when taken with food, and this is probably due largely to the inhibitory effect of food on gastric emptying. Drug effects can be reduced dramatically or even abolished if gastric emptying is retarded by food (Kojima et al., 1971). In contrast, absorption is more rapid and toxicity can be greatly increased when drugs are given orally in the same dose in dilute rather than concentrated solutions, and this effect has been attributed in part to rapid gastric emptying (Borowitz et al., 1971). A striking example of an absorption interaction involving gastric emptying is shown in Fig. 1. Aminopyrine apparently inhibits gastric emptying in rabbits and is absorbed very slowly when given alone. Barbital itself has no significant effect on gastric emptying but it antagonizes the inhibitory action of amidopyrine and greatly increases the rate of absorption of aminopyrine (Goto et al., 1972).

We have been particularly interested in interactions caused by drug-induced changes in the rate of gastric emptying. Paracetamol was chosen as a model drug for absorption studies since it is a weak acid (pK_a 9.5) that is largely un-ionized in both gastric and intestinal fluids, and the rate of absorption in man is directly related to the gastric emptying rate (Heading et al., 1973). Propantheline and metoclopramide delay and accelerate gastric emptying respectively, and their effects on the absorption of an oral dose of 1.5 g of paracetamol were investigated (Nimmo et al., 1973).

Simultaneous measurements of gastric emptying rate and paracetamol absorption were made in six convalescent hospital patients on separate occasions before and after i.v. injection of 30 mg of propantheline. As expected, the mean half-life of gastric emptying was prolonged by propantheline from 25 ± 9 to 152 ± 38 min, and there was a significant reduction in

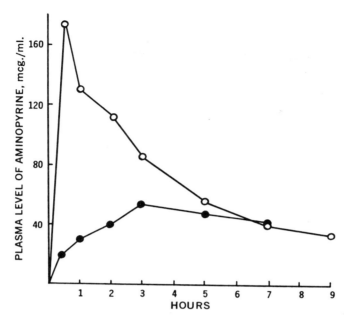

FIG. 1. Plasma concentrations of aminopyrine in rabbits following an oral dose of 225 mg/kg alone (●) and together with 85 mg/kg of barbital (○). From Goto, S., et al. (1972): *J. Pharm. Sci. 61*, 945.

the rate of paracetamol absorption (Fig. 2). The mean peak plasma concentration of paracetamol was reduced from 26.3 ± 4 to 17.5 ± 5 µg/ml and the mean time taken to reach peak concentrations was prolonged from 70 ± 10 to 160 ± 13 min. The 0 to 12 hr urinary excretion of total unchanged and

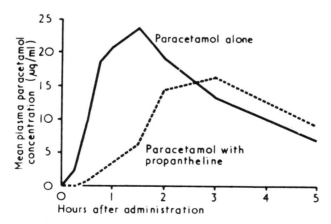

FIG. 2. Inhibitory effect of propantheline (30 mg i.v.) on the absorption of 1.5 g of paracetamol in six patients. From Nimmo, J., et al. (1973): *Brit. Med. J. 1*, 587.

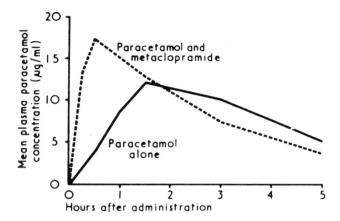

FIG. 3. Increased rate of paracetamol absorption after 10 mg of metoclopramide i.v. Five healthy volunteers received 1.5 g of paracetamol with and without metoclopramide. From Nimmo, J., et al. (1973): *Brit. Med. J. 1*, 587.

conjugated paracetamol was reduced by propantheline from 880 ± 83 to 536 ± 73 mg, but total amount excreted in 24 hr was unchanged. Propantheline therefore delayed gastric emptying and slowed down the rate of paracetamol absorption but did not reduce the total amount absorbed.

In contrast, metoclopramide (10 mg i.v.) significantly increased the rate of paracetamol absorption in five healthy volunteers who were known to be

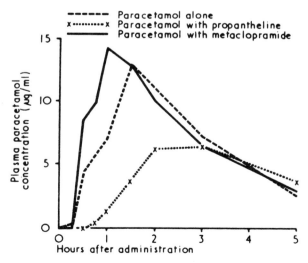

FIG. 4. Effects of propantheline (30 mg i.v.) and metoclopramide (10 mg i.v.) on the absorption of oral doses of 1.5 g of paracetamol in a 22-year-old man. From Nimmo, J. et al. (1973): *Brit. Med. J. 1*, 587.

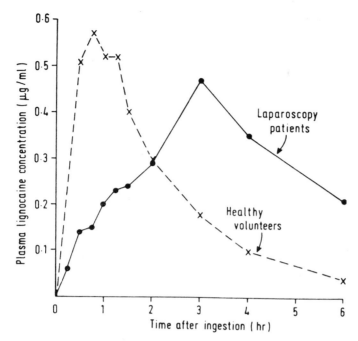

FIG. 5. Mean plasma lignocaine concentrations after ingestion of 400 mg of lignocaine hydrochloride in seven unanesthetized healthy volunteers and 12 laparoscopy patients premedicated with 0.6 mg of atropine i.m. From Adjepon-Yamoah, K. K., et al. (1973): *Brit. J. Anaesth. 45,* 143.

slow absorbers of the drug (Fig. 3). The mean maximum plasma concentration of paracetamol was increased from 12.5 ± 6 to 20.5 ± 4 $\mu g/ml$ and the mean time to peak concentrations decreased from 120 ± 25 to 48 ± 12 min. The effects of propantheline and metoclopramide on paracetamol absorption in the same individual are shown in Fig. 4.

Propantheline and metoclopramide have also been shown to retard and accelerate, respectively, the absorption of tetracycline and pivampicillin in man (Gothoni et al., 1972). On the other hand, propantheline and metoclopramide seemed to have the completely opposite effect on the absorption of digoxin (Manninen et al., 1973). The mean serum digoxin concentration in 11 patients on long-term therapy fell from 0.72 to 0.46 ng/ml when 10 mg of metoclopramide was taken three times daily for 10 days, and in another group of 13 patients the mean digoxin concentration rose from 1.02 to 1.33 ng/ml after 15 mg of propantheline three times a day for a similar period. This paradox could be explained by rather slow dissolution and absorption of digoxin or absorption from a limited area of the intestine. Rapid gastrointestinal transit induced by metoclopramide could reduce the effective time for dissolution and absorption whereas propantheline would have the reverse effect. Similar observations have been made with riboflavin, the absorption of which is delayed by propantheline, although the total amount absorbed is greatly increased (Levy et al., 1972). However, there is an alternative explanation for the digoxin interaction since the blood samples for digoxin estimation were taken 24 hr after the last dose. The lower digoxin concentrations at 24 hr observed with metoclopramide could actually have been due to more *rapid* absorption with lower levels later in the elimination phase. Similarly, the serum digoxin concentrations would obviously be higher at 24 hr if absorption were *delayed* by propantheline. This effect can be seen clearly with the paracetamol interactions shown in Figs. 2 and 3.

We have also observed a striking delay in the absorption of oral lignocaine in patients premedicated with 0.6 mg of atropine i.m. prior to laparoscopy (Adjepon-Yamoah et al., 1973). The mean peak plasma concentration of lignocaine occurred at 45 min in healthy volunteers, but was delayed until 3 hr in the patients (Fig. 5). Subsequent studies have shown that atropine alone significantly delays the absorption of orally administered lignocaine and that absorption is inhibited further by laparoscopy and anesthesia (Adjepon-Yamoah, *unpublished*). Similarly, desmethylimipramine delays the absorption of phenylbutazone (Consolo et al., 1970), and these interactions are probably due to changes in the rate of gastric emptying. Other mechanisms may also be involved, however. For example, changes in gastrointestinal motility and peristalsis could modify tablet disintegration and dissolution and increase or decrease the contact between drug and absorbing epithelium.

SUMMARY

The absorption of drugs from the gastrointestinal tract is a complex process that is influenced greatly by physiological and physicochemical factors. Absorption interactions are often unpredictable, and one drug may enhance the absorption of a second drug but interfere with the absorption of a third drug. Drugs are absorbed much more slowly from the stomach than from the small intestine and absorption may often be limited by the rate of gastric emptying. Atropine, propantheline, and metoclopramide alter the rate of gastric emptying in man and can have significant effects on the rate of absorption of other drugs. Many other therapeutic agents influence gastrointestinal motility and gastric emptying and could cause absorption interactions through a similar mechanism.

REFERENCES

Adjepon-Yamoah, K. K., Scott, D. B., and Prescott, L. F. (1973): Impaired absorption and metabolism of oral lignocaine in patients undergoing laparoscopy. *Brit. J. Anaesth. 45,* 143–147.

Ambre, J. J., and Fischer, L. J. (1973): Effect of coadministration of aluminium and magnesium hydroxides on absorption of anticoagulants in man. *Clin. Pharmacol. Therap. 14*, 231–237.

Barr, W. H., Adir, J., and Garrettson, L. (1971): Decrease in tetracycline absorption in man by sodium bicarbonate. *Clin. Pharmacol. Therap. 12*, 779–784.

Barrowman, J. A., D'Mello, A., and Herxheimer, A. (1973): A single dose of neomycin impairs absorption of vitamin A (Retinol) in man. *Europ. J. Clin. Pharmacol. 5*, 199–202.

Bianchine, J., Calimlim, L. R., Morgan, J. P., Dujuvne, C. A., and Lasagna, L. (1971): Metabolism and absorption of L-3,4 dihydroxyphenylalanine in patients with Parkinson's disease. *Ann. N.Y. Acad. Sci. 179*, 126–140.

Binnion, P. F., and McDermott, M. (1972): Bioavailability of digoxin. *Lancet 2*, 592.

Binns, T. B. (1971): The absorption of drugs from the alimentary tract, lungs and skin. *Brit. J. Hosp. Med. 6*, 133–142.

Borowitz, J. L., Moore, P. F., Yim, G. K. W., and Miya, T. S. (1971): Mechanism of enhanced drug effects produced by dilution of the oral dose. *Toxicol. Appl. Pharmacol. 19*, 164–168.

Brodie, B. B. (1964): Physico-chemical factors in drug absorption. In: *Absorption and Distribution of Drugs* (ed. T. B. Binns), pp. 16–48, Williams and Wilkins, Baltimore.

Chaput de Saintonge, D. M., and Herxheimer, A. (1973): Sodium bicarbonate enhances the absorption of propantheline in man. *Europ. J. Clin. Pharmacol. 5*, 239–242.

Consolo, S., Morselli, P. L., Zaccala, M., and Garattini, S. (1970): Delayed absorption of phenylbutazone caused by desmethylimipramine in humans. *Europ. J. Pharmacol. 10*, 239–242.

Cooke, A. R., and Hunt, J. N. (1970): Absorption of acetylsalicylic acid from unbuffered and buffered gastric contents. *Amer. J. Dig. Dis. 15*, 95–102.

Curwain, B. P., and Holton, P. (1972): The effects of isoprenaline and noradrenaline on pentagastrin-stimulated gastric acid secretion and mucosal blood flow in the dog. *Brit. J. Pharm. 46*, 225–233.

Danysz, A., and Wisniewski, K. (1970): Control of drug transport through cell membranes. *Materia Medica Polona 2*, 35–44.

Gibaldi, M., and Grundhofer, B. (1973): Enhancement of intestinal absorption of a quaternary ammonium compound by salicylate and trichloroacetate. *J. Pharm. Sci. 62*, 343–344.

Gothoni, G., Pentikainen, P., Vapaatalo, H. I., Hackman, R., and Bjorksten, K. A. (1972): Absorption of antibiotics: Influence of metoclopramide and atropine on serum levels of pivampicillin and tetracycline. *Ann. Clin. Res. 4*, 228–232.

Goto, S., Tsuzuki, O., and Iguchi, S. (1972): Relationship between enhancement of plasma level of aminopyrine by barbital and stomach emptying pattern. *J. Pharm. Sci. 61*, 945–947.

Haass, A., Lüllmann, H., and Peters, T. (1972): Absorption rates of some cardiac glycosides and portal blood flow. *Europ. J. Pharmacol. 19*, 366–370.

Heading, R. C., Nimmo, J., Prescott, L. F., and Tothill, P. (1973): The dependence of paracetamol absorption on the rate of gastric emptying. *Brit. J. Pharmacol. 47*, 415–421.

Kekki, M., Pyörälä, K., Mustala, O., Salmi, H., Jussila, J., and Siurala, M. (1971): Multicompartment analysis of the absorption kinetics of warfarin from the stomach and small intestine. *Int. J. Clin. Pharmacol. 2*, 209–211.

Kojima, S., Smith, R. B., and Doluisio, J. T. (1971): Drug absorption V: Influence of food on oral absorption of phenobarbital in rats. *J. Pharm. Sci. 60*, 1639–1641.

Levine, R. R. (1970): Factors affecting gastrointestinal absorption of drugs. *Digest. Dis. 15*, 171–188.

Levy, G., Gibaldi, M., and Procknal, J. A. (1972): Effect of an anticholinergic agent on riboflavin absorption in man. *J. Pharm. Sci. 61*, 798–799.

Levy, G., and Rao, B. K. (1972): Enhanced intestinal absorption of riboflavin from sodium alginate solution in man. *J. Pharm. Sci. 61*, 279–280.

Magnussen, M. P. (1968): The effect of ethanol on the gastrointestinal absorption of drugs in the rat. *Acta Pharmacol. Toxicol. 26*, 130–144.

Manninen, V., Apajalahti, A., Melin, J., and Karesoja, M. (1973): Altered absorption of digoxin in patients given propantheline and metoclopramide. *Lancet 1*, 398–401.

Neuvonen, P. J., Gothoni, G., Hackman, R., and Björksten, K. Interference of iron with the absorption of tetracyclines in man. *Brit. Med. J. 4*, 532–534.

Nimmo, J., Heading, R. C., Tothill, P., and Prescott, L. F. (1973): Pharmacological modification of gastric emptying: Effects of propantheline and metoclopramide on paracetamol absorption. *Brit. Med. J. 1*, 587–589.

Rivera-Calimlim, L. (1972): Effect of chronic drug treatment on intestinal membrane transport of ^{14}C-L-DOPA. *Brit. J. Pharm. 46,* 708–713.

Robinson, D. S., Benjamin, D. M. and McCormack. J. J. (1970): Interaction of warfarin and non-systemic gastrointestinal drugs. *Clin. Pharmacol. Therap. 12,* 491–495.

Siurala, M., Mustala, O., and Jussila, J. (1969): Absorption of acetylsalicylic acid by a normal and an atrophic gastric mucosa. *Scand. J. Gastroent. 4,* 269–273.

Webb, D. I., Chodos, R. B., Mahar, C. Q., and Falcon, W. W. (1968): Mechanism of vitamin B_{12} malabsorption in patients receiving colchicine. *New Engl. J. Med. 279,* 845–850.

Drug Interactions, edited by P. L. Morselli,
S. Garattini, and S. N. Cohen. Raven Press,
New York © 1974

Gastrointestinal Drug Absorption:
Effects of Antacids

Aryeh Hurwitz

*Clinical Pharmacology-Toxicology Center, Departments of Medicine and Pharmacology,
University of Kansas Medical Center, Kansas City, Kansas 66103*

INTRODUCTION

Antacids are among the most widely consumed drugs used in the treatment of serious organic disease and nonspecific complaints. Since they are available without prescription, many patients take antacids without their physician's knowledge or concern. Since most antacids are primarily nonabsorbed, they have been regarded to be devoid of any significant pharmacological action. In studies of antacids, it has been shown that this assumption is not true and that the interactions of antacids with other orally ingested drugs may be of clinical significance. The present report will describe studies in animals, *in vitro* and in people that have explored the interactions of antacids with other drugs. Some of the mechanisms of these interactions will be discussed and others are still being explored and are not well understood. Also, some of the experimental findings in animals await verification in man to confirm their significance.

METHODS

Swiss-Webster mice or Sprague-Dawley rats were used. After an overnight fast, they were given three hourly doses of water or antacid by gastric intubation, 0.02 ml/10 g for the mice and 0.5 ml for the rats. With the third dose of water or antacid, the animals were given the drug whose absorption was studied, again by gastric intubation. Blood samples were obtained by orbital sinus puncture in mice and from the tail artery or heart of the rats. When gastric contents were examined, the stomach and its contents were isolated with ligatures prior to excision. In the human studies, patients and their parents, where applicable, were thoroughly informed of the nature of the experiments and after consent was obtained, they were given other agents either with or without antacids. Blood samples were obtained from the antecubital vein. In the studies of isolated muscle, strips were obtained from normal animal and human gastric tissue and suspended in Tyrode's solution at pH 6.8 in the presence or absence of aluminum chloride. Acetylcholine was applied as indicated and contractions monitored with a transducer and recorder. Drug assays and details of the procedures are given in the original publications cited.

RESULTS

Pentobarbital

Pentobarbital is a rapidly absorbed acidic drug with a pK_a of 7.9. When given with magnesium hydroxide, the drug is present in a basic environment that keeps it in the ionized form and depresses its absorption (Fig. 1) (1). Aluminum hydroxide delays pentobarbital absorption more than magnesium hydroxide, but by a totally different mechanism. Aluminum hydroxide retards gastric emptying and retains more of the pentobarbital in the stomach from which absorption is much slower than from the small bowel. This effect of aluminum hydroxide can be shown to be due to the trivalent aluminum

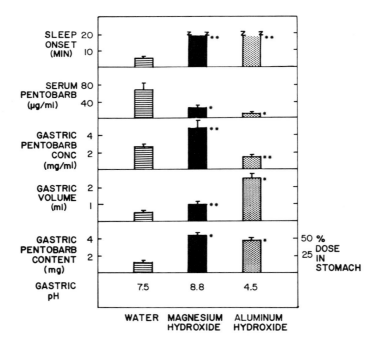

FIG. 1. Effect of aluminum hydroxide gel and milk of magnesia on absorption of sodium pentobarbital. The rats were given 0.5 ml of water, milk of magnesia (magnesium hydroxide), or aluminum hydroxide gel by gastric tube at 2 hr, 1 hr, and immediately prior to gastric administration of sodium pentobarbital, 75 mg/kg. Rats were killed after 20 min. There were six rats in each group. Data adapted from Hurwitz, A., and Sheehan, M. B. (1971): *J. Pharmacol. Exp. Ther.* 179, 124. *$p < 0.001$. **$p < 0.05$.

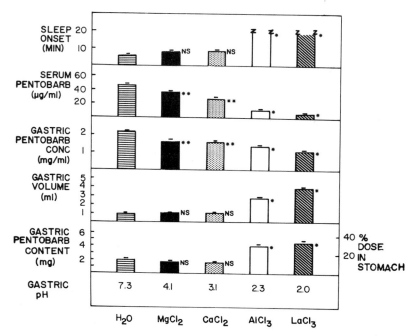

FIG. 2. Effect of magnesium chloride, calcium chloride, aluminum chloride, and lanthanum chloride on absorption of sodium pentobarbital. The rats were given 0.5 ml of water or a 0.2 M solution of the salts indicated by gastric tube at 2 hr, 1 hr, and immediately prior to gastric administration of sodium pentobarbital 75 mg/kg. Rats were killed after 20 min. Mean levels are given ±SE. There were five or six rats in each group. Data adapted from Hurwitz, A., and Sheehan, M. B. (1971): *J. Pharmacol. Exp. Ther. 179*, 124. *p < 0.001. **p < 0.02.

ion and is produced by another trivalent cation, lanthanum, but not by calcium or magnesium (Fig. 2). These effects of magnesium hydroxide and aluminum hydroxide in delaying pentobarbital absorption and onset of sleep in rats have been shown to result from delayed absorption but not from irreversible trapping in the gut, since, when ^{14}C-pentobarbital was given orally, an equal amount of isotope was excreted in the urine in the presence or absence of antacids.

Sulfadiazine

Sulfadiazine, like pentobarbital, is a weakly acidic drug whose pK_a is 6.5. As was found with sodium pentobarbital, the absorption of freely soluble sodium sulfadiazine is retarded by both magnesium hydroxide and aluminum hydroxide, presumably by similar mechanisms (2). In contrast, aluminum hydroxide does not affect the absorption of the free-acid form of sulfadiazine, whereas blood sulfa levels are raised fivefold by its adminis-

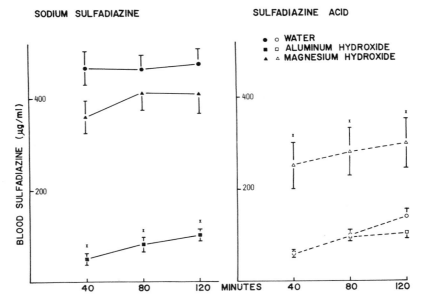

FIG. 3. Effect of pretreatment with aluminum hydroxide gel and magnesium hydroxide gel on gastrointestinal absorption of sulfadiazine sodium and acid. The rats were given 0.5 ml of water, aluminum hydroxide gel, or magnesium hydroxide gel by gastric tube at 2 hr, 1 hr, and immediately prior to gastric administration of sodium sulfadiazine or sulfadiazine acid at a sulfa dose of 500 mg/kg. Blood sulfa levels are given $\pm$SE; five animals in each group; X, $p < 0.025$. Data adapted from Hurwitz, A. (1971): *J. Pharmacol. Exp. Ther. 179*, 485.

tration together with magnesium hydroxide (Fig. 3). Dissolution, rather than gastric emptying is the rate-limiting step in the absorption of sulfadiazine acid and the solubility of this drug in hydrochloric acid is increased three to 25 times in the presence of magnesium hydroxide. Thus, by administering antacids with two different forms of a single drug, sulfadiazine, its blood levels after gastric administration can either be lowered or raised by fivefold in rats.

Quinine

Quinine is a weak base whose pK_a is 8.4. When dissolved in 0.05 N hydrochloric acid and administered to rats by gastric intubation, the absorption of this drug is depressed by aluminum hydroxide which causes delayed gastric emptying (Table 1) (2). Since basic drugs shift from ionized to un-ionized form as the pH is raised, magnesium hydroxide would be expected to cause quinine to become more lipid soluble and more rapidly absorbed. This was not found to be so. In fact, the absorption of quinine is depressed and blood levels lowered to less than one half control values by magnesium hydroxide.

TABLE 1. *Effect of aluminum hydroxide and magnesium hydroxide on gastrointestinal absorption of quinine[a]*

	Effect of pretreatment		
	Water (8)[b]	Aluminum hydroxide (8)	Magnesium hydroxide (8)
Plasma quinine level (μg/ml)	5.51 ± 0.60^c	3.04 ± 0.52^d	2.56 ± 0.31^e
Gastric volume (ml)	0.86 ± 0.09	2.55 ± 0.19^e	1.71 ± 0.11^e
Concentration of quinine in super-natant (mg/ml)	0.95 ± 0.07	0.48 ± 0.03^e	0.08 ± 0.00^e
Amount of quinine in precipitate (mg)	0.46 ± 0.07	1.39 ± 0.12^e	5.14 ± 0.22^e
Gastric quinine content (mg)	1.19 ± 0.14	2.36 ± 0.16^e	5.23 ± 0.22^e
Quinine dose in stomach (%)	9	18	37
Gastric pH	3.6 ± 0.3	4.4 ± 0.1^e	8.7 ± 0.04^e

[a] All determinations were made 30 min after administration of quinine by gastric intubation. Quinine sulfate was dissolved in 0.05 N HCl and given at a dose of 100 mg/kg in a volume of 0.5 ml/100 g.
[b] Number of animals in each group in parentheses.
[c] $\pm$SE.
[d] $p < 0.01$.
[e] $p < 0.001$.
Data from Hurwitz, A. (1971): *J. Pharmacol. Exp. Ther. 179,* 485.

The cause of depressed absorption is the poor solubility of quinine in high pH with precipitation of this drug. A very low concentration remains in solution and absorption is much slower (Table 1).

Isoniazid

Isoniazid is a freely water-soluble drug, which is uncharged in the stomach throughout the pH range encountered. It is rapidly absorbed from the small intestine and, therefore, any drug that delays gastric emptying such as aluminum hydroxide slows the absorption of isoniazid in rats. The combination antacid, magaldrate, has but a slight effect on isoniazid absorption. Aluminum hydroxide affects isoniazid absorption in man in a manner similar to its effect in rats. In eight of ten tuberculous patients, aluminum hydroxide lowered peak isoniazid levels with the mean shifting from 5.6 to 4.3 μg/ml ($p < 0.02$). First-hour levels and areas under the concentration-time curve were decreased (Fig. 4) (3). Delayed gastric emptying and intestinal absorption would be expected to result in a lower area under the concentration-time curve for drugs such as isoniazid that are extensively metabolized during hepatic passage. The depressed peak isoniazid levels in patients when given aluminum hydroxide may be of clinical significance, since it has been shown that, for this drug, peak levels rather than sustained plasma levels

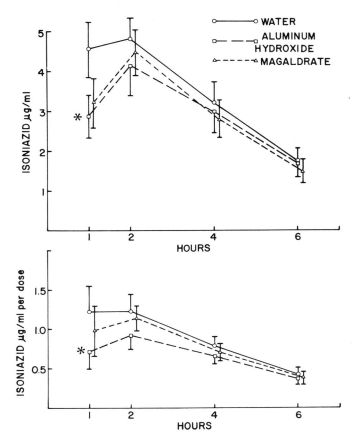

FIG. 4. Effects of antacid pretreatment on plasma isoniazid levels in 10 patients with tuberculosis. Top panel: Plasma isoniazid levels. Bottom panel: Plasma isoniazid levels per dose expressed as μg/ml per mg isoniazid/kg body weight. Levels given $\pm$ SE. *$p <$ 0.05. Data analyzed by paired t test. From Hurwitz, A., and Schlozman, D. L. (1974): *Amer. Rev. Resp. Dis. 109,* 41.

correlate with therapeutic efficacy, especially in intermittent dosage regimens.

Ampicillin

Since ampicillin is an antibiotic with a short half-life, alterations in its absorption should result in marked changes in blood levels. In the mouse, with a $T^{1}/_{2}$ for i.v. sodium ampicillin of 0.35 hr, ampicillin trihydrate and sodium ampicillin are both slowly and incompletely (30%) absorbed after gastric administration. Magnesium hydroxide depresses ampicillin absorption in mice, lowering peak levels after a dose of 50 mg/kg from 11 μg/ml to 5 μg/ml. Aluminum hydroxide, magaldrate, calcium carbonate, and sodium bicarbonate slightly and inconsistently depress absorption in mice. The laxatives magnesium sulfate and sodium sulfate lower ampicillin levels in mice but not to the same extent as magnesium hydroxide. Like cathartics, bethanechol is a drug that induces intestinal hypermotility and diarrhea, but, in contrast, it hastens and increases ampicillin absorption. After intravenous administration of 500 mg sodium ampicillin to 14 men with respiratory infections, the mean terminal half-life of the drug was 1.13 hr. An equal dose of ampicillin trihydrate given orally gave a mean peak level of 2.65 μg/ml at 2.1 hr with only 32.5% of the dose absorbed in 5 hr. The half-life had not reached the terminal T$\frac{1}{2}$ of 1.13 hr by 5 hr after oral ampicillin trihydrate administration and mean serum ampicillin levels of 0.34 μg/ml were still measurable after a 13-hr overnight fast, indicating that gastrointestinal absorption of this drug is slow and incomplete in man. In a crossover study in these patients, aluminum hydroxide gel and magaldrate had no effect on the absorption of ampicillin. In contrast to their effect in depressing the absorption of rapidly and completely absorbed drugs such as isoniazid, the absorption of a slowly and incompletely absorbed drug such as ampicillin is not affected by antacids. The mechanism of magnesium hydroxide depression of ampicillin absorption in mice is poorly understood but probably of no clinical significance in man, since this antacid is not taken in large doses by patients because of its cathartic properties.

Aluminum Hydroxide

Retarded drug absorption in the presence of aluminum hydroxide due to delayed gastric emptying is a recently described phenomenon that has been further explored. When isolated smooth muscle strips from rats or normal human surgical specimens were suspended in Tyrode's solution at pH 6.8 and exposed to increasing concentrations of acetylcholine (10^{-5} to 10^{-2} M), increasing contractile tone was demonstrated. Aluminum chloride, 5×10^{-4} M, inhibited these contractions by more than 50% (Fig. 5), an effect shared by another trivalent cation, lanthanum (4). The concentration of aluminum, 5×10^{-4} M, was threefold lower than that achieved in vivo in the stomach of rats given aluminum hydroxide. Aluminum chloride, 5×10^{-4} M, applied to the mucosal surface of the stomach inhibited contractions evoked by serosally applied acetylcholine. Aluminum inhibition of gastrointestinal smooth-muscle contraction is associated with changes in the fluxes of calcium which occur during excitation-contraction coupling (5).

The effects of antacids on gastric emptying in leukemic children with no gastrointestinal disease were studied. Since antacids are frequently given in an attempt to prevent steroid ulcers in this population, the study was felt to be of therapeutic importance. Using a gamma camera, the rate of disap-

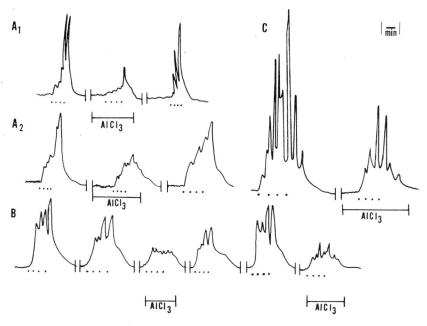

FIG. 5. Effect of AlCl$_3$ (0.5 mM) on the acetylcholine cumulative dose responses (10^{-5}, 10^{-4}, 10^{-3}, 10^{-2} M) of isolated smooth muscle strip from human antrum. Recordings A$_1$, A$_2$, B, and C represent a smooth-muscle strip without mucosal layer from noninvolved areas obtained from three different patients (A, B, C) undergoing gastric surgery for peptic ulcer disease. Intervals 10 min between responses. Dots = increasing doses of acetylcholine chloride. (A$_1$ from lesser, A$_2$ from greater curvature of the stomach of patient A.) From Hava, M., and Hurwitz, A. (1973): *Europ. J. Pharmacol. 22,* 156.

TABLE 2. *Effects of antacids on gastric volumes, pH, and aluminum concentrations in the rat*

	Water	Maalox®	Amphojel®
Volume (ml)	0.29 ± 0.03	1.8 ± 0.3^a	4.0 ± 0.2^a
pH	2.2 ± 0.2	7.4 ± 0.1^a	4.7 ± 0.2^a
Aluminum conc. (M)	<0.001	<0.001	0.015 ± 0.002^a

Ten rats per group. Measurements on gastric contents made 20 min after the third hourly dose of 1 ml water or antacid by gastric intubation.

^{a} $p < 0.001$ by Student's *t* test.

Data from Hava, M. and Hurwitz, A. (1973): *Europ. J. Pharmacol. 22,* 156.

pearance of 200 μC ^{51}Cr sodium chromate from the stomach was monitored. In the first five patients so studied, aluminum hydroxide slowed the mean maximal emptying rate from $5.1 \pm 0.8\%$ per min to $1.8 \pm 0.7\%$ per min (6). Aluminum hydroxide caused 83.6% of the radioisotope to be retained in the stomach at times corresponding to 50% emptying after water. A combination antacid containing both aluminum and magnesium retarded gastric emptying less than aluminum hydroxide alone. In animal studies that confirmed the relative effects of various antacids on gastric emptying, the concentration of aluminum in solution in their stomachs as measured by atomic absorption spectroscopy was at least 15-fold lower in the presence of combination antacid, which raised pH to a higher level, than in the presence of aluminum hydroxide gel alone (Table 2).

DISCUSSION

The foregoing studies and those of others have shown that antacids may alter the rate and amount of absorption of other orally administered drugs. Antacids do this if they affect the rate-limiting steps in absorption, which may vary from one drug to another. For highly soluble and rapidly absorbed drugs, such as pentobarbital, sodium sulfadiazine, quinine, and isoniazid, their passage from the stomach into contact with the absorptive surface of the proximal small bowel is the rate-limiting step in their absorption. Therefore, antacids such as aluminum hydroxide that delay gastric emptying slow the rate of absorption and onset of pharmacological action of these agents. If the drugs have a high rate of elimination and undergo significant metabolism during hepatic passage, this delay in gastrointestinal absorption will not only reduce peak levels but will also lower areas under the concentration-time curve for unchanged drug, as was shown for isoniazid, thereby potentially reducing its therapeutic efficacy. Similar effects of other agents which alter gastric emptying have been shown. Consolo et al. (7) ascribed delayed absorption of phenylbutazone in men given desmethylimipramine to delayed gastric emptying due to the anticholinergic effect of the latter drug. Propantheline delays absorption of acetaminophen and accelerated absorption is caused by metoclopramide (8). In this study the authors were unable to document any effect of aluminum hydroxide on the absorption of acetaminophen, but did not comment on whether or not the antacid had any effect on gastric emptying, such as we have shown.

Although delayed isoniazid absorption in man, which is of probable clinical significance, was found in the presence of aluminum hydroxide, we have been unable to confirm the animal findings of delayed pentobarbital absorption in man, using subjective evaluations of sleep as criteria of hypnotic effect. In another study, patients receiving both antacids and hypnotics did not complain of diminished hypnotic effectiveness (M. Levy, *personal communication*). In this survey, aluminum hydroxide gel was not studied apart from other antacids. Perhaps patients requiring antacids get relief of pain which helps them sleep and those not requiring antacid may feel bloated and uncomfortable when given the antacids. These two conflicting effects would mask the hypnotic effect of pentobarbital in man. The clinical significance of the interaction between antacids and pentobarbital in man has not been demonstrated.

The ability of antacids to alter drug absorption in animals and man by affecting their solubility and dissolution is well recognized. Sulfonamide absorption in patients was shown to be enhanced by antacids more than 30 years ago (9). Tetracycline is poorly absorbed in the presence of aluminum hydroxide, presumably due to chelation (10). Sodium bicarbonate, which raises pH without releasing polyvalent cations, also delays tetracycline absorption, evidently by a different mechanism. In the presence of sodium bicarbonate, tetracycline dissolution is reduced, delaying its absorption (11). In the case of drugs that are slowly and incompletely absorbed and for which chemical interaction, such as, complexation, chelation, or altered solubility cannot be shown, there is less likelihood of a significant interaction with antacids in the gastrointestinal tract. An example is ampicillin, which is slowly and incompletely absorbed and which is absorbed to a similar extent in the presence or absence of aluminum hydroxide or magaldrate in patients.

Magnesium-aluminum hydroxide antacid was found not to affect plasma warfarin levels when both agents were given together (12). In this study the first blood sample was obtained 6 hr after drug administration, by which time the effects of delayed gastric emptying, if any, would have been missed. Also, retarded drug absorption, if not the result of irreversible binding in the gut, would be of no clinical significance for a drug with a long half-life (42 hr for warfarin) if all the drug were eventually absorbed. This would result in similar steady-state blood levels on a multiple dosing schedule.

Further possible drug-antacid interactions are currently being studied in animals and man in an attempt to define those of clinical significance and to evaluate further mechanisms that will enable clinicians and pharmacologists to predict and anticipate such interactions. Those interactions that have been documented thus far occur due to changes in the amount of free drug in solution as affected by dissolution, chelation, or complexation, to changes in ionization of the drug caused by pH shifts, or to changes in gastrointestinal function, especially gastric emptying. Potential interactions due to changes in drug stability as pH is raised, as may occur with penicillins, or to other cation-induced changes in gastrointestinal physiology such as in transit time, stirring of intestinal contents, or cell membrane permeability, are possibilities that are currently being studied.

ACKNOWLEDGMENTS

Supported by U.S. Public Health Service grant GM 15956 from the National Institutes of Health. The author is recipient of U.S. Public Health Service Research Career Development Award GM 70250.

REFERENCES

1. Hurwitz, A., and Sheehan, M. B. (1971): *J. Pharmacol. Exp. Ther. 179*, 124.
2. Hurwitz, A. (1971): *J. Pharmacol. Exp. Ther. 179*, 485.
3. Hurwitz, A., and Schlozman, D. L. (1974): *Amer. Rev. Resp. Dis. 109*, 41.
4. Hava, M., and Hurwitz, A. (1973): *Europ. J. Pharmacol. 22*, 156.
5. Hava, M., and Hurwitz, A. (1973): *Pharmacologist 15*, 171.
6. Vats, T. S., Hurwitz, A., Robinson, R. G., and Herrin, W. (1973): *Pediat. Res. 22*, 340.
7. Consolo, S., Morselli, P. L., Zacala, M., and Garratini, S. (1970): *Europ. J. Pharmacol. 10*, 239.
8. Nimmo, J., Heading, R. C., Tothill, P., and Prescott, L. F. (1973): *Brit. Med. J. 1*, 587.
9. Peterson, O. L., and Finland, M. (1942): *Amer. J. Med. Sci. 204*, 581.
10. Waisbren, B. A., and Hueckel, J. S. (1950): *Proc. Soc. Exp. Biol. Med. 73*, 73.
11. Barr, W. H., Adir, J., and Garrettson, L. (1971): *Clin. Pharmacol. Therap. 12*, 779.
12. Robinson, D. S., Benjamin, D. M., and McCormack, J. J. (1971): *Clin. Pharmacol. Therap. 12*, 491.

Drug Interactions, edited by P. L. Morselli,
S. Garattini, and S. N. Cohen. Raven Press,
New York © 1974

Decreased Serum Concentrations of Rifampicin When Given with PAS Orally*

Gunnar Boman

Department of Clinical Pharmacology, Huddinge University Hospital and Department of Thoracic Medicine, Karolinska Hospital, Stockholm, Sweden

INTRODUCTION

Modern chemotherapy of tuberculosis always includes a combination of two or three antituberculous drugs given during a period of 1.5 to 2 years. Interactions between the drugs combined may give unwanted effects. Rifampicin (RMP), called rifampin in the United States, is a semisynthetic antibiotic which has been widely accepted as a major antituberculous drug the last few years.

MATERIAL AND METHODS

Patients

Sixty-nine tuberculous patients participated in the study. All had normal kidney and liver function. None of the patients had earlier received RMP.

Drugs

On separate days, single oral doses of the following drugs were given in an arbitrary order during 1 week: (a) RMP alone, (b) aminosalicylic acid (PAS) alone, (c) isoniazid (INH) alone, (d) RMP + PAS, and (e) RMP + INH. In the last 14 patients, the administration of PAS and RMP + PAS was omitted. RMP was never given on 2 subsequent days. Commercial preparations were used. Ten milligrams of RMP per kilogram body weight were given in the form of capsules Rifadin. A dose of PAS-granulate corresponding to 0.2 g active substance per kilogram body weight was administered. Tablets of Tibinide were given in a dose of 10 mg INH/kg body weight. All drugs were taken on an empty stomach after fasting overnight and drug intake was supervised. A light breakfast was served 30 to 60 min

---

*This is a synopsis of an original article submitted for publication elsewhere.

later. No other drugs were administered during the study and for at least 24 hr before.

Four of the patients were given an intravenous infusion of sodium-PAS during 2 hr, starting 2 to 6 hr after an oral dose of RMP. Eight to 11 blood samples were drawn before, during, and after the infusion. Three other patients were given an oral dose of PAS-granulate after the evening meal and an oral dose of RMP the next morning. Venous blood was drawn before and at 2, 4, 6, and 8 hr after drug intake.

Assay of Drugs

RMP was determined by a microbiological agar diffusion method, using paper discs as diffusion centers. *Sarcina lutea* was used as test strain. PAS (up to 5.0 mg/ml serum) and INH (up to 100 μg/ml) did not inhibit the growth. No antibacterial activity was found in the blank samples, nor in serum from patients treated with PAS or INH. All concentrations are expressed as "rifampicin," although *Sarcina lutea* is also sensitive to the main desacetylated metabolite of RMP (1).

Concentrations of PAS in whole blood were measured colorimetrically according to Lehmann (2). Plasma concentrations of INH were determined spectrophotometrically according to Maher et al. (3). None of the methods was influenced by addition of RMP to blank samples, nor by samples from patients treated with RMP.

Calculations

The half-lives of RMP and INH were calculated from the disposition rate constants (k), obtained by least-squares regression analysis from the descending slope, assuming first-order kinetics. Regression lines with correlation coefficients (r) less than 0.98 were not accepted. Due to different reasons, mainly delayed peak concentrations and technical errors, k could not be calculated after all doses.

In 18 patients where k could be calculated for both RMP and RMP with PAS, the area under the serum concentration curve (AUC) was calculated by the trapezoidal rule from a plot of concentration versus time on linear coordinates. The "rest area" was calculated by dividing the 8-hr concentration by k.

RESULTS

It is apparent from Fig. 1 that the serum concentrations of RMP were markedly reduced when RMP was given with PAS orally. The differences were highly significant at all time points. Thus, at 2 hr the mean concentration of RMP was reduced from 7.6 to 2.7, at 4 hr from 6.4 to 3.1, at 6 hr from 4.6 to 2.9 and 8 hr after the dose from 3.1 to 2.1 μg/ml. The majority of

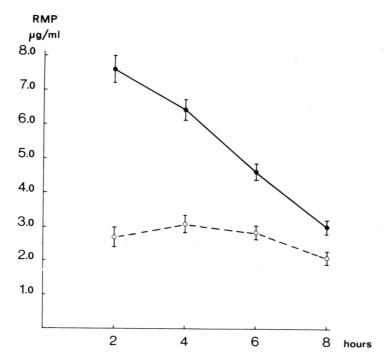

FIG. 1. Mean serum concentrations of RMP after a single oral dose of 10 mg/kg body weight, given alone (●——————●) and after simultaneous oral administration of PAS (0.2 g/kg body weight) (○— — — — —○). Standard error within bars.

patients had an apparent peak value at 2 hr when RMP was given alone. By contrast the mean peak concentration of RMP with PAS was found at 4 hr and individual patients did not reach their highest observed RMP value until 6 or 8 hr after the combined dose. Even if this delay was taken into consideration, a highly significant difference in the peak levels was found (Table 1). The observed mean peak concentrations were less than half the

TABLE 1. *RMP peak serum concentrations—effect of simultaneous oral administration of PAS or INH*

	Observed peak conc.		
	Mean ± SE	Range	
	RMP μg/ml		Signif.
RMP with PAS	3.8 ± 0.3	0.4– 8.8	
			$p < 0.001$
RMP alone	8.0 ± 0.4	1.8–17.5	
			N.S.
RMP with INH	7.8 ± 0.3	2.2–14.5	

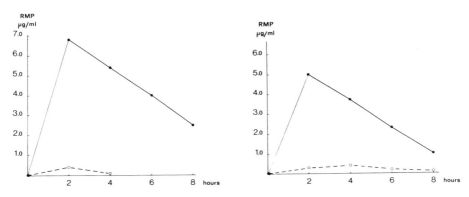

FIG. 2. RMP serum concentration in patient No. 37 (left) and in patient No. 59 (right) after a single oral dose (10 mg/kg body weight), given alone (●————●) and after simultaneous oral administration of PAS (0.2 g/kg body weight) (○— — — — —○).

original values, when RMP was given together with PAS. In 18 patients available for comparison the mean AUC^∞ was reduced from 65.8 for RMP alone to 34.3 $\mu g/ml \cdot h$ for RMP with PAS, a significant decrease ($p <$ 0.001). This result must be interpreted cautiously in view of the large "rest areas" observed in some of the patients. The pronounced effect of PAS on the RMP concentrations in some patients is illustrated in Fig. 2.

No obvious effect of i.v. infusion of PAS on the serum concentrations of RMP could be observed, although the PAS concentrations reached up to 387 $\mu g/ml$. An oral dose of PAS approximately 12 hr before intake of the RMP dose did not appreciably decrease the RMP concentrations.

Using the criteria already described, serum half-life values for RMP given together with PAS could only be calculated for 22 of the 55 patients, mainly due to delayed peak concentrations or nonexponential curves. The mean half-life of RMP was found to be 3.6 to 3.8 hr with a 10-fold interindividual variation. No significant difference was found between the half-life of RMP given alone, with PAS, or with INH (Table 2).

TABLE 2. *RMP serum half-life — effect of simultaneous oral administration of PAS or INH*

	RMP serum half-life		
	N	Mean ± SE Range hours	Signif.
RMP with PAS	22	3.8 ± 0.4 1.7– 8.5	
			N.S.
RMP alone	63	3.8 ± 0.3 1.1–10.3	
			N.S.
RMP with INH	65	3.6 ± 0.2 1.0–10.4	

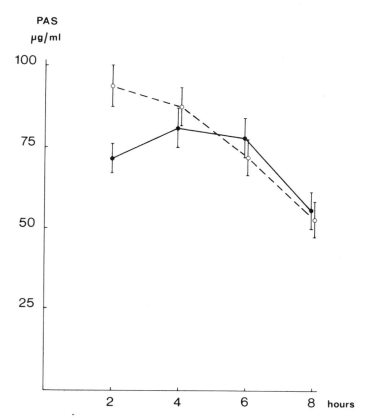

FIG. 3. Mean concentrations of PAS after a single oral dose of 0.2 g/kg body weight, given alone (●————●) and after simultaneous oral administration of RMP (10 mg/kg body weight) (○ − − − − −○). Standard error within bars.

The concentrations of PAS were slightly changed by the simultaneous administration of RMP as illustrated in Fig. 3. When PAS was given with RMP the observed mean peak concentration was found 2 hr after drug intake and was significantly higher than after separate administration. The other differences were not significant. Very marked inter- and intrasubject variations in the concentrations were observed at all time points. The higher PAS concentrations after 2 hr, when PAS was given with RMP, seems to have no clinical importance as the areas were similar.

A possible interaction between RMP and INH has a special interest. Signs of hepatotoxicity are not unusual during RMP treatment and have been attributed to the combination of RMP and INH. However, in our study no significant effect could be demonstrated on the concentrations or half lives of RMP or INH after simultaneous administration of the two drugs.

DISCUSSION

RMP-PAS Interaction

From the data presented, it is evident that PAS reduces the serum concentrations and delays and decreases the peak levels of RMP after simultaneous single-oral-dose administration. The significant reduction of the AUC^∞ after PAS can be interpreted as a decreased fraction of the oral RMP dose entering the systemic circulation or as an increased apparent volume of distribution. Curci et al. (4) have found by equilibrium dialysis that the binding of RMP (20 μg/ml) to bovine serum was reduced from 91 to 78% in the presence of PAS (200 μg/ml). This interaction has not been confirmed in our own experiments with equilibrium dialysis of RMP in human plasma. Oral PAS did not influence the serum half-life of RMP. Intravenous infusions of PAS in a small number of patients did not affect the kinetics of oral RMP. These findings make an effect of PAS on the distribution, metabolism, and elimination of RMP unlikely. Thus, the most plausible explanation is that PAS impairs the gastrointestinal absorption of RMP. Several mechanisms can be proposed.

During long-term treatment PAS has been shown to cause reversible intestinal malabsorption of vitamin B_{12} (5). A single dose of 5 g PAS did not affect the Schilling test (5). Hypocholesterolemia of fat and D-xylose in the presence of normal intestinal mucosa have been observed during prolonged PAS therapy by Halsted and McIntyre (6). They suggest that PAS interferes with intestinal mucosal transport processes. It seems improbable that one or two doses of PAS could induce impressive reduction of RMP absorption by this mechanism. The possibility that PAS alters the physicochemical properties (solubility, dissolution rate, or complex formation) of RMP in the stomach or the intestines has not been ruled out. In this case different galenic preparations of PAS may vary in effect. Another conceivable explanation is that the comparatively large amount of PAS given orally (c. 17 to 23 g incl. constituentia) affects the absorption of RMP in a manner similar to that of food. Solid food prolongs gastric emptying, which influences the rate of drug absorption, regardless of whether they are weak acids, weak bases or undissociated (cf. review in ref. 7). This may explain the delayed and decreased peak concentrations of RMP found in this study. However, the residence time within the entire small intestine must be greatly reduced to decrease the total extent of drug absorbed. Judging from the frequent occurrence of diarrhea in patients treated with PAS, a rapid intestinal transit seems plausible.

CONCLUSIONS

The described interaction between PAS and RMP, resulting in markedly decreased and delayed serum concentrations of the latter, is considered to have significant importance in the treatment of tuberculosis. It is highly unlikely that the observed interaction would diminish during prolonged therapy, particularly as the serum concentrations of RMP tend to decrease by self-induction during continuous treatment (8). Although the mean concentrations of RMP with PAS were well above the minimal inhibitory concentration for *Mycobacterium tuberculosis in vitro,* individual patients may have insufficient concentrations of RMP, running the risk of therapy failure and emergence of RMP-resistant mycobacteria. Thus, RMP and PAS are not considered to be suitable for routine combinations in the chemotherapy of tuberculosis. If an individual patient must be treated with this combination, the drugs should be given with an interval of, say, 8 to 12 hr.

ACKNOWLEDGMENTS

This study was supported by grants from the Swedish National Association against Heart and Chest Diseases, "Carin Tryggers Minnesfond," "Svenska Sällskapet för Medicinsk Forskning," and "Lisa och Johan Grönbergs Stiftelse."

REFERENCES

1. Canetti, G., Djurovic, V., Le Lirzin, M., Thibier, R., and Lepeuple, A. (1970): *Rev. Tuberc. (Paris) 34,* 93.
2. Lehmann, J. (1951): *Scand. J. Clin. Lab. Invest. 3,* 306.
3. Maher, J. R., Whitney, J. M., Chambers, J. S., and Stanonis, D. J. (1957): *Amer. Rev. Tuberc. 76,* 851.
4. Curci, G., Ninni, A., D'Alessio, A., and Iodice, F. (1968): *XIX Congresso Italiano di Tisiologia 3,* 955.
5. Heinivaara, O., and Palva, I. P. (1965): *Acta Med. Scand. 177,* 337.
6. Halsted, C. H., and McIntyre, P. A. (1972): *Arch. Intern. Med. 130,* 935.
7. Levine, R. R. (1970): *Digest. Dis. 15,* 171.
8. Acocella, G., Pagani, V., Marchetti, M., Baroni, G. C., and Nicolis, F. B. (1971): *Chemotherapy (Basel) 16,* 356.

Drug Interactions, edited by P. L. Morselli, S. Garattini, and S. N. Cohen. Raven Press, New York © 1974

Effect of Excretion Changes on Drug Action and Drug Interactions

Marcus M. Reidenberg

Departments of Pharmacology and Medicine, Temple University School of Medicine, Philadelphia, Pennsylvania 19140

INTRODUCTION

Changes in renal function can modify a number of pharmacokinetic processes in the body and thereby lead to unanticipated drug effects or drug interactions.

DRUG EXCRETION

Drug excretion is slowed in patients with impaired renal function. Various methods have been proposed for reducing the usual doses of drugs eliminated from the body by urinary excretion of unmetabolized drug to correct for the delayed excretion in uremia (1–3). This modification of dose is essential for safe, effective use of excreted drugs in patients with impaired renal function.

When a drug is excreted by extrarenal as well as renal pathways, impaired renal function can decrease urinary excretion significantly without necessarily changing the extrarenal excretion rate constant. Thus, the overall elimination rate constant will fall and the major pathway of elimination may shift from renal to extrarenal. Digoxin, for example, is primarily eliminated from the body by urinary excretion in patients with normal renal function. Excretion in feces is a minor pathway. As renal function deteriorates, the urinary excretion of digoxin decreases, whereas the excretion rate in feces remains constant. Thus, fecal losses account for an increasing proportion of the excreted drug and fecal excretion can become the major pathway of digoxin excretion in uremia. (Fig. 1) (4). For these uremic patients, individual variation in the extrarenal elimination rate is important in establishing maintenance dosage requirements and this factor is ignored in the various equations and tables published for calculating digoxin dosage for patients with poor renal function. All such tables assume a constant extrarenal elimination rate represented by a drug half-life of 4.4 days in an anuric patient. We have recently seen a patient with an 8-day half-life for digoxin

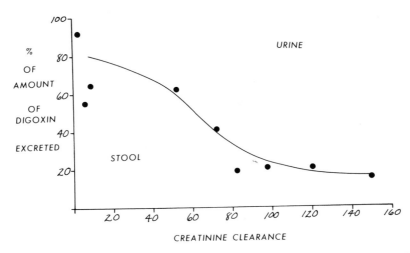

FIG. 1. Ratio of fecal excretion of digoxin to urinary excretion of digoxin following intravenous administration in patients with various degrees of renal function. Data from Bloom
and Nelp (4).

indicating substantial slowing of extrarenal elimination of the drug (5). This
patient had centrolobular necrosis of his liver as well as uremia. The observation indicates that some patients with liver disease can have impaired
extrarenal elimination of digoxin even though the kinetics of digoxin has
been reported as normal in three cirrhotic patients (6).

A major drug interaction involving the kidney is the effect of one drug on
the renal tubular secretion and subsequent excretion of another drug. There
are many examples of this. In general, administration of an organic acid
will slow the tubular secretion of other concurrently given organic acids and
administration of a base will slow the tubular secretion of other bases (2).
Two examples of clinical significance are the slowing of methotrexate excretion by salicylate (7) and the potentiation of the hypoglycemic effect of
acetohexamide by phenylbutazone (8). The phenylbutazone did this by
slowing the excretion of hydroxyhexamide, an active metabolite of acetohexamide.

Another drug interaction affecting drug excretion is the effect of a drug
that changes urine pH on the elimination of any drug that is filtered at the
glomerulus and reabsorbed by nonionic diffusion back into the blood as the
glomerular filtrate passes down the nephron. A change in urine pH that
increases the ionized fraction of the drug in the urine increases the excretion
rate of the drug. This phenomenon has been extensively investigated with
phenobarbital and alkalinization of the urine by Waddell and Butler (9) and
put to use treating patients with phenobarbital poisoning (10).

DRUG METABOLISM

Drug metabolism may be normal or slow in uremic patients depending on the pathway. A list of drugs that have been studied in uremic patients classified by their major pathway of metabolism in man is shown in Table 1.

Hydrolysis of procaine in serum from patients with impaired renal function has been studied in detail. The degree of slowing of the hydrolysis is proportional to the degree of azotemia of the patient. Dialysis of patients

TABLE 1. *Effect of uremia on apparent elimination rate of drugs in man*

Drug	Effect	Reference
Oxidations		
Tolbutamide	None	Glogner (11)
Tolbutamide	None	Reidenberg (12)
Phenobarbital	None	Fabre (13)
Histamine	None	Beall (14)
Phenacetin	None	Prescott (15)
Diphenylhydantoin	None	Letteri (16)
Antipyrine	None	Black (17)
Quinidine	None	Kessler (18)
Propranolol	None	Lowenthal (19)
Vitamin D	Prolonged	Avioli (20)
Reduction		
Cortisol	Prolonged	Englert (21)
Syntheses		
Glucuronide conjugation		
Chloramphenicol	None	Kunin (22)
Acetylation		
Sulfisoxazole	Prolonged	Reidenberg (23)
p-Aminosalicylate	Prolonged	Ogg (24)
Isoniazid	None	Bowersox (25)
Isoniazid	None	Reidenberg (26)
Hydrolyses		
Peptides		
Plasma angiotensinase	None	Osborn (27)
L-Asparaginase	None	Ho (28)
Albumin	None	Wells (29)
Plasma kallikreinogen	None	Colman (30)
Insulin	Prolonged	O'Brien (31)
Insulin	Prolonged	Horton (32)
Insulin	Prolonged	Rabkin (33)
Esters		
Cholinesterase activity	Slowed	Holmes (34)
Cholinesterase activity	Slowed	Simon (35)
Procaine	Prolonged	Reidenberg (36)

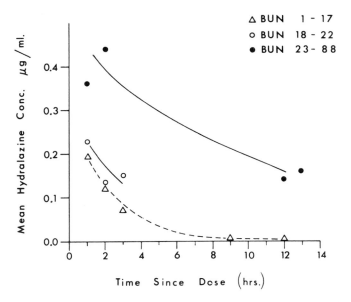

FIG. 2. Mean plasma hydralazine concentrations at various times after an oral dose in outpatients stratified by blood urea nitrogen (BUN). Data from Reidenberg, Drayer, de Marco, and Bello (38).

or plasma did not increase esterase activity. Mixing uremic serum with normal serum appeared to dilute the esterase activity of the normal serum but did not inhibit it. Our conclusion was that the slow hydrolysis is due to a decrease in the amount of enzyme activity in the serum and not to an unexcreted inhibitor being present in the serum (36).

Recently, we have found that plasma concentrations of hydralazine are higher in azotemic patients than in patients with normal renal function (Fig. 2) (37). We have found that uremic patients have plasma isoniazid half-life values within the normal range (26). This confirms the observations of Bowersox (25) but appears to be in disagreement with the observations of Dettli (38).

Observations recently completed on plasma quinidine half-life indicate that the plasma half-life is normal in patients with uremia or with congestive heart failure. These normal results are the findings if one uses an analytical method for quinidine that does not also measure fluorescent quinidine metabolites (18). The older analytical methods used by investigators who have observed prolonged half-life values in patients with these diseases measured metabolites as well as quinidine. These nonspecific methods cannot differentiate slowed metabolism of the drug from normal metabolism with slowed excretion of fluorescent metabolites, the expected consequence of uremia.

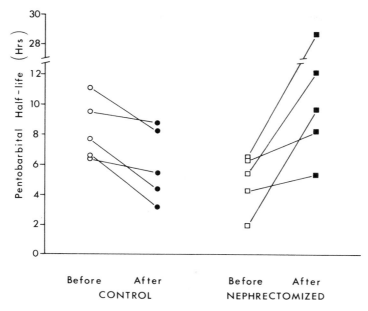

FIG. 3. Plasma half-life values of pentobarbital in dogs. For control animals, before and after refer to a 4-day waiting period. For nephrectomized dogs, "before" refers to period immediately following nephrectomy and before azotemia has occurred; "after" measurements were made on the fourth postoperative day after uremia had developed.

It is interesting that drug oxidations, including barbiturate oxidation, appear normal in uremic patients (Table 1). A study in dogs has produced contrary results. Mongrel dogs were anesthetized with pentobarbital. Those to serve as controls simply had multiple plasma samples drawn and pentobarbital concentrations measured. This was repeated 4 days later. The experimental animals had bilateral nephrectomy while under pentobarbital anesthesia and then multiple blood samples drawn for pentobarbital levels. Thus, this first study was done in animals that were not uremic but had no kidneys. Pentobarbital was given 4 days later, and multiple blood level measurements were made. The analytical method used for pentobarbital was to buffer serum to pH 5.5, extract into heptane with 1.5% isoamyl alcohol, extract back into pH 11 aqueous phosphate buffer, and measure the intensity of fluorescence at 420 nm while exciting at 260 nm (uncorrected) (after Udenfriend, 39). Plasma pentobarbital half-life was estimated graphically. All control animals had shorter half-life values following the second dose than they had after the first, probably indicating microsomal enzyme induction. All of the nephrectomized animals had longer half-life values after the second dose (Fig. 3) (40).

It thus appears that the uremia following acute nephrectomy in the dog is not a representative model of uremia in man for studying drug metabolism.

PLASMA PROTEIN BINDING OF DRUGS

Since drug excretion and drug metabolism can be altered by impaired renal function, modification of dosage of drugs to achieve therapeutic plasma concentrations has been suggested for uremic or azotemic patients. The "biologically active" concentration of a drug is that dissolved in plasma water. However, the methods for measuring plasma concentrations of drugs also include that bound reversibly to plasma proteins. Therefore, it is necessary to know if protein binding of drugs is altered by uremia in order to properly interpret "therapeutic plasma concentrations." The binding of drugs to uremic patients' plasma proteins has been studied (Table 2).

All drugs that are organic acids that have been studied to date have been found to have decreased protein binding in plasma from uremic patients. It would therefore appear prudent to make an allowance for decreased protein binding of drugs that are highly protein-bound organic acids in interpreting plasma concentration measurements of these drugs in uremic patients.

Drugs that are organic bases appear to have a normal fraction bound in plasma from uremic patients (with one excretion). Thus no change in our ideas of the values of therapeutic blood levels for most of these drugs need be made for uremic patients.

TABLE 2. *Effect of uremia on plasma protein binding of some drugs*

Drug	Effect	Reference
Organic acids		
Congo Red	Decreased	Ehrström (41)
Sulfonamides	Decreased	Scholtan (42)
Thyroxine	Decreased	Arango (43)
Sulfonamides	Decreased	Büttner (44)
Sulfonamides	Decreased	Anton (45)
Diphenylhydantoin	Decreased	Reidenberg (46)
Tryptophane	Decreased	Gulassay (47)
Clofibrate	Decreased	Bridgman (48)
Fluorescein	Decreased	Reidenberg (49)
Organic bases		
Desmethylimipramine	Normal	Reidenberg (46)
Quinidine	Normal	Lunde (50)
Quinidine	Normal	Reidenberg (49)
Dapsone	Normal	Reidenberg (49)
Triamterene	Decreased	Reidenberg (49)
Trimethoprim	Normal	Craig (51)

TISSUE SENSITIVITY IN UREMIA

In addition to pharmacokinetic abnormalities produced by impaired renal function, changes in tissue sensitivity or in drug responses can be seen in uremic patients. Those drugs whose action is dependent on renal function such as diuretics or urographic contrast media will be less effective as renal function deteriorates.

The uremic state also modifies the responses to some drugs that have extrarenal sites of action. Cellular sensitivity to insulin is decreased in uremia. The hypnotic response to barbiturates is increased in uremia (2, pp. 33–35). Uremic patients have a flat dose-response curve when multiple small doses of atropine are given intravenously and the heart rate change is monitored (52).

Uremic patients' erythrocytes appear to be more sensitive to cephalothin's ability to induce a positive direct Coombs' test than erythrocytes from nonuremic patients (53).

SUMMARY

Impaired renal function modifies both pharmacokinetic processes and sensitivity to pharmacologic actions of drugs. Drug excretion and certain pathways of drug metabolism are slowed in uremia. The binding of organic acids to plasma proteins is decreased and allowance must be made for this in interpreting plasma concentration measurements of drugs. A few examples of change in extrarenal tissue sensitivity to drugs in uremic patients are known and listed. Patients with impaired renal function should have ordinary treatment programs modified for them to correct for their abnormal pharmacokinetic processes or abnormal pharmacologic responses. Both safety and efficacy can thereby be increased for these people.

ACKNOWLEDGMENTS

This work was supported in part by U.S. Public Health Service grants GM 18279 and RR 349 from the General Clinical Research Centers Branch of the National Institutes of Health. The author is a recipient of Research Career Development Award K4-GM 09766 from the National Institute of General Medical Sciences.

REFERENCES

1. Dettli, L., Spring, P., and Ryter, S. (1971): *Acta Pharmacol. Toxicol. 29*, 211.
2. Reidenberg, M. M. (1971): *Renal Function and Drug Action*, Saunders, Philadelphia.
3. Bennett, W. M., Singer, I., and Coggins, C. H. (1973): *JAMA 223*, 991.
4. Bloom, P. M., and Nelp, W. B. (1966): *Amer. J. Med. Sci. 251*, 133.
5. Reidenberg, M. M., and Katz, M. (1973): *New Engl. J. Med. 289*, 1148.
6. Marcus, F. I., and Kapadia, G. G. (1964): *Gastroenterology 47*, 517.

7. Liegler, D. G., Henderson, E. S., Hahn, M. A., and Oliverio, V. T. (1969): *Clin. Pharmacol. Ther. 10*, 849.
8. Field, J. B., Ohta, M., Boyle, C., and Remer, A. (1967): *New Engl. J. Med. 277*, 889.
9. Waddell, W. J., and Butler, T. C. (1957): *J. Clin. Invest. 36*, 1217.
10. Lassen, N. A. (1960): *Lancet 2*, 338.
11. Glogner, P., Lange, H., and Pfab, R. (1968): *Med. Welt. 52*, 2876.
12. Reidenberg, M. M. (1973): *Proc. Fifth Internat. Cong. Pharmacol.*, Vol. 3, p. 175, Karger, Basel.
13. Fabre, J., Freudenreich, J. de, Duckert, A., Pitton, J. S., Rudhardt, M., and Virieux, C. (1967): *Helv. Med. Acta 33*, 307.
14. Beall, G. N., and Van Arsdel, P. P. (1960): *J. Clin. Invest. 39*, 676.
15. Prescott, L. F. (1969): *Clin. Pharmacol. Ther. 10*, 383.
16. Letteri, J. M., Mellk, H., Louis, S., Kutt, H., Durante, P., and Glazko, A. (1971): *New Engl. J. Med. 285*, 648.
17. Black, M., *personal communication.*
18. Kessler, K. M., Lowenthal, D. T., Gibson, T., Warner, H., and Reidenberg, M. M. (1974): *New Engl. J. Med. 290*, 706.
19. Lowenthal, D. T., Briggs, W. A., Gibson, T. P., Matusik, E., and Demaree, G. (1973): *Pharmacologist 15*, 188.
20. Avioli, L. V., Birge, S., Lee, S. W., and Slatopolsky, E. (1968): *J. Clin. Invest. 47*, 2239.
21. Englert, E., Brown, H., Willardson, D. G., Wallach, S., and Simons, E. L. (1958): *J. Clin. Endocr. 18*, 36.
22. Kunin, C. M., Glazko, A. J., and Finland, M. (1959): *J. Clin. Invest. 38*, 1498.
23. Reidenberg, M. M., Kostenbauder, H., and Adams, W. (1969): *Metabolism 18*, 209.
24. Ogg, C. S., Toseland, P. A., and Cameron, J. S. (1968): *Brit. Med. J. 2*, 283.
25. Bowersox, D. W., Winterbauer, R. H., Stewart, G. L., Orme, B., and Barron, E. (1973): *New Engl. J. Med. 289*, 84.
26. Reidenberg, M. M., Shear, L., and Cohen, R. V. (1973): *Amer. Rev. Resp. Dis. 108*, 1426.
27. Osborn, E. C., Jerums, G., and Jupp, B. A. (1968): *Cardiovasc. Res. 2*, 33.
28. Ho, D. H. W., Thetford, B., Carter, C. J. K., and Frei, E. (1970): *Clin. Pharmacol. Ther. 11*, 408.
29. Wells, J. V. (1969): *Clin. Sci. 37*, 221.
30. Colman, R. W., Mason, J. W., and Sherry, S. (1969): *Ann. Int. Med. 71*, 763.
31. O'Brien, J. P., and Sharp, A. R., Jr. (1967): *Metabolism 16*, 76.
32. Horton, E. S., Johnson, C., and Lebovitz, H. E. (1968): *Ann. Intern. Med. 68*, 63.
33. Rabkin, R., Simon, N. M., Steiner, S., and Colwell, J. A. (1970): *New Engl. J. Med. 282*, 182.
34. Holmes, J. H., Nakamoto, S., and Sawyer, K. C., Jr. (1958): *Trans. Amer. Soc. Artif. Intern. Organs 4*, 16.
35. Simon, N. M., del Greco, F., Dietz, A. A., and Rubinstein, H. M. (1969): *Trans. Amer. Soc. Artif. Intern. Organs 15*, 328.
36. Reidenberg, M. M., James, M., and Dring, L. G. (1972): *Clin. Pharmacol. Ther. 13*, 279.
37. Reidenberg, M. M., Drayer, D., deMarco, A. L., and Bello, C. T. (1973): *Clin. Pharmacol. Ther. 14*, 970.
38. Dettli, L., and Spring, P. (1973): In: *Pharmacology and The Future of Man, Proceedings of the Fifth International Congress on Pharmacology*, Vol. 3, p. 170, S. Karger, Basel.
39. Udenfriend, S., Duggan, D. E., Vasta, B. M., and Brodie, B. B. (1957): *J. Pharmacol. Exper. Ther. 120*, 26.
40. Wishner, W., Salganicoff, L., and Reidenberg, M. M., *unpublished observations.*
41. Ehrstrom, M. C. H. (1937): *Acta Med. Scand. 91*, 191.
42. Scholtan, W. (1961): *Arzneimittelforsch. 11*, 707.
43. Arango, G., Mayberry, W. E., Hockert, T. J., and Elveback, L. R. (1968): *Mayo Clinic Proc. 43*, 503.
44. Buttner, H., Portwick, F., Manzke, E., and Staudt, N. (1969): *Klin Wschr 42*, 103.
45. Anton, A. H., and Corey, W. T. (1971): *Acta Pharmacol. Toxicol. 29* (Suppl. 3), 134.
46. Reidenberg, M. M., Odar-Cederlof, I., von Bahr, C., Borgå, O., and Sjoqvist, F. (1971): *New Engl. J. Med. 285*, 264.
47. Gulassay, P. F., Peters, J. H., and Schoenfeld, P. (1971): *Abstracts of Fifth Ann. Meeting, Amer. Soc. Nephrology*, p. 29 (1971).

48. Bridgman, J. F., Rosen, S. M., and Thorp, J. M. (1972): *Lancet 2,* 506.
49. Reidenberg, M. M., and Affrime, M. (1973): *Ann. N.Y. Acad. Sci. 226,* 115.
50. Lunde, P. K. M. (1973): *Proc. Fifth Internat. Congr. Pharmacol. 3,* 201.
51. Craig, W. A., and Kunin, C. M. (1973): *Ann. Int. Med., 78,* 491.
52. Lowenthal, D. T., and Reidenberg, M. M. (1972): *Proc. Soc. Exper. Biol. Med. 139,* 390.
53. Molthan, L., Reidenberg, M. M., and Eichman, M. F. (1967): *New Engl. J. Med. 277,* 123.

Drug Interactions, edited by P. L. Morselli,
S. Garattini, and S. N. Cohen. Raven Press,
New York © 1974

Genetic and Environmental Factors Influencing Drug Metabolism

Daniel W. Nebert and Joseph R. Robinson

Section on Developmental Pharmacology, Laboratory of Biomedical Sciences, National Institute of Child Health and Human Development, National Institutes of Health, Bethesda, Maryland 20014

In our laboratory we are studying the regulation of enzyme "activity," i.e., what causes enzyme "activity" to increase or decrease in response to certain exogenous stimuli. Rather than studying soluble enzymes such as tyrosine aminotransferase or glutamine synthetase, where one can isolate and purify a protein and then equate immunoprecipitable radioactivity with *de novo* enzyme synthesis, we are involved in a more complex system: a membrane-bound multicomponent enzyme system which is of major importance in the metabolism of not only numerous endogenous lipophilic substrates such as steroids, cholesterol, bilirubin, and fatty acids, but is essential in the metabolism of most xenobiotics. These exogenous substrates include everything from hair sprays, hexachlorophene, and body deodorants to polycyclic hydrocarbons, herbicides, wood terpenes, insecticides, and many drugs (1, 2). I would like first to review briefly the currently accepted characteristics of the mono-oxygenase enzyme systems, secondly to describe some studies we have done with inbred mice in which we have determined certain genetic differences in drug metabolism between different strains of mice, thirdly to suggest that we may be able to predict in cell culture what will happen to the drug in man or in the intact animal, and lastly to show data indicating that the genetic differences in drug metabolism between strains of mice most likely represent a difference at the regulatory rather than the structural gene locus.

When one speaks of mono-oxygenase "activity," this denotes the integrity of an electron chain flowing between several membrane-bound components. Reducing equivalents are supplied by NADPH and perhaps NADH, and one atom of molecular oxygen is incorporated into the hydrophobic substrate to render an intermediate or product which is more polar and hence more readily conjugable and excreted from the body (1, 2). Any compound possessing a sufficiently high chloroform-to-water partition ratio will be attracted to the lipoidal membrane and then will be metabolized; these enzyme systems therefore metabolize most xenobiotics, as well as steroids, hemin, bilirubin, indoles, thyroxine, sympathomimetic amines, and fatty

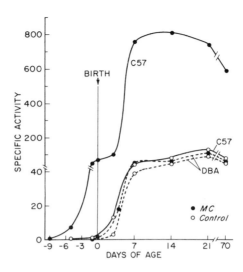

FIG. 1. Hepatic levels of the constitutive aryl hydrocarbon hydroxylase activity and of the enzyme system in response to MC treatment of C57BL/6N and DBA/2N mice as a function of age (6). Each *closed circle* depicts the mean hydroxylase specific activity from the individual livers of six to 15 mice 24 hr after the intraperitoneal administration of 80 mg of MC per kg of body weight. Each *open circle* represents the mean enzyme activity from the individual livers of five to 12 mice 24 hr before treatment of corn oil only. The standard deviation of each group was always less than 25% and usually less than 15% of the mean specific activity. The closed circles depicting the hepatic oxygenase activity prior to birth represent the average specific activity found in five or more individual livers from a litter of fetuses whose mother had received intraperitoneally 80 mg of MC per kg of body weight 24 hr before. The closed circles on day "0" indicate the mean hepatic levels of the enzyme from individual mice born within 24 hr after their mother had received the dose of MC. In this figure the enzyme is expressed as *specific activity*, units per mg of liver homogenate protein. *One unit* of aryl hydrocarbon hydroxylase activity is defined (6, 7) as that amount of enzyme catalyzing per min at 37°C the formation of hydroxylated product causing fluorescence equivalent to that of 1 pmole of 3-hydroxybenzo[a]pyrene. The specific activity of duplicate samples varied less than 10%. The enzyme assay was carried out as previously described (6) with 0.40 to 1.0 mg of tissue protein per 1.0 ml of reaction mixture. The mice were fed normal laboratory chow *ad libitum* until the time of sacrifice. All experiments were begun at approximately the same time of day.

acids (1, 2). These mono-oxygenase "activities" are extremely sensitive to differences in sex, age, strain, and species and to differences in the hormonal or nutritional state of the animal (1). Certain of the "activities" vary by as much as fivefold between 8:00 A.M. and 8:00 P.M., i.e., there may be an important circadian rhythmicity. Any environmental factors such as cigarette smoke, insecticides, or even cedar or pine wood bedding (3) used in animal cages may change what one might consider the "control enzyme activity."

It used to be said (1) that there were two well-defined classes of microsomal enzyme "inducers." There are now at least four classes of compounds that distinctly differ in their mechanisms by which they stimulate mono-oxygenase "activities." One class, exemplified by the polycyclic hydrocarbons, "induces," or stimulates, a rise in the "activity" of several mono-oxygenases. Virtually all tissues, with the possible exception of nervous tissue and the adrenal cortex, may possess these inducible enzyme "activities." Maximally induced activity is attained 1 to 2 days after a single dose. There is little, if any, proliferation of the endoplasmic reticulum. The second class, typified by phenobarbital and more than 200 other compounds, affects not only membrane-bound mono-oxygenases but mitochondrial-bound and cytosol enzymes as well. The effect is primarily in the liver. Hepatic biliary excretion is also increased. Maximally induced activity usually requires 3 to 7 days of continuous doses of phenobarbital. There is a marked proliferation of the smooth endoplasmic reticulum as determined by electron microscopy (1). Another class of mono-oxygenase "inducers" includes a group of steroids, the best one of which is pregnenolone-16α-carbonitrile (4). A fourth class of inducers is the biogenic amines, such as tryptamine or isoproterenol, in cell culture (5). If liver cells in culture (5) or intact animals (1) are given several "types" of inducers, you will find that the mono-oxygenase "activity" reached is often the sum of each of the levels maximally induced by a single inducer. Thus, each of these classes of inducers appears to be acting through some distinctly different mechanism.

Figure 1 shows the extent of induction of a hepatic mono-oxygenase "activity"—in this case aryl hydrocarbon (benzo[a]pyrene) hydroxylase—as a function of the age of inbred mice. The basal enzyme activity in the C57BL/6N mouse is detectable several days prior to birth in hepatic fetal liver, rises rapidly during the first week of life, and declines after the weaning period. The cause for this physiological rise in enzyme activity is unknown but is probably related to such clinical entities as neonatal hyperbilirubinemia and the Gray Syndrome, in which the newborn, and especially the premature, has for some reason not acquired the necessary microsomal enzymes for metabolizing bilirubin and choloramphenicol, respectively. If one gives to the pregnant C57BL/6N mother a single intraperitoneal dose of 3-methylcholanthrene (MC)[1] and then assays the fetal liver 24 hr later, there is a marked stimulation of enzyme activity, detectable as early as 9 days prior to birth. This inducibility rises as a function of age during the perinatal period, reaching a peak at 1 to 3 weeks of age and declining slightly in the adult. The basal enzyme in the DBA/2N mouse and the activity after MC treatment are about the same. In other words, the DBA/2N mouse never develops the capacity to respond to this foreign stimulus.

With C57BL/6N and DBA/2N inbred mice (6–8), the hydroxylase

---

[1] Abbreviations used are: MC, 3-methylcholanthrene; BA, benz[a]anthracene; B6, the C57BL/6N inbred mouse strain; D2, the DBA/2N inbred mouse strain; and TCDD, 2,3,7,8-tetrachlorodibenzo-p-dioxin.

induction in liver and in several other tissues was as great as the responsive B6 parent in the F_1 generation and also in offspring of the backcross between the F_1 and the dominant parent. In offspring of the backcross between the F_1 and the recessive DBA/2N parent and in offspring of the F_2 generation, however, MC treatment caused a bimodal distribution in which approximately 50 and 75% of the animals, respectively, possessed the inducible enzyme. The noninducible enzyme activity was not different from control values. The hydroxylase induction did not segregate with coat color or sex. Incidentally, phenobarbital induces the hydroxylase activity to the same extent in either strain of mice (6–8); here, then, is further evidence that phenobarbital and polycyclic hydrocarbons differ in their mode of action as inducers. Therefore, we can say that expression of hydroxylase induction by aromatic hydrocarbons between these two strains segregates as a single autosomal dominant trait (6–8). This finding affords an exciting experimental model especially for pharmacology or toxicology, because certain drugs can cause disturbances in hormonal or nutritional balance or can be otherwise toxic to the animal. We therefore can distinguish between specific effects related to the enzyme induction process and nonspecific phenomena – simply by studying littermates of the F_2 generation or from the backcross between the F_1 heterozygote and the recessive inbred parent. Accordingly, we have studied genetic differences in the susceptibility to chemically initiated carcinogenesis (9–11) and in the cytochrome or monooxygenase active site (12–17). However, these areas of study will not be covered in this report.

Figure 2 shows the transplacental induction of this enzyme by MC in F_2 offspring prior to birth. The MC was administered intraperitoneally to the pregnant (B6D2)F_1 mother on day 19 or 20, and 24 hr later the hydroxylase activity in the placenta, fetal bowel, and fetal liver of 10 offspring was determined. In this experiment, there were seven of the 10 progeny in which the hydroxylase activity in placenta, fetal bowel, and fetal liver was inducible, and there were three of the 10 that had virtually no response to the inducer MC. It is interesting to note that if the placental enzyme was inducible, so was the hydroxylase in the fetal bowel and fetal liver from that individual, and vice versa. Even though there are "responsive" animals in this uterus and even though the mother has the inducible enzyme, the "nonresponsive" animals in the uterus still fail to respond. Therefore, although the "nonresponsive" animal is filled with MC and although the enzyme is actively metabolizing MC, a failure of response at the genetic level persists.

This brought to mind a study we did about 4 years ago in collaboration with the National Naval Medical Center Obstetrics Department (19). We found (Fig. 3) a strong correlation between aryl hydrocarbon hydroxylase induction in the placenta and a history of cigarette smoking during pregnancy. The correlation was not absolute, because we found a number of

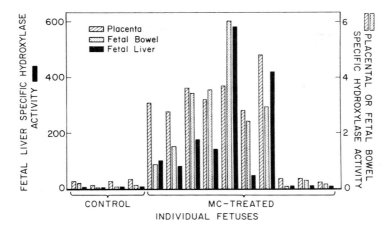

FIG. 2. Placental, fetal bowel, and fetal liver aryl hydrocarbon hydroxylase activities in (B6D2)F$_2$ fetuses from a MC-treated (B6D2)F$_1$ mother (18). The MC was administered as a single intraperitoneal dose (80 mg/kg body weight) in corn oil to the mouse at about 19 or 20 days' gestational age, and the enzyme activities were determined 24 hr later. A control pregnant (B6D2)F$_1$ mouse received corn oil alone. The specific hydroxylase activities are expressed as units per mg of tissue protein for placenta and fetal bowel and in units per mg of microsomal protein for fetal liver.

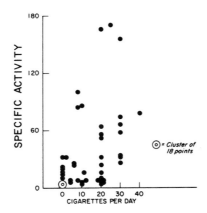

FIG. 3. Human placental aryl hydrocarbon hydroxylase activity as a function of the number of cigarettes smoked daily during the pregnancy (19). The correlation coefficient $r = 0.53$ ($p < 0.001$). Of 59 placentas assayed, 35 were obtained from women who claimed to have smoked between two and 40 cigarettes daily during gestation until the day of parturition, and 24 were obtained from women who claimed to be nonsmokers. The specific hydroxylase activities are expressed as pmoles of 3-hydroxybenzo[a]pyrene formed per 20 min per mg of whole placenta homogenate (19).

pack-a-day smokers who had virtually no enzyme detectable, and we found several nonsmokers who had quite significant amounts of the enzyme. Perhaps these nonsmokers had a charcoal-broiled steak the night before delivery, followed a bus on the way to the hospital, or were continually exposed to cigarette smoking within their household. These differences might also be explained by the brand of cigarettes smoked or by the extent to which they inhaled the smoke. A remaining possibility is that these differences reflect genetic differences in the expression of aryl hydrocarbon hydroxylase induction by aromatic hydrocarbons in man. Evidence to support this possibility has recently come from C. R. Shaw's laboratory (20), where they suggest that the hydroxylase induction in human lymphocyte cultures exposed to MC is controlled by two alleles at the same locus.

We have now studied more than 12 strains and appropriate crosses between many of these strains (21). The initial finding was that the expression of hydroxylase induction in crosses between C57BL/6N and DBA/2N (6–8) or between C57BL/6J and DBA/2J (22) is fully dominant. The expression in F_1 offspring from C3H/HeJ and DBA/2J (22) or from C3H/HeN and DBA/2N (21) is codominant, or additive; in other words, it is gene-dose dependent (21, 22). In offspring from the "responsive" C57BL/6N crossed with the "nonresponsive" AKR/N, hydroxylase induction is totally suppressed—presumably because of some specific interaction between these two strains. When the "responsive" C3H/HeN, BALB/cAnN, or C57BL/6J is crossed with the "nonresponsive" AKR/N, hydroxylase induction is fully expressed in the F_1 offspring; this has led us to propose (21) a minimum of two, but quite possibly three, genes controlling the expression of hydroxylase induction. Hence, we have all of the possible combinations a geneticist would ever hope to study, which we are investigating further with the use of cell culture and *in vivo* systems. Moreover, we have found that this *Ah* locus is not just associated with aryl hydrocarbon hydroxylase induction in the mouse, but is associated with the metabolism of more than a dozen substrates, including other carcinogenic and noncarcinogenic polycyclic hydrocarbons, *p*-nitroanisole, 7-ethoxycoumarin (15), and perhaps naphthalene, zoxazolamine, and diphenylhydantoin (*manuscripts in preparation*).

As reviewed recently by Milunsky and Littlefield (23), it is now possible by means of tissue culture techniques to study human skin, fibroblasts, white cells, or amniotic fluid cells in culture. The enzyme defects quite accurately reflect the homozygote or heterozygote state in the tissue of the intact animal. This has led to the possible *in utero* diagnosis of more than four dozen inborn errors in metabolism and has led to a much better molecular understanding of these diseases during the past several years. Likewise, when tumor cells removed from a patient or an animal are grown in culture, the responses of these cells to various chemotherapeutic agents in culture may simulate the responses of the tumor to those drugs *in vivo* (24); it is

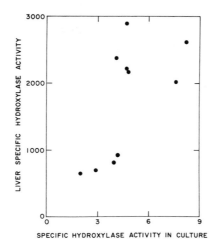

FIG. 4. Aromatic hydrocarbon-inducible aryl hydrocarbon hydroxylase activity in liver microsomes as a function of aromatic hydrocarbon-inducible hydroxylase activity in fetal cell cultures among 10 inbred strains of mice (18). Each *closed circle* represents the mean of 10 individual enzyme determinations in liver microsomes from one inbred strain of mice treated with MC (80 mg/kg body weight) 24 hr before sacrifice, and the mean of six individual enzyme determinations in cultured secondary fetal cells derived from the same strain of mice and treated for 16 to 24 hr with 13 μM BA. The correlation coefficient r is 0.64 (0.02 < p < 0.05). The aromatic hydrocarbon-nonresponsive strains included DBA/2N, NZW/BLN, NZB/BLN, and AKR/N; the aromatic hydrocarbon-responsive strains included C57BL/6N, C3H/HeN, BALB/cAnN, CBA/HN, AL/N, and N:GP(SW). The gestational age of fetuses used for preparing the cultures, the density of cells seeded, and the rate of growth of the cultured cells were kept as similar as possible (25). Maintenance of the animals, preparation of the liver microsomes, and performance of the hydroxylase assay are previously described (6–8).

hoped that certain cancers can be successfully treated in this manner. With the use of cell culture, therefore, can one predict any toxic or teratogenic effects of a drug in a given individual?

Figure 4 shows that, for each of 10 strains of mice, there exists a good correlation between the aromatic hydrocarbon-inducible hydroxylase activity in liver and the inducible enzyme activity in cells derived from fetuses of the same mouse strain. In the four relatively "nonresponsive" strains, the hydroxylase activity in BA-treated cultures often rose by as much as two- to threefold, compared with control enzyme levels. In the six "responsive" strains, the magnitude of enzyme induction was about three- to 10-fold. The kinetics of hydroxylase induction in fetal cell cultures of four mouse strains by BA in the growth medium has been previously illustrated (25).

Figure 5A shows that B6 inbred mice are more susceptible to excessive doses of MC than are D2 mice. The time required for 50% of the group to die was approximately 6.3 days for the B6 strain and 8.5 days for the D2

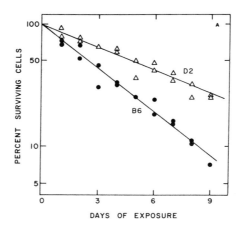

FIG. 5A. Toxicity of aromatic hydrocarbon administration to C57BL/6N (B6) and DBA/2N (D2) mice *in vivo* (18). MC at an intraperitoneal dose of 500 mg/kg body weight was administered daily to groups of 30 mice, and the number of survivors was recorded each day. We have found (26) similar results with intraperitoneal benzo[a]pyrene and 7,12-dimethylbenz[a]anthracene administered to several other "responsive" and "nonresponsive" inbred strains.

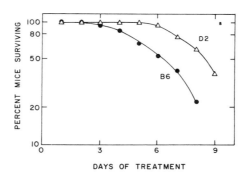

FIG. 5B. Cytotoxicity of 20 μM benzo[a]pyrene in primary cultures derived from whole fetuses of C57BL/6N (B6) or DBA/2N (D2) mice (18). The growth medium was exchanged daily with fresh benzo[a]pyrene-containing medium, and the number of surviving cells was compared daily with the number of cells in cultures grown without benzo[a]pyrene. Duplicate dishes of control and experimental cultures from either strain were harvested daily for cell counts.

strain. The time necessary for 50% of another aromatic hydrocarbon-"nonresponsive" strain, AKR/N, to die was about 8.8 days (not shown). Figure 5B illustrates that the toxicity of aromatic hydrocarbons to B6 and D2 mice *in vivo* is also manifest in fetal cell cultures from these two inbred strains. In this particular experiment, the time at which 50% of the cells have survived continuous exposure to 20 μM benzo[a]pyrene was about

2.6 days for B6 cultures and about 4.8 days for D2 cultures. Alkali-extractable phenolic metabolites parallel the amount of hydroxylase activity in fetal cultures from these two inbred strains (25); thus, the accumulation of hydroxylated benzo[a]pyrene (27, 28) and/or epoxides that then react covalently with cellular macromolecules presumably accounts for the toxicity *in vivo* and in cell culture. The 3,4-epoxybenzo[a]pyrene has recently been identified as the intermediate that interacts with DNA in hamster liver (29).

It might be possible to assess teratogenicity of certain drugs with the use of a similar cell culture experimental system (18). The experiments should include: (i) determination of differences in teratogenicity of a xenobiotic between two inbred strains or species of animals; (ii) demonstration via metabolism of the compound *in vivo* that either detoxification or potentiation of the xenobiotic is related to the teratogenic effect; (iii) measurement of the same differences in metabolism of the xenobiotic in cultures derived from fetal cells, fibroblasts, leukocytes, or amniotic fluid cells; (iv) development of quantitative methods in cell culture (i.e., cell plating efficiency, chromosomal breaks, changes in DNA, RNA, or protein synthesis, metabolite formation, etc.) for predicting the teratogenic index of the compound in other strains or species of animals (18).

The experimental difficulties are numerous. It is shown in Fig. 2 that the metabolism of a drug can differ among the fetal, placental, and maternal tissues. Thus, for example, if the teratogenic form of a drug is a long-lived intermediate, this form may be generated in the maternal tissues and may flood the fetal tissues by way of the maternal-fetal circulation. On the other hand, if the teratogenic form of a drug is a short-lived, extremely reactive intermediate, the interaction of this form with cellular macromolecules in each fetal cell would depend upon the metabolic generation of the intermediate in each cell. The complexity of growing various types of cells in culture must also be appreciated. Enzyme activities and presumably metabolism of xenobiotics may be influenced by (i) the type of culture medium and serum used (5, 23); (ii) the pH as a determinant of cellular growth and contact inhibition (30, 31); (iii) cell generation time and cell cycle (32, 33); (iv) senescence in culture (33, 34); (v) degree of cell confluency (33, 35, 36); (vi) enzyme changes during gestation (7, 33, 37, 38); (vii) differences in enzyme levels between one tissue and another of the same animal (7, 8, 23, 33, 39–41). In spite of these experimental difficulties, it should be possible in the future to predict the teratogenic effects of certain drugs by studying their metabolism in fetal cell culture and by quantitating the effects of a drug or its metabolites on the cell cultures. Likewise, various human pharmacogenetic disorders (42, 43) may be detectable in cell culture such that a patient's response to a certain drug might be predicted with the use of cultured fibroblasts, leukocytes, amniotic fluid cells, or fetal cells derived from that particular individual.

Most recently we have investigated TCDD, an extremely potent inducer of aryl hydrocarbon hydroxylase activity. Compared with the dose of MC required for inducing the hydroxylase activity, the dose of TCDD required is about 30,000 times less (44). Even at massive intraperitoneal doses of MC or β-naphthoflavone until death (45), the hydroxylase induction or formation of a new spectrally distinct CO-binding hemoprotein — cytochrome P_1450 — does not occur in the D2 mouse or in other genetically "nonresponsive" inbred strains. If the inducing property of TCDD is considerably greater than its lethal effects, as compared with MC or β-naphthoflavone, we reasoned that TCDD may be an effective compound for testing the capacity of mono-oxygenase induction or cytochrome P_1450 formation in the "nonresponsive" mouse.

Table 1 shows the response of these mono-oxygenase activities in the liver and kidney of MC- or TCDD-treated B6 and D2 mice. As reported before (15), MC induces the hepatic hydroxylase, O-de-ethylase, O-demethylase, and N-demethylase activities in B6 mice but not in D2 mice. TCDD caused rises in these four enzyme activities that were about the same in B6 and D2 mice (45, 46). The same phenomenon was found in the kidney for the hydroxylase and the O-de-ethylase. The O-demethylase and N-demethylase activities were not detectable in the kidney, most likely because the assay involves a colorimetric determination of product formation, whereas the hydroxylase and O-de-ethylase activities rely on the more sensitive fluorescent determination (15) of product formation. We also found (45) evidence for the spectrally distinct CO-binding hemoprotein in liver, kidney, bowel, lung, and skin of TCDD-treated B6 and D2 mice and in MC-treated B6 mice, but not in MC-treated D2 mice.

These data suggest that the aromatic hydrocarbon "responsiveness" trait is associated with regulatory gene(s) and that the D2 mouse has the structural gene, i.e. the capacity for induction of these mono-oxygenase activities and for cytochrome P_1450 formation. The regulatory gene product may be a "receptor site" for the inducer. Perhaps a deficient "receptor site" in the D2 mouse is made to function by an inducing compound of sufficiently high affinity (i.e. TCDD). Perhaps MC and β-naphthoflavone would also work at higher doses — if they were not lethal to the animal. This may explain why there is significant inducible hydroxylase activity in fetal cell cultures derived from D2 mice or other "nonresponsive" strains (18, 25), since the cells are directly exposed to optimal concentrations of BA in the growth medium. Alternatively, however, TCDD may effect induction of these mono-oxygenases and formation of this new cytochrome by means of some other (e.g. posttranscriptional) mechanism.

In conclusion, we have shown that genetic differences in drug metabolism in the mouse are accurately reflected in fetal cell culture. The genetically mediated increase in hydroxylase induction is correlated with cytotoxicity

TABLE 1. *Effect of 3-methylcholanthrene or 2,3,7,8-tetrachlorodibenzo-p-dioxin on mono-oxygenase activities in liver and kidney of C57BL/6N or DBA/2N mice*

| Strain | Treatment in vivo | Mono-oxygenase activity[a] | | | | | |
| | | Liver | | | | Kidney | |
		Hydroxylase	O-De-ethylase	O-Demethylase	N-Demethylase	Hydroxylase	O-De-ethylase
B6	control	310	1.8	0.4	6.9	0.30	<.01
D2	control	230	1.1	0.6	6.1	0.15	<.01
B6	MC	1860	11.2	2.1	16.7	22	.06
D2	MC	210	1.1	0.5	6.7	0.36	<.01
B6	TCDD	2060	21.2	1.8	20.1	61	.05
D2	TCDD	1970	27.6	2.7	18.3	48	.08

[a] As described previously in detail (15) the specific activities of each of the four mono-oxygenases — aryl hydrocarbon hydroxylase, 7-ethoxycoumarin O-de-ethylase, *p*-nitroanisole O-demethylase, and 3-methyl-4-methylaminoazobenzene N-demethylase — are expressed in units per milligram of microsomal protein.

in fetal cell culture and with a shortened survival time in the animal. The genetic predisposition of each fetal tissue, each individual fetus, the placenta, and perhaps the maternal liver and other maternal tissues all may be important in the metabolism (either enhancement or inactivation of drugs) and therefore in the toxicity, teratogenicity, or carcinogenicity of certain drugs or other xenobiotics. The genetic expression of aromatic hydrocarbon "responsiveness" appears to be controlled by one or more regulatory genes rather than alterations at the structural locus.

ACKNOWLEDGMENT

The valuable technical assistance of L. L. Bausserman, F. M. Goujon, and N. Considine is greatly appreciated.

REFERENCES

1. Conney, A. H. (1967): *Pharmacol. Rev. 19*, 317.
2. Daly, J. W., Jerina, D. M., and Witkop, B. (1972): *Experientia 28*, 1129.
3. Vesell, E. S. (1967): *Science 157*, 1057.
4. Lu, A. Y. H., Somogyi, A., West, S., Kuntzman, R., and Conney, A. H. (1970): *Arch. Biochem. Biophys. 152*, 457.
5. Gielen, J. E., and Nebert, D. W. (1972): *J. Biol. Chem. 247*, 7591.
6. Nebert, D. W., Goujon, F. M., and Gielen, J. E. (1972): *Nature New Biol. 236*, 107.
7. Nebert, D. W., and Gielen, J. E. (1972): *Fed. Proc. 31*, 1315.
8. Gielen, J. E., Goujon, F. M., and Nebert, D. W. (1972): *J. Biol. Chem. 247*, 1125.
9. Nebert, D. W., Benedict, W. F., Gielen, J. E., Oesch, F., and Daly, J. W. (1972): *Mol. Pharmacol. 8*, 374.
10. Benedict, W. F., Considine, N., and Nebert, D. W. (1973): *Mol. Pharmacol. 9*, 266.
11. Nebert, D. W., Benedict, W. F., and Kouri, R. E. *(in press):* In: *Model Studies in Chemical Carcinogenesis,* P. O. Ts'o and J. A. Dipaolo, eds., Marcel Dekker, Inc., New York.
12. Nebert, D. W., Gielen, J. E., and Goujon, F. M. (1972): *Mol. Pharmacol. 8*, 651.
13. Goujon, F. M., Nebert, D. W., and Gielen, J. E. (1972): *Mol. Pharmacol. 8*, 667.
14. Nebert, D. W., and Kon, H. (1973): *J. Biol. Chem. 248*, 169.
15. Nebert, D. W., Considine, N., and Owens, I. S. (1973): *Arch. Biochem. Biophys. 157*, 148.
16. Nebert, D. W., Robinson, J. R., and Kon, H. (1973): *J. Biol. Chem. 248*, 7637.
17. Nebert, D. W., Heidema, J. K., Strobel, H. W., and Coon, M. J. (1973): *J. Biol. Chem. 248*, 7631.
18. Nebert, D. W. (1973): *Clin. Pharmacol. 14*, 693.
19. Nebert, D. W., Winker, J., and Gelboin, H. V. (1969): *Cancer Res. 29*, 1763.
20. Kellermann, G., Luyten-Kellermann, M., and Shaw, C. R. (1973): *Amer. J. Human Genet. 25*, 327.
21. Robinson, J. R., Considine, N., and Nebert, D. W. *(in press): J. Biol. Chem.*
22. Thomas, P. E., Kouri, R. E., and Hutton, J. J. (1972): *Biochem. Genet. 6*, 157.
23. Milunsky, A., and Littlefield, J. W. (1972): *Ann. Rev. Med. 23*, 57.
24. Ogawa, M., Bergsagel, D. W., and McCulloch, E. A. (1973): *Blood 41*, 7.
25. Nebert, D. W., and Bausserman, L. L. (1970): *J. Biol. Chem. 245*, 6373.
26. Robinson, J. R., Felton, J. S., and Nebert, D. W. *(in press): Mol. Pharmacol.*
27. Gelboin, H. V., Huberman, E., and Sachs, L. (1969): *Proc. Nat. Acad. Sci. USA 64*, 1188.
28. Benedict, W. F., Gielen, J. E., and Nebert, D. W. (1972): *Int. J. Cancer, 9*, 435.
29. Wang, I. Y., Rasmussen, R. E., and Crocker, T. T. (1972): *Biochem. Biophys. Res. Commun. 49*, 1142.

30. Ceccarini, C., and Eagle, H. (1971): *Proc. Nat. Acad. Sci. USA 68*, 229.
31. Nigra, T. P., Martin, G. R., and Eagle, H. (1973): *Biochem. Biophys. Res. Commun. 53*, 272.
32. Eagle, H. (1965): *Science 148*, 42.
33. Nebert, D. W., and Gelboin, H. V. (1968): *J. Biol. Chem. 243*, 6250.
34. Robbins, E., Levine, E. M., and Eagle, H. (1970): *J. Exp. Med. 131*, 1211.
35. DeLuca, C., and Mitowsky, H. M. (1964): *Biochim. Biophys. Acta 89*, 208.
36. DeMars, R. (1964): *Nat. Cancer Inst. Monogr. 13*, 181.
37. Leroy, J. G., Dumon, J., and Raermecker, J. (1970): *Nature 226*, 553.
38. Nebert, D. W., and Bausserman, L. L. (1971): *Ann. N.Y. Acad. Sci. 179*, 561.
39. Uhlendorf, B. W., and Mudd, S. H. (1968): *Science 160*, 1007.
40. Shih, V. E., and Littlefield, J. W. (1970): *Lancet 2*, 45.
41. Shih, V. E., and Schulman, J. D. (1970): *Clin. Chim. Acta 27*, 73.
42. La Du, B. M. (1972): *Ann. Rev. Med. 23*, 453.
43. Vesell, E. S. (1972): *N. Engl. J. Med. 287*, 904.
44. Poland, A., and Glover, E. (1974): *Mol. Pharmacol. 10*, 349.
45. Poland, A. P., Glover, E., Robinson, J. R., and Nebert, D. W. (1974): *J. Biol. Chem. 249*, in press.
46. Nebert, D. W., Robinson, J. R., and Poland, A. P. (1973): *Genetics 74*, s193.

Drug Interactions, edited by P. L. Morselli,
S. Garattini, and S. N. Cohen. Raven Press,
New York © 1974

Metabolic Activation of Acetaminophen, Furosemide, and Isoniazid to Hepatotoxic Substances

Jerry R. Mitchell and David J. Jollow

Laboratory of Chemical Pharmacology and Experimental Therapeutics Branch, National Heart and Lung Institute, National Institutes of Health, Bethesda, Maryland 20014

INTRODUCTION

Since the pioneering work of the Millers in the United States and of Magee and colleagues in England, it has become increasingly evident that many chemical carcinogens bring about their effects by combining covalently with DNA and other tissue macromolecules. The carcinogen may react directly but more commonly combines only after metabolic activation to chemically reactive metabolites, which then link covalently with tissue macromolecules (1–5).

Studies on the mechanism of formation of carcinogenic metabolites in the body have shown that chemically inert substances can be converted to reactive metabolites by a variety of different reactions. For example, secondary amines such as N-methyl-4-aminoazobenzene, primary amines including β-naphthylamine and aminobiphenyl, and acetylated primary amines including 2-acetylaminofluorene are N-hydroxylated by either cytochrome P-450 enzymes or amine N-oxidase (1, 2, 4, 6). Dialkylnitrosamines are N-demethylated by cytochrome P-450 enzymes to monoalkylnitrosamines, which then apparently rearrange to unknown active metabolites that act like alkyl carbonium ions (3). Pyrrolizidine alkaloids are thought to be dehydrogenated to chemically reactive pyrrole derivatives (7). Polycylic hydrocarbons and furano compounds such as aflatoxins undergo epoxidation by cytochrome P-450 enzymes to form potent reactants (8). Similar reactions have also been implicated in the formation of chemically reactive metabolites that cause other kinds of toxicity such as liver necrosis (3, 7, 8, 10).

TOXICITY BY THERAPEUTIC AGENTS

The realization that the enzyme pathways responsible for the metabolic activation of many carcinogens are the same microsomal mixed-function oxidases that normally metabolize most drugs led Brodie to speculate that drug-induced tissue lesions might also be mediated through the covalent binding of active metabolites (11). The lack of reactivity of most chemically stable drugs and the frequent localization of tissue damage only in those organs or to those animal species having the necessary drug-metabolizing enzymes supported this view.

Evaluation of this possibility, however, has been difficult. Potential therapeutic agents that reproducibly cause pathological lesions in animal toxicity tests are rarely marketed for clinical use. Moreover, most active drug metabolites produce their effects by combining reversibly with receptor sites. Thus, their pharmacologic activity usually can be evaluated simply by measuring the concentration of the metabolite in plasma (12). But when the response is tissue damage caused by the covalent binding of chemically reactive metabolites to tissue macromolecules, rarely can the relationship between the plasma level of the metabolite and the severity of the lesion be determined. Indeed, with highly reactive metabolites, little or none ever reaches the plasma.

How then can one readily determine the formation of such chemically unstable and reactive metabolites? It seemed possible that there might be a relationship between the severity of the lesion and the amount of covalently bound metabolite for any particular drug. The covalent binding of the reactive metabolite could then be used as an index of the formation of the metabolite. Furthermore, this parameter might well be the most reliable estimate of the availability of the metabolite *in situ* for causing tissue damage, since much of the metabolite often decomposes or is further metabolized before it can be isolated in body fluids or urine. Thus, one approach to the problem would be to determine whether radiolabeled drugs administered to animals over a wide dose range are covalently bound to macromolecules in target tissues that subsequently become necrotic.

CORRELATION OF COVALENT BINDING WITH NECROSIS

We have used this approach to implicate toxic metabolites as mediators of the hepatic necrosis produced by such commonly administered drugs as acetaminophen (paracetamol), acetanilide, and furosemide. These hepatotoxins covalently bind to tissue macromolecules. Since they are chemically stable substances, the finding of a covalent linkage with macromolecules of their target tissue, the liver, indicates that they are converted in the body to reactive alkylating or arylating agents. Moreover, autoradiograms showed that the binding occurred preferentially in the necrotic areas of the liver (13). Covalent binding was also measured quantitatively by extraction of tissue proteins with organic solvents or by isolation of the radiolabeled material bound to single amino acids (13, 14). Both covalent binding and hepatic necrosis after ^{3}H- or ^{14}C-labeled acetaminophen and ^{3}H- or ^{35}S-labeled

TABLE 1. *Effect of treatments on* in vivo *covalent binding of acetaminophen (pHAA) to mouse tissue protein*

Treatment	Dose of pHAA	Severity of liver necrosis after pHAA[a]	Covalent bound ^{3}H-acetaminophen[b]	
			Liver	Muscle
	(mg/kg)		(nmol/mg protein)	
None	375	1–2+	1.02 ± 0.17	0.02 ± 0.02
Piperonyl butoxide	375	0	0.33 ± 0.05	0.01 ± 0.01
Cobaltous chloride	375	0	0.39 ± 0.11	0.01 ± 0.03
ANIT	375	0	0.11 ± 0.06	0.01 ± 0.02
Phenobarbital	375	2–4+	1.60 ± 0.10	0.02 ± 0.02
None	750	3–4+	1.89 ± 0.15	0.04 ± 0.03
Piperonyl butoxide	750	0 or 1+	0.78 ± 0.16	0.04 ± 0.02
Cobaltous chloride	750	0 or 1+	0.85 ± 0.15	0.03 ± 0.03
Phenobarbital	750	4+	2.08 ± 0.12	0.01 ± 0.01

[a] Severity of liver necrosis (1+ to 4+) taken from ref. 15.
[b] Covalently bound ^{3}H-acetaminophen determined 2 hr after ^{3}H-acetaminophen, i.p. Values are means ±SE of at least four experimental or eight control observations. (Data from refs. 13 and 15.)

furosemide were dose dependent, and the peak level of binding preceded the development of histologically recognizable necrosis by a few hours (13–16). Pretreatment of animals with inducers of metabolism, such as phenobarbital, or with inhibitors of metabolism, such as piperonyl butoxide, cobalt chloride, or α-naphthylisothiocyanate (ANIT), similarly altered the rate of metabolism of the hepatotoxins, the severity of hepatic necrosis and the extent of hepatic binding of radiolabeled metabolites. These relationships are illustrated in Table 1.

ENZYME PATHWAY TO TOXIC METABOLITE

Since both the hepatic necrosis and the covalent binding of the toxic metabolites to liver tissue were decreased by inhibitors of cytochrome P-450 enzymes, it seemed likely that the formation of the toxic metabolites might be catalyzed by microsomal cytochrome P-450 systems. Rather than attempting to isolate the highly reactive metabolites of acetaminophen and furosemide, enzyme-dependent covalent binding to hepatic microsomes *in vitro* was used as an index of the formation of the presumed toxic metabolites (14, 17). The binding followed Michaelis-Menten kinetics, and treatments that altered hepatic damage and covalent binding *in vivo* similarly influenced covalent binding *in vitro,* as illustrated in Fig. 1. Binding was dependent on temperature, oxygen, NADPH, time, and enzyme concentration. It was inhibited by a carbon monoxide–oxygen (9:1) atmosphere and by an antibody preparation against NADPH-cytochrome c reductase,

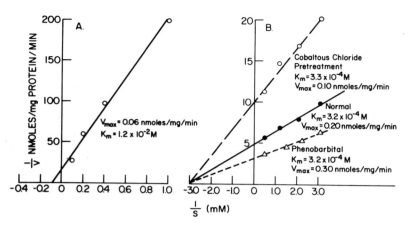

FIG. 1. Double reciprocal plots of mixed-function oxidase-dependent ³H-acetaminophen binding to microsomal protein *in vitro*. (A) Plot for acetaminophen incubated with rat liver microsomes and cofactors for 12 min. Values are means of at least four incubations; SEM were less than ±7%. (B) Plot for acetaminophen incubated for 12 min with cofactors and microsomes from normal mice or from mice pretreated with cobaltous chloride or phenobarbital. Values are means of at least four incubations; SEM were less than ±6%. (Data from ref. 17.)

demonstrating that the toxic pathways for both acetaminophen and furosemide involved cytochrome P-450 mixed-function oxidases.

These results presented something of a dilemma. The most likely activation of acetaminophen would seem to be N-hydroxylation similar to that for another N-acetylarylamine, 2-acetylaminofluorene (2). However, it is commonly believed that the N-oxidation of N-alkylarylamines is not catalyzed by a cytochrome P-450-mediated oxidation (18) and some reports have appeared that carbon monoxide does not inhibit N-hydroxylation of 2-acetylaminofluorene (19, 20). Since a role for cytochrome P-450 in the N-hydroxylation of N-acetylarylamines was crucial to the hypothesis that the toxic metabolite of acetaminophen (*p*-hydroxyacetanilide) was an N-hydroxy derivative, the N-hydroxylation of N-acetylarylamines was further investigated, using 2-acetylaminofluorene and *p*-chloroacetanilide as model compounds (6, 21). A carbon monoxide–oxygen (9:1) atmosphere clearly inhibited N-hydroxylation of both compounds as did pretreatment of the animals with cobaltous chloride. Furthermore, a specific antibody preparation against purified NADPH–cytochrome c reductase isolated from rat liver microsomes inhibited the N-hydroxylation of 2-acetylaminofluorene and *p*-chloroacetanilide. Thus, it appears that at least some N-acetylarylamines can be N-oxidized by cytochrome P-450 mixed-function oxidases. Although conclusive proof of the nature of the toxic metabolite of acetaminophen must await the isolation or capture of the reactive intermediate, other evidence also supports the premise that the toxic metabolite is an

N-hydroxy derivative. A comparison of the hepatotoxicity of structural analogues of acetaminophen (parahydroxyacetanilide) has shown that substitution of a methyl group onto the nitrogen of acetaminophen completely prevents the hepatic necrosis. Since ortho-hydroxyacetanilide also failed to produce liver necrosis, a direct oxidation of acetaminophen to the potentially reactive quinone-imine form is unlikely. In addition, an examination of the metabolites of acetaminophen did not reveal the presence of a dihydrodiol or catechol. Thus, no evidence was found to implicate the intermediacy of an epoxide as the toxic metabolite (22). Moreover, the electron-donating ability of the amino and hydroxyl group substituents on the phenyl ring of acetaminophen makes it improbable that an epoxide metabolite could be the reactive hepatotoxin (cf. 8).

The most likely activation of furosemide, on the other hand, would seem to be an epoxidation of the furan ring similar to that proposed for the carcinogenic and hepatotoxic aflatoxins (9). Furosemide radiolabeled with tritium in the furan moiety was shown to bind covalently to hepatic microsomes in the presence of oxygen and NADPH to the same extent as furosemide radiolabeled specifically with ^{35}S in the sulfonamide portion. Thus, the bound metabolite consists of the entire furosemide molecule. The covalent linkage apparently occurs through the furan moiety. Mild acid hydrolysis of furosemide splits the molecule into its methylfuran and chlorocarboxy-sulfonamide parts. When the protein-furosemide conjugates were similarly hydrolyzed, the binding of the furan-radiolabeled furosemide was unchanged, whereas most of the binding of the sulfonamide-radiolabeled furosemide was lost. In addition, a comparison of the hepatotoxicity of analogues of furosemide has shown that the pathological lesion can be reproduced by such simple furans as hydroxymethylfuran. Moreover, pretreatment with phenobarbital shifts the zone of necrosis produced by furosemide and hydroxymethylfuran from centrilobular-midzonal to entirely midzonal without significantly increasing the size of the necrotic areas. A similar effect of phenobarbital on the hepatic necrosis produced by ngaione, a furano sesquiterpene, has also been reported (23). Interestingly, phenobarbital also fails to potentiate the hepatocarcinogenicity of aflatoxins (24). Presumably phenobarbital is inducing detoxifying pathways as much as toxifying ones *in vivo,* since phenobarbital pretreatment greatly enhances the covalent binding of furosemide to microsomes *in vitro* but not *in vivo.* Thus, considerable evidence implicates a furan metabolite, probably an epoxide, as the toxic substance. As with acetaminophen, however, final proof must await the isolation of the reactive intermediate.

DOSE THRESHOLD FOR TOXICITY

In view of the striking correlation between the severity of hepatotoxicity and the extent of covalent binding by the toxic metabolite of acetamino-

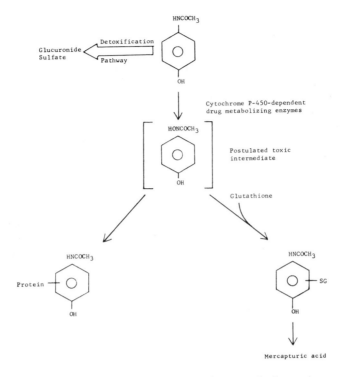

FIG. 2. Pathways of acetaminophen metabolism.

phen, it was surprising to find that significant covalent binding did not occur until over 60% of the acetaminophen had been eliminated from the liver (13). Glutathione was depleted from the liver of animals receiving acetaminophen because it combined with a minor metabolite of the drug and formed a readily excreted mercapturic acid (22, 25, 26). Thus, the possibility arose that the toxic metabolite of acetaminophen ordinarily is detoxified by reacting preferentially with glutathione (Fig. 2). After the liver is depleted of glutathione, however, the metabolite no longer can be inactivated by this pathway and thus combines with liver macromolecules essential to the life of hepatocytes.

Consistent with this view, the effects of various pretreatments that alter the availability of glutathione also altered hepatic necrosis and covalent binding of acetaminophen. Depletion of glutathione by diethyl maleate pretreatment dramatically potentiated acetaminophen-induced hepatic necrosis and covalent binding (25). Conversely, treatment with cysteine, a precursor of glutathione (27), decreased both the hepatotoxicity and covalent binding. Since neither diethyl maleate nor cysteine inhibited the metabolism of acetaminophen, they apparently altered the hepatic damage via their effect on glutathione availability (25).

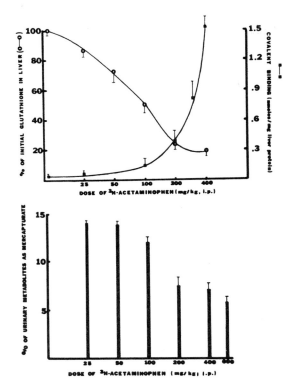

FIG. 3. Relationship *in vivo* between the concentration of glutathione in the liver, the formation of an acetaminophen-glutathione conjugate (measured in urine as acetamino-phen-mercapturic acid), and covalent binding of an acetaminophen metabolite to liver proteins. Several doses of ³H-acetaminophen were administered i.p. to hamsters and glutathione concentrations and covalent binding of radiolabeled material were deter-mined 3 hr later. An additional group of hamsters were treated similarly and urinary metabolites were collected for 24 hr. (Data from refs. 22 and 26.)

By correlating the formation of the acetaminophen-glutathione conjugate *in vivo* with covalent binding and hepatic damage, an electrophilic metabo-lite, presumably N-hydroxy-N-acetyl-*p*-hydroxyaniline, was shown to be detoxified by preferentially combining with the nucleophilic glutathione (22, 25, 26). For example, covalent binding and liver necrosis occurred only after doses of acetaminophen sufficiently large to exceed the availability of glutathione for detoxification (Fig. 3). Similarly, when glutathione con-centrations in the liver were compared with the extent of covalent binding at various times after the administration of acetaminophen, significant bind-ing occurred only after glutathione was markedly depleted (25).

Studies carried out with the model hepatotoxin, bromobenzene, also demonstrate a relationship between hepatic necrosis, hepatic glutathione, and hepatic covalent binding of the toxic epoxide metabolite of bromo-

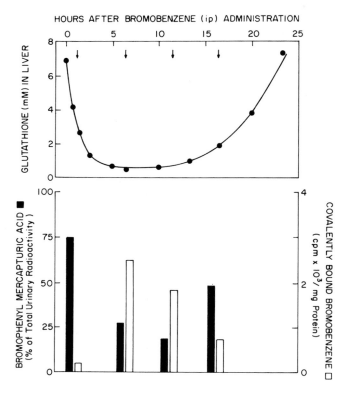

FIG. 4. Relationship *in vivo* between the concentration of glutathione in the liver, the formation of a bromobenzene-glutathione conjugate (measured in urine as bromophenyl-mercapturic acid) and covalent binding of a bromobenzene metabolite to liver proteins. Nonradioactive bromobenzene (10 mmoles/kg) was administered i.p. to rats and the depletion of glutathione from the liver was determined. ^{14}C-Bromobenzene (50 μC, 11.8 mC/mmole) was administered i.v. to additional bromobenzene-treated rats at the time intervals marked with arrows. Urinary metabolites were collected for 12 hr. The rats were then sacrificed and the extent of ^{14}C-bromobenzene bound to liver protein was determined. (Data from ref. 28.)

benzene (28, 29). By correlating the formation of the bromobenzene-glutathione conjugate *in vitro* and *in vivo* with covalent binding and hepatic damage, the toxic metabolite was shown to be detoxified by preferentially combining with glutathione (Fig. 4). The collective data in animals, therefore, indicate that glutathione may be essential for the protection of thiol and other nucleophilic groups in cell macromolecules from a variety of toxic drug metabolites and other alkylating agents.

The significance of glutathione in protecting man from acetaminophen-induced liver injury is yet uncertain, but it probably is responsible for the remarkable safety of the drug after usual therapeutic doses. Since the toxic metabolite of acetaminophen combines preferentially with glutathione after nontoxic doses, measurement of the acetaminophen-glutathione conjugate excreted in urine as a mercapturic acid can be used to estimate the formation of the toxic metabolite of acetaminophen in humans. In 12 patients the amount of mercapturate formed was always about 4% of the administered dose over a dose range from 600 to 1800 mg, demonstrating that the availability of glutathione was never limiting after these therapeutic doses (30). In addition, phenobarbital pretreatment of these patients for 5 days increased the amount of acetaminophen excreted as a mercapturate from 4% to about 7.5% of the therapeutic doses, indicating an increased formation of the toxic metabolite after phenobarbital induction but again without exceeding the availability of glutathione at these doses. These data suggest that the hepatic injury after acetaminophen overdosage might be increased in humans receiving inducers such as phenobarbital. In fact, a retrospective study of patients suffering from acetaminophen-induced hepatic necrosis has confirmed this view (31). Because acetaminophen-induced hepatic damage and covalent binding in animals is prevented, but not reversed, by a variety of exogenously administered nucleophiles such as cysteine, cysteamine, and dimercaprol (25, 30), these substances may provide a possible rationale for treatment of overdosed patients seen early after poisoning.

The hepatic necrosis produced by furosemide also exhibited a dose threshold for toxicity (14, 16). No covalent binding or necrosis occurred until a dose of 100 mg/kg was exceeded. But furosemide, unlike the halobenzenes and acetaminophen, does not deplete the liver of glutathione. Thus, the reason for the threshold is unclear, but preliminary evidence suggests that it may be due to saturation by the drug of the reversible binding sites of plasma proteins either alone or in combination with the saturation of the active renal secretory systems (32). More free furosemide is then available to the liver for metabolism.

In summary, the concept of a dose threshold for toxicity is an important one for drug-induced liver injury. If a wide range of drug doses is not examined in studies of liver damage, insight into the mechanism of the injury will often be impossible.

HEPATOTOXICITY AFTER THERAPEUTIC DOSES OF DRUGS

Let us turn to another important facet of this problem. Does the concept of drug metabolism as a cause of toxicity apply only to drugs given in huge overdoses or could it also explain important hepatic drug reactions seen clinically after such drugs as isoniazid and iproniazid? Three of our recent clinical studies may have shed some light on this complex problem.

First was a prospective study in which 250 patients receiving isoniazid were examined monthly for serum glutamic oxaloacetate transaminase (SGOT) and bilirubin elevations (33). About 20% showed abnormal values that subsided while the patients continued to take isoniazid. Measurement of 6-hr plasma concentrations of isoniazid in these patients failed to show a correlation between slow rates of metabolism (acetylation) and abnormal liver function tests. Although some investigators have reported such a correlation in a small number of patients (34), other studies also failed to find a correlation between isoniazid hepatic injury and slow acetylation of isoniazid (35, 36). In our study no anti-isoniazid antibodies were found and no correlation was seen between hepatic injury and antinuclear antibodies measured at the end of the study.

The second study was a retrospective analysis of 224 patients with possible isoniazid-related hepatic injury (37). These patients were part of a special surveillance program carried out by the U.S. Public Health Service on 13,000 recipients of isoniazid to determine the actual incidence of isoniazid-related hepatic injury. Some of the important findings of this study were (a) isoniazid-related liver injury was indistinguishable biochemically (S.G.O.T., bilirubin, alkaline phosphatase) and morphologically from iproniazid-induced liver damage or from other causes of acute hepatocellular injury such as viral hepatitis; (b) no clinical evidence for a hypersensitivity mechanism was apparent; (c) about 50% of the patients with hepatic reactions were residents of Honolulu and of Oriental ancestry — accordingly, as many as 90% of this group would be expected genetically to be fast acetylators of isoniazid (38).

These observations led to the third study. Twenty-one patients with apparent isoniazid hepatitis were phenotyped into fast and slow acetylators of isoniazid, using the sulfamethazine method (39). A striking 88% incidence of fast acetylators was found (unpublished).

For this reason, acetylisoniazid and isopropylisoniazid (iproniazid) were given to rats, mice, and hamsters to see if they would produce hepatic necrosis (40). Rare, scattered single cell necrosis was seen occasionally in normal animals, but after pretreatment with phenobarbital, a marked hepatitis occurred with doses above 200 mg/kg. This necrosis was prevented by simultaneous treatment with inhibitors of drug metabolism, such as cobaltous chloride, aminotriazole, and piperonyl butoxide. When the metabolism of isoniazid and its acetyl and isopropyl analogues was examined in rats, very little isoniazid was hydrolyzed, whereas 40 to 50% of the administered acetylisoniazid or isopropylisoniazid was hydrolyzed to isonicotinic acid and the respective free hydrazine derivative.

Since many hydrazines are known to be potent hepatotoxins, carcinogens, and mutagens (41, 42), the hepatotoxicity of various hydrazines was examined in animals (40). After phenobarbital pretreatment, acetylhydrazine and isopropylhydrazine produced a striking midzonal and centrilobular necrosis at doses as low as 15 mg/kg. However, only rare single cell necrosis was seen even after LD_{50} doses of hydrazine, methylhydrazine, ethylhydrazine, and n-propylhydrazine. The necrosis produced by acetylhydrazine and isopropylhydrazine was prevented by pretreatment of

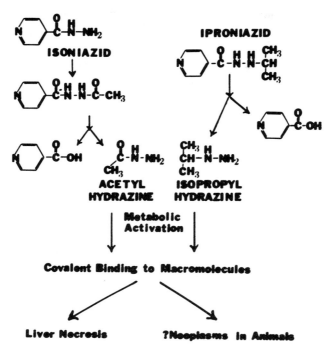

FIG. 5. Proposed metabolic activation pathways for isoniazid, acetylisoniazid, and iso-propylisoniazid (iproniazid).

animals with inhibitors of drug metabolism such as cobaltous chloride, aminotriazole, and piperonyl butoxide.

As further proof that acetylisoniazid was converted in the body to a chemically reactive metabolite, ^{14}C-acetyl-labeled acetylisoniazid was administered to rats. A large amount of covalent binding of the radiolabeled material (about 1 nmole/mg protein) was found in liver, the target organ. This binding was increased by pretreatment with phenobarbital and markedly decreased by pretreatment with cobaltous chloride or aminotriazole. However, no covalent binding occurred after acetylisoniazid if the radiolabel was in the pyridine ring, indicating that the reactive metabolite came only from the acetylhydrazine moiety.

Thus, metabolic activation of the liberated hydrazines satisfactorily accounts for the hepatic necrosis produced by acetylisoniazid and iso-propylisoniazid in animals (Fig. 5). A possible explanation, therefore, is provided for the increased incidence of isoniazid hepatitis in humans with fast acetylator phenotype, since human fast acetylators of isoniazid produce more acetylisoniazid than do slow acetylators (Table 2).

Other clinical observations also make this hypothesis an attractive one.

TABLE 2. *Twenty-four hour urinary excretion of isoniazid and metabolites in nine humans receiving isoniazid (5 mg/kg, p.o.)*

Acetylator phenotype	INH[a]	INH Hydrazones	AcINH[b]	INA Derivatives[c]	Acetyl hydrazine produced[d]
	(% of dose)				(mmoles/70 kg man)
Fast (4)	2.8 ± 0.4	3.6 ± 0.4	45.3 ± 4.2	48.3 ± 3.8	1.2 ± 0.10
Slow (5)	11.9 ± 1.1	21.7 ± 4.9	34.8 ± 2.4	31.6 ± 5.1	0.8 ± 0.13

[a] INH—isoniazid.
[b] AcINH—acetylisoniazid.
[c] Isonicotinic acid and isonicotinyl glycine.
[d] The amount of acetyl hydrazine produced was calculated assuming that all of the isonicotinic acid and isonicotinyl glycine arose by hydrolysis of acetylisoniazid. This has been demonstrated in other human studies (43, 44).

For example, the increased incidence of isoniazid liver injury in patients concomitantly receiving rifampin (45, 46), an excellent inducer of human drug metabolizing enzymes (47), might be due to an increased activation of acetylhydrazine to its toxic form. Similarly, the apparently increased incidence of isoniazid hepatitis when isoniazid is administered alone, in contrast to its administration with *p*-aminosalicylic acid (PAS), might be explained by an inhibition of the acetylation of isoniazid by PAS (48).

In view of the possible clinical implications, however, it should be noted that this work at present is only an hypothesis for the mechanism of isoniazid hepatitis in humans. Confirmation must await more definitive metabolic studies in patients.

METABOLIC ACTIVATION, HEMOLYSIS AND BONE MARROW INJURY

Although this chapter has dealt primarily with hepatotoxic drugs, we anticipate that the metabolic activation of compounds to toxic substances may eventually be implicated in the pathogenesis of a wide variety of tissue lesions induced by drugs and by environmental pollutants. For example, it is well known that 7,12-dimethylbenzanthracene causes leukopenia, thrombocytopenia, and bone marrow aplasia (49). Recent studies have shown that the severity of the syndrome produced by 7,12-dimethylbenz-anthracene could be reduced by the inhibitors of drug metabolism, SKF 525-A or 7,8-benzoflavone (50). Since 7,12-dimethylbenzanthracene is not metabolized by bone marrow preparations of rats, it seems likely that a metabolite formed in the liver mediates the toxicity.

Repeated injections of benzene also produce bone marrow aplasia in rats. The lesion is prevented when the metabolism of benzene is altered by a variety of pretreatments (SKF 525-A, piperonyl butoxide, phenobarbital) (51). Although the finding that phenobarbital pretreatment protects against benzene-induced bone marrow damage has led investigators to propose that benzene itself is the toxic agent (52), this seems unlikely since pretreatments such as cobaltous chloride and aminotriazole, which inhibit the synthesis of cytochrome P-450 in rats, block the metabolism of benzene and markedly reduce the bone marrow damage *(unpublished results)*. Thus, it seems likely the bone marrow aplasia caused by benzene is mediated by an unknown active metabolite.

Another example of metabolic activation is drug-induced methemoglobinemia and hemolysis. Aromatic amines including aniline are known to cause methemoglobinemia by being converted to phenylhydroxylamines, which on oxidation to their nitroso derivatives and subsequent reduction back to the phenylhydroxylamines promote the formation of methemoglobin (53, 54). In addition, certain aniline-derivative drugs also cause hemolysis, especially in patients having a genetic deficiency in erythrocyte glucose-6-phosphate dehydrogenase (55). ^{51}Cr-labeled rat erythrocytes injected intravenously into rats have been used to measure the effects of drugs on hemolysis (30, 56, 57). After the intraperitoneal administration of aromatic amines, such as aniline, *p*-phenetidine, and *p*-chloroaniline, the rate at which ^{51}Cr declined in blood was greatly increased, confirming that these compounds induced hemolysis in rats. The hemolysis is apparently caused by metabolites rather than by the parent amines, since these compounds in incubation mixtures had no effect on erythrocyte survival. Moreover, pretreatment of rats with carbon tetrachloride, which decreased the metabolism of the aromatic amines, prevented the hemolysis induced *in vivo*.

The corresponding N-acetylated derivatives, namely acetanilide, phenacetin, and *p*-chloroacetanilide, also caused hemolysis in this system, although to a lesser degree than did the free amines. The hemolysis produced by the acetylated amines was prevented by pretreatment of the rats with *bis-p*-nitrophenyl phosphate, which inhibits deacetylation (58). In contrast, the administration of the deacetylase inhibitor did not prevent the hemolysis induced by the free amines. These results suggest that these analgesic drugs require metabolic transformation in two steps in order to cause hemolysis, presumably deacetylation and N-hydroxylation (30, 56, 57). In the past, the same active intermediate was thought to cause both hemolysis and methemoglobinemia. However, phenobarbital pretreatment of rats increases the methemoglobinemia but decreases the hemolysis caused by acetanilide and aniline, whereas pretreatment with an inhibitor of metabolism, piperonyl butoxide, evokes exactly the opposite effects (30, 56, 57). These results clearly demonstrate that methemoglobinemia and drug-induced hemolysis are mediated by different active metabolites and suggest that methemoglobinemia is not a prerequisite for hemolysis.

PERSPECTIVE

A major obstacle in the development of new drugs is the fact that potentially useful therapeutic agents occasionally cause pathological lesions in man and animals. In studying the mechanisms of drug-induced toxicity, three major questions must be considered. First, is the toxicity caused by the drug itself or is it caused by a metabolite? Second, does the toxic drug or its metabolite exert its effect by combining reversibly or covalently with tissue components? Third, what factors affect the severity of the lesion after the toxic drug or its metabolite reacts with intracellular sites? Although little is known about the third set of factors above, considerable progress has been made in elucidating those factors that control the formation and fate of toxic drug metabolites. A better understanding of these factors may lead to more rational approaches to the design of nontoxic therapeutic agents in the future.

REFERENCES

1. Miller, E. C., and Miller, J. A. (1966): *Pharmacol. Rev. 18,* 805.
2. Miller, J. A. (1970): *Cancer Res. 30,* 559.
3. Magee, P. N., and Barnes, J. M. (1967): *Adv. Cancer Res. 10,* 163.
4. Weisburger, J. H., and Weisburger, E. K. (1973): *Pharmacol. Rev. 25,* 1.
5. Mitchell, J. R., and Jollow, D. J. (1973): Third International Conference on Liver Diseases: Drugs and the Liver, Freiburg, Germany.
6. Thorgeirsson, S. S., Jollow, D. J., Sasame, H. A., Green, I., and Mitchell, J. R. (1973): *Mol. Pharmacol. 9,* 398.
7. Mattocks, A. R. (1973): *Proc. 5th Int. Congr. Pharmacology,* Vol. 2, Karger, Basel.
8. Daly, J. W., Jerina, D. M., and Witkop, B. (1972): *Experientia 28,* 1129.
9. Swenson, D. H., Miller, J. A., and Miller, E. C. (1973): *Biochem. Biophys. Res. Commun. 53,* 1260.
10. Recknagel, R. O. (1967): *Pharmacol. Rev. 19,* 145.
11. Brodie, B. B. (1967): In: *Drug Responses in Man,* p. 188, Churchill, London.
12. Brodie, B. B., and Mitchell, J. R. (1973): In: *Biological Effects of Drugs in Relation to their Plasma Concentrations* (D. S. Davies and B. N. C. Prichard, eds.) Macmillan, London.
13. Jollow, D. J., Mitchell, J. R., Potter, W. Z., Davis, D. C., Gillette, J. R., and Brodie, B. B. (1973): *J. Pharmacol. Exp. Ther. 187,* 195.
14. Potter, W. Z., Nelson, W. L., Thorgeirsson, S. S., Sasame, H., Jollow, D. J., and Mitchell, J. R. (1973): *Fed. Proc. 32,* 305.
15. Mitchell, J. R., Jollow, D. J., Potter, W. Z., Davis, D. C., Gillette, J. R., and Brodie, B. B. (1973): *J. Pharmacol. Exp. Ther. 187,* 185.
16. Mitchell, J. R., Potter, W. Z., and Jollow, D. J. (1973): *Fed. Proc. 32,* 305.
17. Potter, W. Z., Davis, D. C., Mitchell, J. R., Jollow, D. J., Gillette, J. R., and Brodie, B. B. (1973): *J. Pharmacol. Exp. Ther. 187,* 202.
18. Ziegler, D. M., Jollow, D., and Cook, D. E. (1971): In: *Flavins and Flavoproteins,* p. 507 (H. Kamin, ed.), University Park Press, Baltimore.
19. Matsushima, T., and Weisburger, J. H. (1972): *Biochem. Pharmacol. 21,* 2043.
20. Weisburger, H., and Weisburger, E. K. (1971): In: *Handbook of Experimental Pharmacology: Concepts in Biochemical Pharmacology,* Vol. 28, part 2 (B. B. Brodie and J. R. Gillette, eds.), p. 312, Springer-Verlag, New York.
21. Hinson, J., Mitchell, J. R., and Jollow, D. J. (1974): *Fed. Proc. 33,* 573.
22. Jollow, D. J., Thorgeirsson, S. S., Potter, W. Z., Mitchell, J. R., Gillette, J. R., and Brodie, B. B. (1973): *Fed. Proc. 32,* 305.

23. Seawright, A. A., and Hedlicka, J. (1972): *Brit. J. Exp. Path. 53,* 242.
24. Judah, J. D., McLean, A. E. M., and McLean, E. K. (1970): *Amer. J. Med. 49,* 609.
25. Mitchell, J. R., Jollow, D. J., Potter, W. Z., Gillette, J. R., and Brodie, B. B. (1973): *J. Pharmacol. Exp. Ther. 187,* 211.
26. Potter, W. Z., Jollow, D. J., Thorgeirsson, S. S., and Mitchell, J. R. *(in press): Pharmacology.*
27. Boyland, E., and Chasseaud, L. F. (1967): *Biochem. J. 104,* 95.
28. Jollow, D. J., Mitchell, J. R., Zampaglione, N., and Gillette, J. R. *(in press): Pharmacology.*
29. Zampaglione, N., Jollow, D. J., Mitchell, J. R., Stripp, B., Hamirck, M., and Gillette, J. R. (1973): *J. Pharmacol. Exp. Ther. 187,* 218.
30. Mitchell, J. R., Jollow, D. J., Gillette, J. R., and Brodie, B. B. (1973): *Drug Metab. Dispos. 1,* 418.
31. Wright, N., and Prescott, L. F. (1973): *Scot. Med. J., 18,* 56.
32. Weihe, M., Potter, W. Z., Nelson, W. L., Jollow, D. J., and Mitchell, J. R. *(in press): Tox. Appl. Pharmacol.*
33. Thorgeirsson, U. P., Potter, W. Z., Thorgeirsson, S. S., Black, M., Wijsmuller, G., Woolpert, S. F., Jollow, D. J., and Mitchell, J. R. (1973): *Fed. Proc. 32,* 305.
34. Lal, S., Singhal, S. N., Burley, D. M., and Crossley, G. (1972): *Brit. Med. J. 1,* 148.
35. Smith, J., Tyrrell, W. F., Gow, A., Allan, G. W., and Lees, A. W. (1972): *Chest 61,* 587.
36. Raisfeld, I. H., and Feingold, M., *(in press): Gastroenterology.*
37. Black, M., Mitchell, J. R., Zimmerman, H., Ishak, K., and Epler, G. (1973): *Gastroenterology 65,* A-4/528.
38. Kalow, W. (1962): *Pharmacogenetics,* W. B. Saunders Co., Philadelphia, Pa.
39. Rao, K. V. N., Mitchison, D. A., Nair, N. G. K., Prema, K., and Tripathy, S. P. (1970): *Brit. Med. J. 3,* 495.
40. Snodgrass, W., Potter, W. Z., Timbrell, J., Jollow, D. J., and Mitchell, J. R. (1974): *Clin. Res. 22,* 323A.
41. Back, K. C., and Thomas, A. A. (1970): *Ann. Rev. Pharmacol. 10,* 395.
42. Druckrey, H. (1973): *Xenobiotica 3,* 271.
43. Yard, A. S., McKennis, H., Jr. (1962): *Pharm. Chem. 5,* 196.
44. Peters, J. H., Miller, K. S., and Brown, P. (1965): *J. Pharmacol. Exp. Ther., 150,* 298.
45. Lees, A. W., Allan, G. W., Smith, J., Tyrrell, W. F., and Fallon, R. J. (1971): *Tubercle 52,* 182.
46. Lees, A. W., Allan, G. W., Smith, J., Tyrrell, W. F., and Fallon, R. J. (1972): *Chest 61,* 579.
47. Remmer, H., Schoene, B., and Fleischmann, R. A. (1973): *Drug Metab. Dispos. 1,* 224.
48. Tiitinen, H. (1969): *Scand. J. Resp. Dis. 50,* 281.
49. Phillips, F. S., Sternberg, S. S., and Marquardt, H. (1973): *Proc. 5th Int. Congr. Pharmacol. 2,* 75.
50. Suria, A., Mitchell, J. R., Stripp, B., Jollow, D., and Gillette, J. R. (1971): *Pharmacologist 13,* 241.
51. Mitchell, J. R. (1971): *Fed. Proc. 30,* 2044.
52. Ikeda, M., and Ohtsuji, H. (1971): *Toxicol. Appl. Pharmacol. 20,* 30.
53. Kiese, M. (1966): *Pharmacol. Rev. 18,* 1091.
54. Uehleke, H. (1973): *Proc. 5th Int. Congr. Pharmacol.,* Vol. 2, Karger, Basel.
55. Beutler, E. (1969): *Pharmacol. Rev. 21,* 73.
56. DiChiara, G., Hinson, J. A., Potter, W. Z., Jollow, D. J., and Mitchell, J. R. (1973): *Fed. Proc. 32,* 305.
57. DiChiara, G., Potter, W. Z., Jollow, D. J., Mitchell, J. R., Gillette, J. R., and Brodie, B. B. (1972): *Proc. 5th Int. Congr. Pharmacol.,* p. 57.
58. Heymann, E., Krisch, K., Buch, H., Buzello, W. (1969): *Biochem. Pharmacol. 18,* 801.

Drug Interactions, edited by P. L. Morselli,
S. Garattini, and S. N. Cohen. Raven Press,
New York © 1974

Inhibition of Drug Metabolism in Man

L. Skovsted, J. M. Hansen, M. Kristensen, and L. K. Christensen

Copenhagen University Medical School, Gentofte Hospital, Copenhagen, Denmark

A great number of drugs have been shown to increase hepatic drug metabolism by inducing the synthesis of the liver microsomal enzyme system. It is well documented that the administration of such drugs may accelerate the metabolism of other drugs. The clinical importance of this effect has appeared from many studies.

Animal experiments and *in vitro* experiments have shown that one drug may also inhibit the biotransformation of another drug. Cook et al. (8) observed that SKF 525-A (β-diethylamino-ethyl-diphenyl-propylacetate) prolongs the effect of many drugs and this effect was shown to be due to inhibition of drug metabolism by Brodie (3). Many studies have followed trying to explain the mechanism of this inhibitory action of SKF 525-A (1). Several other examples of inhibition of drug metabolism in animals have been reported (24).

Drug-induced depression of biotransformation of other drugs do also occur in man. This type of interaction indeed has important therapeutic implications.

We reported in 1963 on three cases of hypoglycemic attacks in tolbutamide-treated diabetics caused by the concurrent administration of sulfaphenazole. It was shown (Fig. 1) that the sulfonamide caused a pronounced increase in the serum level of tolbutamide. Serum tolbutamide half-life determinations were carried out after i.v. injection of 1 g of the drug. The administration of a daily dose of 1 to 2 g of sulfaphenazole to three volunteers for 7 days caused an increase in tolbutamide half-life from a mean of 4 hr to a mean of 27 hr. In man tolbutamide is known to be metabolized to a hydroxymethyl derivative. The latter is further oxidized to a carboxy compound [1-butyl-3-(*p*-carboxy) phenylsulfonylurea], which is the major metabolite. Both derivatives have a serum half-life of about 20 to 30 min. They are both found in the urine, which contains, however, only negligible amounts of unchanged tolbutamide.

On one occasion we had the opportunity of performing a few experiments on a sample of human liver tissue (20). In Fig. 2, it is shown that the liver slices transform some of the tolbutamide to carboxytolbutamide and hydroxytolbutamide. After the addition of 16 mg of methyl-sulfaphenazole to 100 ml of incubation mixture, however, no appreciable amounts of the

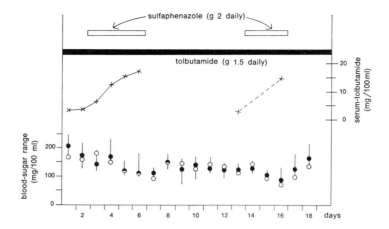

FIG. 1. Sulfaphenazole-induced increase in serum tolbutamide and lowering of blood-sugar values. The mean of five daily determinations is indicated by ● and the fasting blood sugar by ○.

two metabolites could be detected. This may be an indication that the block is in the first oxidation step. In humans, Schulz and Schmidt (29) found serum half-lives of hydroxymethyltolbutamide and carboxytolbutamide to be 35 and 20 min, respectively. These values remained unchanged after prior administration of sulfaphenazole. These results give more direct evidence that the block is primarily in the oxidation of tolbutamide to hydroxytolbutamide.

The value of the half-life will be proportional to the distribution volume of tolbutamide and inversely proportional to the amount of the free, non-protein-bound form of the drug. In four persons, the mean distribution volumes (V_d) of tolbutamide before and after giving sulfaphenazole were 11.7 and 16% of the body weight respectively. This 35% increase in V_d may consequently not explain the observed several hundred percent increase in the half-life of tolbutamide.

In ultrafiltration experiments, the percentage of nonprotein-bound tolbutamide was found to increase from 3.6 to 7.5% after addition of 13.2 mg sulfaphenazole per 100 ml serum. Evidently this increase will tend to lower the serum half-life of tolbutamide. Administration of 2 g of sulfaphenazole a day results in a blood concentration of 6 to 10 mg of the sulfonamide per 100 ml.

It seems clear that the main cause of the sulfaphenazole-induced hypoglycemia is an accumulation of tolbutamide. The fact that a much higher than normal proportion of this increased amount of serum tolbutamide will be unbound by protein may possibly contribute to the hypoglycemia.

Sulfaphenazole also inhibits the metabolism of diphenylhydantoin. In

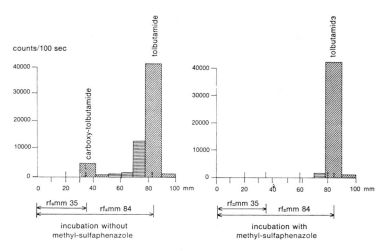

FIG. 2. Effect of methylsulfaphenazole on tolbutamide metabolism by slices of human liver.

two patients the half-life was tripled, and in another five patients a daily dose of 2 g sulfaphenazole for 4 to 5 days caused a change in the steady-state concentration of serum diphenylhydantoin from a mean of 7.5 mg per liter to a mean of 14 mg per liter.

In the above mentioned and in the following studies, the test drugs were always given intravenously. The half-life of tolbutamide in blood was evaluated after giving 0.75 or 1 g intravenously and the plasma concentrations were measured by the procedure of Spingler (33). The half-life of diphenylhydantoin was determined by giving an intravenous injection of 100 mg of diphenylhydantoin to which 20 μC 4-^{14}C-diphenylhydantoin had been added.

In 10 normal controls, the half-life of diphenylhydantoin was determined twice at 8- to 10-day intervals. The reproducibility of tolbutamide half-lives were evaluated in a similar manner. In both cases the variation coefficient was found to be about 10%.

So far as other sulfonamides are concerned, it was found by Hansen and Siersbek-Nielsen of our group that sulfamethizole also impairs drug metabolism. A daily dose of 4 g of sulfmethizole given to six volunteers for 7 days caused a significant change in tolbutamide half-life from a mean of 5.7 hr to a mean of 9.2 hr and a significant decrease in plasma clearance from 17.0 ± 5.4 to 10.5 ± 1.2 ml per min ($p < 0.02$), the distribution volume being unchanged. The same dose of sulfamethizole given to eight persons inhibited diphenylhydantoin metabolism causing an increase in the half-life from a mean of 11.9 to 19.8 hr and a change in plasma clearance from 43.9 ± 17.1 to 28.0 ± 9.3 ml per min ($p < 0.01$). The plasma steady-state level of diphenylhydantoin increased from 21 to 28 mg per liter. Sulfamethizole in the above cited dose was also found to prolong the half-life of warfarin (60 mg given i.v.) in two patients from initial values of 67 and 62 hr to 100 and 85 hr, respectively.

Studies on the effect of other sulfonamides are in progress. Also sulfadiazine and sulfamethoxazole seem to have some inhibitory effect on drug metabolism (Table 1).

The next drug to be discussed is phenylbutazone. This compound may cause enzyme induction in animals. In some cases this induction is preceded by an inhibitory effect (5). In man, it has been found to stimulate aminopyrine metabolism (4). According to our observations, phenylbutazone also has a pronounced and sustained inhibitory effect on drug metabolism. In six patients a 400 to 800 daily dose of phenylbutazone caused an increase in the mean half-life of tolbutamide from 4.5 to 10.5 hr. Oxyphenylbutazone has a similar effect. Phenylbutazone (0.1 g a day for 5 days) was given to 21 patients causing an increase in the mean diphenylhydantoin half-life value from 14.5 to 22 hr. In two patients, the serum concentration of diphenylhydantoin rose from 10 to about 20 mg per liter.

In 1966, we observed that bishydroxycoumarin in therapeutic dosage is a potent inhibitor of diphenylhydantoin metabolism (16). In two patients, the anticoagulant increased the mean half-life from 9 to 36 hr. In six patients, the mean steady-state plasma concentration increased from 5 to 14 mg per liter.

Tolbutamide metabolism is also inhibited by bishydroxycoumarin (19). A mean increase (eight patients) in tolbutamide half-life from 4.5 to 18 hr was observed (20). Similarly the steady-state blood concentration of tolbutamide was 3 to 4 doubled after giving bishydroxycoumarin. The latter also caused an increase in chlorpropamide half-life from about 36 to 89 hr and the serum level of chlorpropamide was approximately doubled (20).

An in vitro inhibition of rat and human liver microsomal mixed-function oxidase by bishydroxycoumarin and other coumarin derivatives was later observed by Deckert and Remmer (11).

The fourth drug to be discussed is chloramphenicol. Dixon and Fouts (12) have shown that chloramphenicol decrease the rate of metabolic transformation of hexobarbitone, acetanilide, codeine, and aminopyrine in mice. In vitro experiments showed an inhibitory effect of a noncompetitive nature on the microsomal drug-metabolizing enzyme system from the liver of mice.

We found that chloramphenicol (2 g a day) retards the biotransformation of tolbutamide (causing an increase in the mean half-life from 5.5 to 15 hr), diphenylhydantoin (causing an increase in the mean half-life from 12.5 to 29 hr) and bishydroxycoumarin (increasing the mean half-life from 8.5 to 25.5 hr). In accord with these results, the mean plasma levels of tolbutamide rose from 7.5 to 14 mg per 100 ml and those of diphenylhydantoin from 2 to 10 mg per liter serum (7).

Mouritsen and Faber in our laboratory observed that the above mentioned dose of chloramphenicol inhibits the transformation of cyclophosphamide to its biologically active metabolite in four patients. The mean plasma half-life was in this case prolonged from 7.5 to 11 hr.

Recently, we have observed that clofibrate (in a dose of 2 g daily for 14 days) inhibits the metabolism of tolbutamide, diphenylhydantoin, and Dicumarol. The mean plasma half-life of tolbutamide increased from 6 to 11 hr (three persons). The corresponding value for diphenylhydantoin was an increase in half-life from 12 to 20.5 hr (five patients). A change in plasma concentration of diphenylhydantoin from 3.2 to 5.8 mg per liter (five patients) was observed. Clofibrate changed the mean half-life of Dicumarol from 11.5 to 18 hr (three patients).

From the above observations and experiments, it appears that sulfaphenazole, sulfamethizole, phenylbutazone, oxyphenylbutazone, bishydroxycoumarin, chloramphenicol, and clofibrate may in certain instances potently prolong the effect of other drugs. It seems reasonable to assume that this effect is due to a retardation of hepatic drug metabolism. As far as chloramphenicol (12) is concerned, such inhibition has been observed during *in vitro* animal experiments. This drug has also been shown to inhibit the microsomal drug-metabolizing enzyme in liver tissue from man.

In the majority of our studies the inhibition effect has been documented by an increase in half-life values as well as by a rise in plasma steady-state concentrations of the drugs metabolized. Changes in the distribution volume of these drugs were comparatively small and could not explain the observed increases in the half-lives. In fact, the plasma clearance of a drug (calculated from V_d and the half-life) is more informative than its half-life value.

The inhibitory compounds mentioned have in some of the cases caused a decrease in the protein binding of the test drugs. This will tend to increase their metabolic transformation and may result in an underestimation of the inhibitory effect as evaluated from measurement of half-lives, plasma clearance rates, and plasma steady-state levels.

Our studies were prompted by the clinical observation of patients with drug-induced tolbutamide and diphenylhydantoin intoxication. For that reason, we have primarily been interested in the metabolic fate of these two drugs. Supplementary studies on the effects of the inhibitory drugs described by us, including the effect on the transformation of antipyrine, are in progress.

The finding of a decrease in the urinary excretion of drug metabolites may be taken as further evidence of inhibition of drug biotransformation. Thus Kristensen (20) found that sulfaphenazole given to seven patients receiving a 1 g dose of tolbutamide caused a mean decrease of the cumulated 24-hr excretion of carboxytolbutamide from 800 to 250 mg.

Hansen et al. (17) observed in our laboratory that the anticonvulsive drug

TABLE 1. *Inhibition of drug metabolism as evaluated by increase in plasma half-lives*

Inhibitory substance	Dose per day	Number of days given	Drug metabolized	Mean half-life (hr)		n	Reference
				Before giving inhibitor	After giving inhibitor		
Sulfaphenazole	2 g	8	Tolbutamide	4.0	27.5	3	(6), (20)
	2 g	7	Diphenylhydantoin (DPH)	7.8	31.9	5	(A.o.)
	2 g	7	Chlorpropamide	35.0	90.0	6	(20)
Sulfamethizole	4 g	7	Tolbutamide	5.7	9.2	6	(A.o.)
	4 g	7	DPH	11.9	19.8	8	(A.o.)
	4 g	7	Warfarin	64.8	92.2	2	(A.o.)
Sulfadiazine	4–6 g	7	Tolbutamide	3.5	5.5	4	(20)
	4 g	7	DPH	8.8	16.3	5	(A.o.)
Sulfamethoxazole			Tolbutamide	5.8	9.0	5	(13)
Phenylbutazone	0.6 g	8	Tolbutamide	4.5	10.5	6	(20)
	0.1 g	5	DPH	14.5	22.3	21	(2)
Oxyphenylbutazone	0.3 g	7	Tolbutamide	4.8	12.0	5	(20)
	0.6 g	7	DPH	10.5	27.5	7	(A.o.)
Bishydroxycoumarin	50 mg	7	Tolbutamide	5.0	17.5	8	(20)
		7	DPH	9.3	39.2	2	(16)
		7	Chlorpropamide	36.5	89.0	2	(19)
Chloramphenicol	2 g	10	Tolbutamide	5.5	14.7	3	(7)
	2 g	10	DPH	12.5	29.0	3	(7)
	2 g	6	Bishydroxy-coumarin	8.5	25.5	4	(7)
	2 g	12	Cyclophospha-mide	7.5	11.2	4	(A.o.)
	1.5–3 g		Chlorpropamide	33.0	108.0	5	(27)

Drug	Dose	Days	Drug affected			n	Ref.
Clofibrate	2 g	14	Tolbutamide	6.0	11.0	3	(A.o.)
		14	DPH	12.0	20.5	5	(A.o.)
		14	Bishydroxy-coumarin	11.5	18.0	3	(A.o.)
Novobiocin		10	Tolbutamide	5.5	9.8	4	(A.o.)
		9	DPH	9.8	15.8	3	(A.o.)
Disulfiram	300 mg	7	DPH	11.0	15.7	6	(A.o.)
			Warfarin				(28)
	7 mg/kg	4	Antipyrine	14.0	23.0	7	(36)
Phenyramidol	1.2 g	4	Bishydroxy-coumarin	21.0	46.0	4	(30)
	300 mg	5	DPH	26.0	55.0	5	(32)
	1.2 g	4	Tolbutamide	7.0	18.0	3	(31)
Benzodiazepine	30 mg	7	Antipyrine	13.0	16.0	6	(36)
Sulthiame	200–800 mg	7–13	DPH	11.0	19.5	4	(17)
Allopurinol	5 mg/kg	14	Antipyrine	11.6	19.1	6	(35)
	5 mg/kg	14	Bishydroxy-coumarin	50.0	152.0	6	(35)
Nortriptyline	0.6 mg/kg	8	Antipyrine	8.4	20.7	6	(35)
	0.6 mg/kg	8	Bishydroxy-coumarin	35.0	106.0	6	(35)
Sulfamethoxazole and trimethoprim	2 g 0.4 g	7	DPH	12.8	19.2	6	(A.o.)
Phenprocoumon	1 mg	7	DPH	9.9	14.0	5	(A.o.)

(A.o.) Author's observation.

sulthiame prolongs the diphenylhydantoin serum half-life (from a mean of 11 hr to a mean of 19 hr) and gives a rise in plasma steady-state concentration of diphenylhydantoin (from a mean of 11 mg to a mean of 22 mg per liter). Olesen and Jensen (26) found, however, no decrease in the urinary excretion of the parahydroxy metabolite of the parent compound. This discrepancy has thus far remained unexplained.

The mechanism by which these inhibitors exert their effect is not understood. Even *in vitro* experiments have not given any complete answer to the problems connected with inhibition of drug metabolism.

Several other examples of the inhibition of the biotransformation of one drug by another in man have been reported (Table 1). Kutt et al. (21) described an inhibitory effect of isoniazide and para-aminosalicylic acid on diphenylhydantoin metabolism. Olesen (25) and Kiørbo (18) observed that diphenylhydantoin transformation was inhibited by disulfiram and this drug will also have such effect on the metabolism of antipyrine (36) and warfarin (28).

Salomon and Schrogie (30–32) found that the muscle relaxant phenyramidol retards the biotransformation of diphenylhydantoin, of tolbutamide, and of warfarin.

Vesell et al. (35) described the inhibitory property of allopurinol and of nortriptyline on drug metabolism. These substances prolong the plasma half-lives of antipyrine and of bishydroxycoumarin. Experiments in our laboratory have shown that allopurinol administered for up to 8 weeks does not cause any change in the biotransformation of diphenylhydantoin.

The demonstration by Gram and Overø (15) that certain neuroleptics inhibit the metabolism of tricyclic antidepressants is also noteworthy.

The inhibitory drugs described by us caused an inhibition of drug metabolism in every subject tested. Certainly the degree of inhibition, however, varied considerably from person to person. As far as the inhibitory property of phenylbutazone is concerned Andreasen et al. (2) in our laboratory found large individual variations in the prolongation of the diphenylhydantoin half-life at identical plasma phenylbutazone levels. The inhibitory effect was also observed even if the inhibitory drug had been given for months. Any indication of a biphasic phenomenon with a change of an inhibitory to an enzyme inducing effect was never noticed.

Shortly after giving sulfaphenazole, phenylbutazone, bishydroxycoumarin, and chloramphenicol, a pronounced decrease in the slope of the blood disappearance curves of the test drugs was observed. Since the inhibitory drugs do not cause any considerable change in distribution volume of the test drugs, this observation may be considered an indication of a rapid onset of the inhibitory effect, and the changes of the slopes can not be due to redistributional phenomena.

Clearly, these examples of inhibited drug metabolism are of considerable clinical importance. Several cases of severe, even life-threatening, drug

TABLE 2. *Examples of serious drug-intoxication cases caused by inhibition of drug biotransformation*

Intoxicating drug	Inhibitory substance	Signs of toxicity	Reference
Tolbutamide	Sulfaphenazole	Hypoglycemic collapse (2 cases)	(6)
Tolbutamide	Phenylbutazone	Hypoglycemic collapse	(A.o.)
Tolbutamide	Bishydroxycoumarin	Hypoglycemic collapse	(20)
Tolbutamide	Chloramphenicol	Hypoglycemic collapse	(7)
Chlorpropamide	Phenylbutazone	Hypoglycemic collapse (2 cases)	(9), (34)
Chlorpropamide	Bishydroxycoumarin	Hypoglycemic collapse	(A.o.)
Diphenylhydantoin	Isoniazid, Para-aminosalicylic acid	Cerebellar symptoms (13 cases)	(21)
Diphenylhydantoin	Bishydroxycoumarin	Vertigo, anorexia (2 cases)	(16)
Diphenylhydantoin	Phenylbutazone	Vertigo, anorexia, vomitus, irreversible cerebellar damage (2 cases)	(22), (37)
Diphenylhydantoin	Disulfiram	Cerebellar symptoms (3 cases)	(18)
Diphenylhydantoin	Sulthiame	Vertigo, anorexia, vomitus	(17)
Diphenylhydantoin	Sulfamethizole	Vertigo, cerebellar symptoms (2 cases)	(A.o.), (23)

(A.o.) Author's observation.

intoxication due to interactions of this type have been observed (Table 2).

Probably the true facts of such cases are often not realized. A series of 20 cases of tolbutamide-induced, unexplained hypoglycemic episodes published by other authors has been reviewed (20). In nine of these, satisfactory information about the use of other drugs was given. Two of these patients also received bishydroxycoumarin, and another was treated with chloramphenicol. The inhibitory action of these substances on tolbutamide metabolism may well explain these three cases of hypoglycemic collapse.

In most cases any of the inhibitory drugs mentioned should not be given to persons receiving the drugs listed in Table 1. The data given in this table will indicate which combinations are potentially most dangerous.

Our pharmacotherapeutic armamentarium is now so abundant that such drug combinations may easily be avoided. Anyway, they should not be used unless plasma-drug levels are carefully monitored. In this connection, it should be mentioned that sulfamethoxipyridazin, sulfadimethoxin, sulfametorin, warfarin, and phenindione have been found by us to have no inhibitory effect on the test drugs used by us.

An exaggerated therapeutic effect or any unexpected rise in the plasma concentration of the drugs listed in Table 1 should always cause a thorough questioning concerning a possible intake of one of the interacting inhibitory drugs.

REFERENCES

1. Anders, M. W. (1971): *Ann. Rev. Pharmacol. 11,* 41.
2. Andreasen, P. B., Frøland, A., Skovsted, L., Andersen, S. A., and Hauge, M. (1973): *Acta Med. Scand. 193,* 561.
3. Brodie, B. B. (1956): *J. Pharm. Pharmacol. 8,* 1.
4. Chen, W., Vrindten, P. A., Dayton, P. G., and Burns, J. J. (1962): *Life Sci. 2,* 35.
5. Cho, A. K., Hodshon, B. J., and Brodie, B. B. (1970): *Biochem. Pharmacol. 19,* 1817.
6. Christensen, L. K., Hansen, J. M., and Kristensen, M. (1963): *Lancet 2,* 1298.
7. Christensen, L. K., and Skovsted, L. (1969): *Lancet 2,* 1397.
8. Cook, L., and Fellows, E. J. (1954): *J. Pharamcol. Exp. Ther. 112,* 382.
9. Dalgas, M., Christensen, J., and Kjerulf, K. (1973): *Ugeskr. Laeger 127,* 834.
10. Davies, D. S., and Thorgeirson, S. S. (1971): *Acta Pharm. Tox. 29,* 181.
11. Deckert, F. W., and Remmer, H. K. (1972): *Chem. Biol. Interact. 5,* 255.
12. Dixon, L. D., and Fouts, J. R. (1962): *Biochem. Pharmacol. 11,* 715.
13. Dubach, U. C., Buckert, A., and Raaflaub, J. (1966): *Schweitz. Med. Wschr. 96,* 1483.
14. Gillette, J., Sasame, H., and Stripp, B. (1973): *Drug Metab. Dispos. 1,* 164.
15. Gram, L. F., and Overø, K. F. (1972): *Brit. Med. J. 1,* 463.
16. Hansen, J. M., Kristensen, M., Skovsted, L., and Christensen, L. K. (1966): *Lancet 2,* 265.
17. Hansen, J. M., Kristensen, M., and Skovsted, L. (1968): *Epilepsia 9,* 17.
18. Kiorbøe, E. (1966): *Epilepsia 7,* 246.
19. Kristensen, M., and Hansen, J. M. (1967): *Diabetes 16,* 211.
20. Kristensen, M. (1973): Medikament-Medikamentinteraktion, Thesis, Dan. Laegestud. Forlag, Copenhagen.
21. Kutt, H., Winters, W., and Mc Dowell, F. H. (1966): *Neurology 16,* 594.
22. Lund, L. (1971): *personal communication.*
23. Lundberg, P. O., *personal communication.*
24. Mannering, G. J. (1971): In: *Handbuch der experimentellen Pharmakologie,* Vol. 28/2 p. 452, Springer, Berlin.
25. Olesen, O. V. (1966): *Acta Pharm. Tox. 24,* 317.
26. Olesen, O. V., and Jensen, O. N. (1969): *Dan. Med. Bull. 16,* 154.
27. Petitpierre, B., and Fabre, J. (1970): *Lancet 1,* 789.
28. Rothstein, E. (1972): *J. Am. Med. Ass. 221,* 1052.
29. Schulz, E., and Schmidt, F. H. (1970): *Pharmacologia Clinica 2,* 150.
30. Sølomon, H. M., and Schrogie, J. J. (1966): *J. Pharmacol. Exp. Ther. 154,* 660.
31. Sølomon, H. M., and Schrogie, J. J. (1967): *Metabolism 16,* 1029.
32. Sølomon, H. M., and Schrogie, J. J. (1967): *Clin. Pharm. Ther. 8,* 554.
33. Spingler, H. (1957): *Klin. Wochenschr. 35,* 533.
34. Thomsen, P. E. B., Ostenfeld, H. O. L., and Kristensen, M. (1970): *Ugeskr. Laeger 132,* 1722.
35. Vesell, E., Passananti, G. T., and Greene, F. E. (1973): *New Engl. J. Med. 283,* 1484.
36. Vesell, E., and Passananti, G. T. (1973): *Drug Metab. and Dispos. 1,* 402.
37. Wendelboe, J. (1971): *personal communication.*

Drug Interactions, edited by P. L. Morselli,
S. Garattini, and S. N. Cohen. Raven Press,
New York © 1974

Drugs Metabolized by Intestinal Microflora

Peter Goldman, Mark A. Peppercorn, and Barry R. Goldin

*Department of Pharmacology, Harvard Medical School and the Clinical Pharmacology
Unit at the Longwood Area Hospitals, Beth Israel Hospital, Boston, Massachusetts 02215*

INTRODUCTION

The recognition that certain drugs are metabolized by the intestinal microflora calls attention to the possible involvement of the intestinal bacteria in
pharmacokinetic drug interactions. An obvious interaction is one between
a drug metabolized by the flora and an antibiotic. In this kind of interaction
the antibiotic diminishes the flora and hence decreases the metabolism of
the drug. There are, however, indications that exogenous compounds other
than antibiotics can alter the activity and composition of the intestinal flora
of man and experimental animals. Hence where only certain constituents
of the flora are responsible for the metabolism of a drug, alterations of the
flora produced by another drug may be the basis for a drug interaction. In
this review, emphasis will be accorded to studies that demonstrate that two
drugs, salicylazosulfapyridine and L-DOPA, are metabolized by the intestinal microflora and the consequent alterations in metabolism of these compounds that occur when experimental animals or human subjects receive
concomitant antibiotics. These interactions may have some implications
for the clinical pharmacology of these drugs. Other factors that might govern
the mediation of interactions by the flora will also be discussed after a consideration of the evidence that these drugs are indeed metabolized at least
in part by the flora.

L-DOPA[1]

An increased level of dopamine generation within the central nervous system (CNS) is believed to be the mechanism by which L-DOPA exerts its
therapeutic effect in Parkinsonian patients. This view has been questioned
by Calne et al. since the chemical transformation of L-DOPA is rapid
whereas the therapeutic response to the drug may be slow (1). These

---

[1] Abbreviations used are the following: L-DOPA, L-3,4-dihydroxyphenylalanine; *m*-HPAA,
3-hydroxyphenylacetic acid; *p*-HPAA, 4-hydroxyphenylacetic acid; *m*-HPPA, 3-hydroxy-
phenylpropionic acid; HVA, homovanillic acid; Dopac, 3,4-dihydroxyphenylacetic acid; and
SASP, salicylazosulfapyridine.

TABLE 1. *Metabolites of L-DOPA in conventional and germ-free rats*[a]

Compound fed	m-HPAA Conv.	GF	p-HPAA Conv.	GF	HVA Conv.	GF	Dopac Conv.	GF	Dopamine Conv.	GF	m-Tyramine Conv.	GF
L-DOPA (40)[b]	0.8	—	0.4	0.5	1.0	1.9	0.7	1.0	+	+	—	—
Dopamine (100)	4.0	—	0.6	0.08	3.9	1.7	3.0	1.6	+	+	—	—
Dopac (100)	0.2	—	—	—	11.8	6.8	15	13.7	—	—	—	—
DL-m-Tyrosine (150)[c]	48	9.9	—	—	—	—	—	—	—	—	+	+
m-Tyramine (90)[c]	23	9.1	—	—	—	—	—	—	—	—	+	+

[a] Rats in metabolism cages were allowed to eat the compound in their diet for 24 hr. Urines were collected during this 24-hr period and for the following 48 hr. Data shown are average values for two rats given each compound and have been corrected for the amount of these compounds excreted by the rats prior to the feeding of the test compound.

[b] The amount of compound added to the diet of each rat (in milligrams) is shown in parentheses.

[c] Fifty milligrams was fed to the germ-free rats.

+ Indicates that the compound was present but was not quantified.

— Indicates less than 0.5 mg of m-tyramine and m-tyrosine, less than 0.1 mg of dopamine, and less than 0.02 mg of the organic acids.

workers suggested the possibility that the activity of L-DOPA might be due to the presence of some minor metabolites of the drug, e.g., m-tyrosine or m-tyramine and they noted that the dehydroxylation at *para* position of the aromatic ring in similar compounds can be attributed to the intestinal microflora. The role of the intestinal flora in the formation of metabolites of L-DOPA was suggested when it was noted that the elevated levels of m-tyramine and m-hydroxyphenylacetic acid seen in the urine of patients taking L-DOPA were lowered when these patients were also given neomycin (2, 3). Thus m-tyramine, a compound with some pharmacological activity, seems to be formed as the result of the activity of the intestinal microflora.

Germ-free rats make it possible to get additional evidence for deciding which reactions in L-DOPA metabolism can be attributed to the intestinal bacteria. For this purpose, L-DOPA and its metabolites were fed to both germ-free and conventional rats and the metabolites in their urine were determined (4). As shown in Table 1, the quantities of urinary metabolites were generally similar except that m-hydroxyphenylacetic acid was not found in the urine of germ-free rats fed catechols. These data allow conclusions to be drawn about the reactions in the metabolism of L-DOPA that can be attributed exclusively to the intestinal microflora. To make this interpretation, it must be assumed that mammalian enzyme activity is the same in both kinds of rats and that each compound has the same distribution in both germ-free and conventional rats. On this basis, some of the transformations in the L-DOPA pathway found in conventional rats can be assigned to the activity of the intestinal flora. For example, dopamine is converted to m-hydroxyphenylacetic acid in conventional but not in germ-

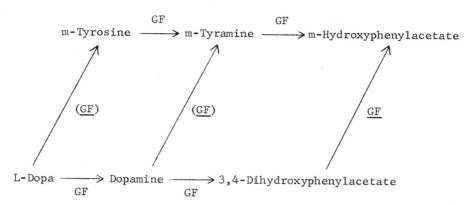

FIG. 1. A transformation that occurs in a germ-free animal is designated by GF, whereas one that does not occur is designated by G̲F̲. A symbol in parenthesis indicates that the designation was obtained by inference from the available data.

free rats suggesting that at least one reaction in this pathway (Fig. 1) is mediated by the intestinal microflora. Since germ-free rats are capable of converting *m*-tyramine to *m*-hydroxyphenylacetic acid, they apparently are unable to convert dopamine to *m*-tyramine. Consistent with this conclusion is the demonstration that rat cecal contents will make this transformation of dopamine when incubated under the anaerobic conditions that might approximate those existing within the intestine (Table 2).

Since *m*-tyrosine has biological activity that might be related to that of L-DOPA, the possibility has been raised that some of the activity of L-DOPA might be due to its conversion to *m*-tyrosine in the animal (3). This conversion requires a dehydroxylation reaction at the *para* position of a substituted catechol; several reactions of this kind can be attributed to the intestinal

TABLE 2. *Bacterial transformation of* L-*DOPA metabolites*[a]

| | Metabolite produced (mg) | | | |
Compound incubated	*m*-HPAA	*m*-HPPA	Dopac	*m*-Tyramine
L-DOPA	0.4	0.3	—	+
Dopamine	—	—	—	+
Dopac	1.8	—	+	—
m-Tyrosine	1.3	0.8	—	—
m-Tyramine	—	—	—	+

[a] Incubation of rat cecal contents with 5 mg of each compound was carried out under anaerobic conditions (4). No evidence was found in any instance for the presence of *p*-HPAA, HVA, dopamine, or *m*-tyrosine.
+Indicates that the compound was present but was not quantified.
— Indicates less than 0.1 mg of *m*-tyramine or less than 0.01 mg for the organic acids.

microflora. Since this kind of reaction has not been found with mammalian enzymes, it would seem that the conversion of L-DOPA to *m*-tyrosine, if it occurs, would be mediated by the flora. Our data with germ-free rats bear on this point. It can be seen that the germ-free rat is capable of transforming *m*-tyrosine to *m*-hydroxyphenylacetic acid. Hence failure to detect *m*-hydroxyphenylacetic acid in the urine of germ-free rats fed L-DOPA can be interpreted as the inability of the germ-free rat to make the conversion from L-DOPA to *m*-tyrosine (4). The capacity of germ-free rats to make some of the transformations normally found in the metabolism of L-DOPA is summarized in Fig. 1.

As a rule, transformations in the metabolism of L-DOPA that occur in conventional but not in germ-free rats can be demonstrated in cultures of rat intestinal contents cultivated under anaerobic conditions. Thus the bacterial transformation from dopamine to *m*-tyramine and from 3,4-dihydroxyphenylacetic acid to *m*-hydroxyphenylacetic acid has been demonstrated (Table 2). Similarly another *p*-dehydroxylation reaction, that necessary for the conversion of L-DOPA to *m*-hydroxyphenylpropionic acid, has been found under these conditions as well as in the conventional rat (4). Although our studies did not reveal any evidence for the conversion of L-DOPA to *m*-tyrosine, the assumptions involved in the experimental approaches to the study of the intestinal flora make it impossible to exclude completely the possibility that this conversion does indeed occur during therapy with L-DOPA.

Our studies and those in Sandler's laboratory implicate the involvement of the flora in specific steps in the metabolism of L-DOPA but these studies do not indicate which constituents of the flora are responsible for these reactions. Caffeic acid, a component of the vegetable matter in the normal diet, undergoes a series of reactions (Fig. 2), the products of which have been demonstrated in the urine of rats and man and in response to the activity of mixed cultures of the microflora of several animal species. These reactions include dehydroxylation at the *para* position of the aromatic ring and decarboxylation of the side chain, reactions which might be considered analogous to some of those occurring in the metabolism of L-DOPA. It is interesting, therefore, that among a representative collection of strains of the bacteria characteristic of the human gastrointestinal tract no single organism, cultivated on artificial media, is capable of more than one reaction in the caffeic acid pathway (5). Data to be presented later indicate the potential hazards of attributing reactions of bacteria in culture to those that these bacteria may perform when they are within the host. These results, however, suggest that metabolic transformations of the kind seen with L-DOPA are apt to be determined by the nature of the constituents of the flora. Thus the potential for altered drug metabolism exists, not only with diminished flora as might be expected from the administration of antibiotics, but also by the introduction of certain drugs or environmental chemicals

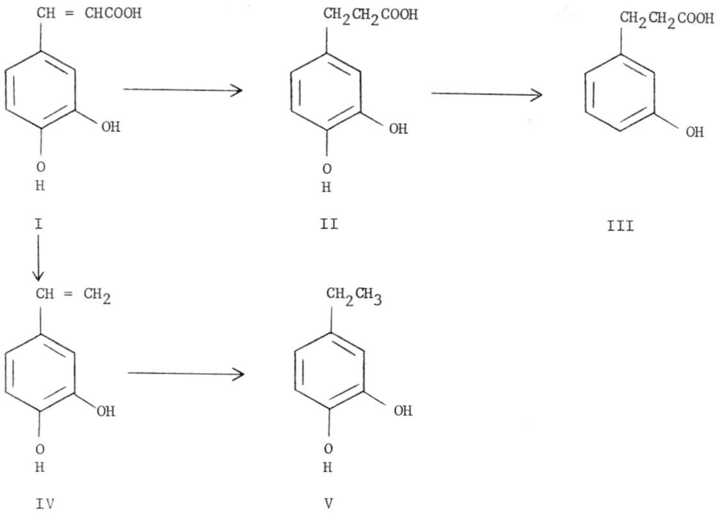

FIG. 2. Metabolism of caffeic acid. Caffeic acid (I) is reduced to dihydrocaffeic acid (II), which is dehydroxylated to 3-hydroxyphenylpropionic acid (III). In another pathway, caffeic acid can be decarboxylated to yield 4-vinylcatechol (IV), which can be reduced to 4-ethylcatechol (V). References to the studies responsible for the elucidation of this pathway are listed in ref. 5.

that affect specific constituents of the flora. We will cite examples of how prolonged feeding of certain compounds metabolized by the flora leads to alterations in the excretion of the metabolites of these compounds. Presumably this occurs as the result of alterations that occur in the flora in response to the continued feeding of the compound.

SALICYLAZOSULFAPYRIDINE

The intestinal flora seems to play a significant role in the metabolism of salicylazosulfapyridine (SASP), a drug regarded as effective therapy in ulcerative colitis as well as effective prophylaxis against relapse for patients with a recent attack of this disease. The drug is 5-aminosalicylate in azo linkage with sulfapyridine (Fig. 3), and these two components of the parent drug and their derivatives are the metabolites recovered when the drug is given to rats and patients.

In contrast to the conventional rat whose excreta contain no SASP, excreta of the germ-free rat contain only SASP and none of its metabolites (Table 3) (6). The metabolism of sulfapyridine and 5-aminosalicylate is the same in both germ-free and conventional rats, indicating that the only difference in SASP metabolism in the two kinds of rats is in the initial reaction. It is therefore possible to attribute this reaction, reduction of the azo bond,

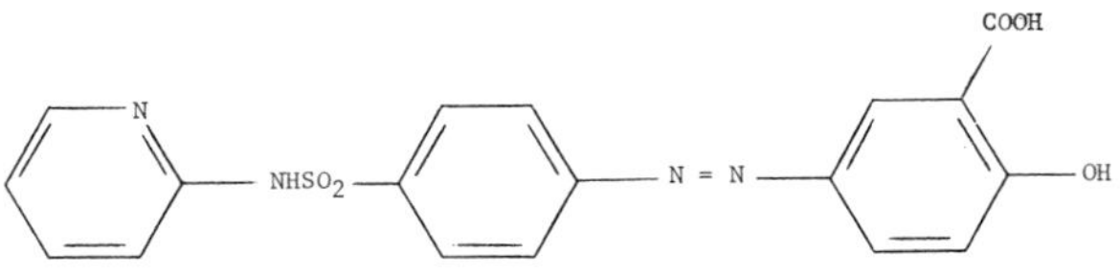

FIG. 3. Salicylazosulfapyridine.

to the activity of the intestinal microflora; further support for this concept is shown by other experiments. As predicted, the concomitant administration of neomycin to a rat getting SASP suppresses the intestinal microflora and allows SASP to be recovered in the feces (Table 4). From the opposite point of view, when a germ-free rat is selectively associated with a bacterial culture capable of reducing the azo bond or is removed from a germ-free environment and is housed in the conventional animal room for a few days, reduction of SASP occurs as in the conventional rat. Thus the animal's capacity to reduce the azo bond is always correlated with the presence of bacteria and the extent of the reduction can be correlated with the amount of intestinal flora (6). Of course, there are many physiological differences between germ-free and conventional animals, and it is possible that a mammalian azo reductase might be induced by the presence of an intestinal flora. It seems unnecessary to invoke this alternative explanation since reduction of the azo bond in SASP was demonstrated in cultures of each of 13 different bacteria characteristic of the gastrointestinal tract of man and rodents. Thus the capacity for this reaction seems to be widespread among intestinal bacteria in contrast to the reactions required in the transformation of aromatic compounds, which seem to be confined only to certain types.

It is curious that SASP should undergo breakdown by the intestinal bacteria at its presumed site of action in the therapy of inflammatory diseases

TABLE 3. *Recovery of SASP and its metabolites in excreta of germ-free and conventional rats[a]*

	Germ-free		Conventional	
	Urine	Feces	Urine	Feces
SASP	1.5[c]	53	0	0
Sulfapyridine[b]	0	0	65	0
5-Aminosalicylate[b]	0	0	55	27

[a] The diet was supplemented with 1% SASP (w/w) for 24 hr and the amount of drug ingested was quantified. Measurements represent the total excreted during the 24 hr of SASP ingestion and for the subsequent 48 hr.
[b] Includes acetylated derivatives.
[c] Numbers indicate percentage of administered dose.

TABLE 4. *The effect of neomycin on the SASP recovered in the intestinal contents of rats*

Average drug intake g/kg/day		Average SASP recovery (range) mg/g			
SASP[a]	Neomycin	Small intestine	Cecum	Colon	Feces
0.14	0.12	0.2 (0.16–0.27)	0[b]	0	0
0.18	0	0.2 (0.13–0.23)	0	0	0
0.23	0.45	0.5 (0.4–0.6)	1.8 (0.7–3.1)	1.4 (0.6–3.2)	1.5 (0.7–2.6)
0.37	0	0.5 (0.1–0.8)	0	0	0
0.6	0.6	0.9 (0.5–1.3)	7.2 (6.3–8.1)	9.8 (7.5–12)	13.9 (7.8–20)
0.7	0	0.6 (0.5–0.7)	0.2 (0–0.4)	0	0

[a] Rats were allowed to eat *ad libitum* a diet containing the two drugs at various levels for at least 4 days prior to sacrifice.

[b] SASP present at a level less than 0.1 mg/g was not detected.

of the large intestine. The site of breakdown suggests that it might be the metabolites of the drug rather than the parent compound that are responsible for the effectiveness of the drug. Sulfapyridine has an antibacterial action, and it is possible that 5-aminosalicylate, a congener of salicylate, might, like other congeners of salicylate, have anti-inflammatory action. Indeed, the original design of SASP by Svartz (7) was based on the assumption that the parent drug would have the two therapeutic activities that could be attributed individually to its constituents.

SASP or its possibly active metabolites may affect inflammatory disease of the colon either by the levels achieved in the body fluids or by the contact that these agents have with the intestinal mucosa. In either mechanism it seems likely that the intestinal microflora can govern drug or metabolite distribution that might in turn determine effectiveness of the drug. The data of Table 4 indicate that SASP is ordinarily not found in the intestine of the rat but that suppression of the intestinal microflora by neomycin permits the recovery of SASP from the colonic contents. Presumably similar alterations in SASP metabolism would occur in patients with their intestinal microflora suppressed by antibiotics, and this might mean different degrees of SASP contact with the diseased colon. Preliminary studies suggest that this is indeed the case. The effect of antibiotics on blood levels of SASP and its metabolites has not yet been examined.

Reduction of the azo bond of SASP by the intestinal flora causes the localization of higher levels of 5-aminosalicylate in the colonic contents than if 5-aminosalicylate itself were given to an animal (8). A relatively greater amount of 5-aminosalicylate is found in the colonic contents of rats when SASP and 5-aminosalicylate are also compared on the basis of parenteral administration. These findings suggest that SASP might serve merely as a vehicle that delivers 5-aminosalicylate to the colon. If an anti-inflammatory agent delivered to the colon in this manner is responsible for the activity of SASP, then a different drug might be designed to deliver 5-aminosalicylate or an even more active anti-inflammatory agent to the colon. In this kind of drug design it might be possible to eliminate the sulfa-pyridine since this portion of the molecule has been implicated as a cause of SASP toxicity. Perhaps after the drug or metabolite distribution associated with the optimal efficacy of SASP is determined, it will be possible to base drug design on these considerations involving the intestinal flora.

CHARACTERIZATION OF THE INTESTINAL MICROFLORA

The administration of antibiotics is an obvious way in which the intestinal flora of man and experimental animals can be altered. But there are other ways as well. It has been shown for example that the fecal flora of an African population differs from that of an English population (9). This difference, which probably arises largely from dietary differences, has been suggested as having a relationship to the greater incidence of colonic cancer in the English population. Different metabolic transformations by flora of the two groups have been suggested as the basis for the actual formation of car-cinogens in the one group (9).

Changes in the intestinal flora occur when the diet is changed as when humans are placed on a chemically defined diet without residue (10). In addition it has been shown that continuous feeding of certain exogenous compounds other than antibiotics can alter the metabolic capacity of the host's microflora. Prolonged feeding of cyclamate, whose transformation to cyclohexylamine is governed by the intestinal flora, results in a higher urinary output of cyclohexylamine (11, 12). This finding, which occurs in both experimental animals and man, can be attributed to a flora that is al-tered in response to continued feeding of cyclamate (11). Whereas the in-creased conversion of cyclohexylamine on prolonged feeding of cyclamate was minimal in two subjects, another had a very striking increase in this conversion. Prolonged feeding of the carcinogen fluorenylacetamide to the rat also causes alterations in the metabolic transformations of derivatives of this compound that can be attributed to the flora (13).

Thus there are examples in the literature where the continued ingestion of foreign compounds can alter the flora of the host as well as its metabolic activity. It has been pointed out that the flora of experimental animals may influence factors in their well-being, such as weight gain or resistance to challenge with experimental infection (14). However, when it is also found that the metabolism and distribution of certain drugs can be affected by the intestinal microflora, this area becomes of more direct interest to the pharmacologist. Germ-free techniques that have been used in these studies on L-DOPA and salicylazosulfapyridine together with a knowledge of the types of chemical transformation that can be attributed to the microflora establish an approach to the determination of whether the microflora can be implicated in the transformations of a given drug. However, the factors that may govern the extent of these transformations in a given host are limited by our knowledge of the microflora itself. Let us turn to the ways that are now available for learning about the flora of an animal.

Techniques have been developed that enable the very fastidious anaerobic organisms that comprise the gastrointestinal microflora to be cultivated in laboratory media (15). These techniques were developed to be used with experimental animals and they require that the samples of the flora be removed from their physiological site within the gastrointestinal tract under anaerobic conditions. These techniques have been extended to the cultivation of the bacteria of human feces. Thus it is now possible to examine metabolic transformations in culture of the anaerobic bacteria isolated from human feces. Caution must be exercised, however, in attributing bacterial transformations of compounds that are observed in culture media to the activity of these bacteria when they are lodged in the host. This is illustrated by studies on the metabolism of caffeic acid. Presumably the urinary metabolites of caffeic acid reflect the metabolic activity of the animal's intestinal flora since these transformations are demonstrable in cultures of the flora and can be diminished in the urine when animals and human subjects are treated with neomycin (16, 17). The demonstration that the germ-free animal is incapable of these transformations (18) further supports the role of the flora when these transformations occur in the conventional animal.

It seemed, therefore, that the metabolism of caffeic acid might serve as a model for defining the relationship between the character of the intestinal microflora of an animal and the metabolism of that compound as revealed by an examination of the animal's urine. For this purpose, germ-free rats were selectively associated with certain types of bacteria characteristic of the rodent gastrointestinal tract; it was then ascertained whether the bacteria were capable of conferring on these animals the capacity to make the transformations of caffeic acid metabolism. In other words, would these bacteria confer selectively on germ-free animals some of the characteristics of the conventional animal?

An examination of the urinary constituents of rats fed metabolites of caffeic acid (Table 5) indicates that association with certain bacteria did enable them to gain the capacity to make some of the metabolic transformations present in the conventional animals. Although the data are not extensive, it seems that the character of these transformations might be related to the type of bacteria that was associated with the rat. However, it is clear that the additional metabolic capacity conferred on the rats by these bacteria do not relate to the metabolic transformations of these bacteria when cultivated on the artificial media used in these studies. This is not surprising since bacteria have a number of mechanisms for altering their metabolism

TABLE 5. *Correlation of metabolic reactions attributed to bacteria in culture or when associated with a germ-free rat*[a]

Bacteria	Dihydrocaffeic acid		m-Hydroxyphenyl-propionic acid		Vinylcatechol		Ethylcatechol.	
	Urine	Medium	Urine	Medium	Urine	Medium	Urine	Medium
S. faecalis	+	+	0	0	0	0	0	0
Lactobacillus sp. 1	0	0	0	0	0	+	0	0
Four intestinal bacteria	tr	+	+	0	0	+	tr	0

[a] The bacteria were examined for their ability to generate the compound shown from its immediate precursor in the scheme shown in Fig. 2 when either grown in culture or when selectively associated with a germ-free rat. +, tr, or 0 indicate respectively the presence, the occasional presence, or the absence of the metabolite in multiple samples of the urine of the animals fed the precursor compound or the medium of bacteria containing the precursor compound. Further experimental details can be found in ref. 18.

in response to alterations in their growth conditions. Furthermore, the bacteria may lodge in portions of the gut where the compound to be metabolized is not well distributed. For example, differences in distribution within the animal between vinylcatechol and the bacteria that metabolize it might account for the failure of vinylcatechol to be metabolized in rats associated with *Lactobacillus* sp. Thus, distribution differences between compound and the intestinal bacteria within the host also might determine the nature of drug interactions that are mediated by the flora.

The distribution of a drug within the animal has long been recognized as a determinant of its metabolic fate and its pharmacological effect, but the distribution of bacteria within the host is a topic that has only recently received attention. It has been fairly common practice to assess the intestinal flora of a human subject by an analysis of his fecal flora. This approach has the advantage of ease of sampling technique but histological sections of the flora of experimental animals done in Savage's laboratory indicate that the constituents of the flora have a rather distinct organization in relation to the mucosa of the host (19). Since it is these bacteria in their natural environment that are probably responsible for the metabolic transformations of pharmacologic interest, it is clear that there is a challenge to learn about these bacteria. Only then will the effect of drugs on these bacteria be understood, and only then will a rational basis be advanced for understanding drug interactions mediated by the flora.

SASP and L-DOPA illustrate the complexities of studying drugs that are metabolized by the flora. Both drugs are considered as effective for their indicated use in therapeutics but unfortunately only in a fraction of patients. Other patients have a variable response; attempted use of these therapeutic agents in some patients must be curtailed because of side effects. Now, of course, these vagaries of therapeutics are general ones and ulcerative colitis is a disease that is particularly noted for its variable course. Hence some of these problems in therapeutics are not surprising. However, it seems worth considering the possibility that some of the variability in the response of different patients to SASP and L-DOPA can be attributed to the variations in their flora. It is difficult to determine the likelihood of this possibility at present because there is no convenient method of assessing the activity of the flora of a patient as it functions *in situ*. Thus, although the flora may be altered in response to dietary changes or the feeding of other exogenous compounds, it is not possible to determine the significance of these alterations of the flora in modifying drug metabolism. The significance of the flora in mediating drug interactions will only be determined by detailed pharmacokinetic studies that relate the distribution of drugs metabolized by the flora and their potentially active metabolites to the therapeutic response of the patient.

SUMMARY

Studies of the metabolism of L-DOPA and SASP in conventional and germ-free rats indicate that certain transformations in the metabolism of these drugs are due exclusively to the activity of the intestinal microflora. With respect to L-DOPA, these reactions include dehydroxylation at the *para* position of both dopamine and 3,4-dihydroxyphenylacetic acid. With SASP it is the initial reaction, reduction of the azo bond, that is governed by the intestinal flora.

When SASP is fed to conventional rats none of the drug is recovered in the urine, feces, or colon; the excreta contain only the products of the azo-bond reduction, 5-aminosalicylate and sulfapyridine, and their metabolites with recoveries of greater than 50%. In germ-free rats, the recovery of SASP itself is greater than 50% and no metabolites of SASP are detectable. When germ-free rats are associated with strains of intestinal bacteria capable of reducing the azo bond in SASP, they gain the capacity to reduce SASP. When the intestinal bacteria of conventional rats are diminished by the feeding of neomycin, unchanged SASP can be recovered in the cecum, colon, and feces. Thus, the metabolism and distribution of drugs metabolized by the intestinal flora can be altered by antibiotics. It has been shown that prolonged feeding of other compounds metabolized by the flora can cause changes in the constituents of the flora as well as changes in the quantities of metabolites caused by the activity of the flora. These findings suggest that the intestinal flora may be responsible for the mediation of drug interactions involving drugs that are metabolized by the flora.

REFERENCES

1. Calne, D. B., Karoum, F., Ruthven, C. R. J., and Sandler, M. (1969): *Brit. J. Pharmacol.* 37, 57.

2. Sandler, M., Karoum, F., Ruthven, C. R. J., and Calne, D. B. (1969): *Science 166*, 1417.
3. Sandler, M., Goodwin, B. L., Ruthven, C. R. J., and Calne, D. B. (1971): *Nature 229*, 414.
4. Goldin, B. R., Peppercorn, M. A., and Goldman, P. (1973): *J. Pharmacol. Exp. Ther. 186*, 160.
5. Peppercorn, M. A., and Goldman, P. (1971): *J. Bact. 108*, 996.
6. Peppercorn, M. A., and Goldman, P. (1972): *J. Pharmacol. Exp. Ther. 181*, 555.
7. Svartz, N. (1942): *Acta Med. Scand. 110*, 577.
8. Peppercorn, M. A., and Goldman, P. (1973): *Gastroenterology 64*, 240.
9. Hill, M. J., Drasar, B. S., Aries, V., Crowther, J. S., Hawksworth, G., and Williams, R. E. O. (1971): *Lancet 1*, 95.
10. Winitz, M., Adams, R. F., Seedman, D. A., Davis, P. N., Jayko, L. G., and Hamilton, J. A. (1970): *Amer. J. Clin. Nutr. 23*, 546.
11. Renwick, A. G., and Williams, R. T. (1972): *Biochem. J. 129*, 869.
12. Drasar, B. S., Renwick, A. G., and Williams, R. T. (1972): *Biochem. J. 129*, 881.
13. Williams, J. R., Grantham, P. H., Marsh III, H. H., Weisburger, J. H., and Weisburger, E. K. (1970): *Biochem. Pharmac. 19*, 173.
14. Dubos, R., Schaedler, R. W., Costello, R., and Hoet, P. (1965): *J. Exp. Med. 122*, 67.
15. Holdeman, L. V., and Moore, W. E. C. (eds.) (1972): *Anaerobic Laboratory Manual*, Virginia Polytechnic Institute Anaerobic Laboratory, Blacksburg, Virginia.
16. Asatoor, A. M., Chamberlain, M. J., Emmerson, B. T., Johnson, J. R., Levi, A. J., and Milne, M. D. (1967): *Clin. Sci. 33*, 111.
17. Dayman, J., and Jepson, J. B. (1969): *Biochem. J. 113*, 11P.
18. Peppercorn, M. A., and Goldman, P. (1972): *Proc. Nat. Acad. Sci. USA 69*, 1413.
19. Davis, C. P., Mulcahy, D., Takeuchi, and Savage, D. C. (1972): *Infect. Immun. 6*, 184.

Drug Interactions, edited by P. L. Morselli,
S. Garattini, and S. N. Cohen. Raven Press,
New York © 1974

Comparative Aspects of Drug Metabolism by Mammalian Lung and Liver: Mixed Function Oxidation and Conjugation Reactions

Theodore E. Gram, Charles L. Litterst, and Edward G. Mimnaugh

Laboratory of Toxicology, National Cancer Institute, National Institutes of Health, Bethesda, Maryland 20014

INTRODUCTION

A common mechanism by which drug action may be terminated *in vivo* is by enzymatic conversion of the active drug to biologically less active metabolites. There is little doubt that from a quantitative standpoint, the liver is the most important organ involved in the metabolism of drugs and other foreign compounds. This is true irrespective of the type of metabolic transformation under consideration: oxidation, conjugation, hydrolysis, etc. However, it is known that many of these enzymatic conversions also occur in extrahepatic tissues, such as, kidney, lung, intestine, skin, placenta, and adrenal. Until recently, drug metabolism in extrahepatic organs had not been studied in detail and it had been generally assumed without validation that the characteristics and behavior of the hepatic and extrahepatic systems were very similar. The present work is a comparative investigation of drug metabolism in mammalian lung and liver and has revealed some minor quantitative differences but great qualitative similarity.

RESULTS

Mixed-Function Oxidase System

Subcellular Distribution of Mixed-Function Oxidases in Lung and Liver

Homogenization conditions for lung and liver were established which provided high yields and specific activities of microsomal enzymes together with relatively minor contamination of the microsomal fractions by mitochondrial marker enzymes and relatively minor disruption of lysosomes. Pooled livers or lungs from adult male New Zealand rabbits (~3 kg) were minced and homogenized in 0.25 M sucrose–50 mM hepes buffer, pH 7.5.

TABLE 1. *The distribution of the MFO system and its components in subcellular fractions of rabbits lung and liver*

Substrate or component	Liver					Lung				
	N	HM	LM	MIC	SOL	N	HM	LM	MIC	SOL
Aniline	18	17	6	57	2	23	15	15	43	4
Benzphetamine	31	7	13	47	2	20	10	13	54	3
Biphenyl	11	9	15	63	2	18	13	10	57	1
NADPH cytochrome c reductase	10	16	9	62	3	8	17	12	62	1
Cytochrome P-450	11	18	10	58	4	6	29	23	37	5

The values presented represent the percent of total activity in all fractions contained in each of the five subcellular fractions, all on a protein or specific activity basis. The abbreviations under each organ represent, respectively: nuclear (N) heavy mitochondrial (HM), light mitochondrial (LM), microsomal (MIC), and soluble (SOL).

The homogenates were strained through gauze and subjected to differential centrifugation yielding five subcellular fractions. These fractions and their designations, chosen for convenience, were as follows

$600 \times g$ for 10 min, pellet (nuclear)
$3,300 \times g$ for 10 min, pellet (heavy mitochondrial)
$10,000 \times g$ for 20 min, pellet (light mitochondrial)
$192,000 \times g$ for 45 min, pellet (microsomal)
$192,000 \times g$ for 45 min, supernatant (soluble)

The distribution of the mixed-function oxidase (MFO) system and its components in subcellular fractions of lung and liver is presented in Table 1. As can be seen, the general pattern of distribution of the MFO components was very similar in liver and lung (1). The microsomal fractions exhibited the highest specific activities, being two to four times higher than any other cell fraction. Unexpectedly high activities were found in the nuclear fractions, especially when expressed on a per gram tissue basis. Electron microscopic analysis revealed that the MFO activity observed in the nuclear and other cell fractions was probably attributable to microsomal contamination. Thus, large numbers of partially disrupted cells including endoplasmic reticulum and microsomal vesicles were observed in both nuclear fractions. Microsomal vesicles were observed in mitochondrial fractions as well.

Relative MFO Activities in Lung and Liver

Turning our attention to the microsomal fractions, the specific activities of the MFO components are given in Table 2. It is of interest that although the cytochrome P-450 content of liver microsomes was almost eight times

TABLE 2. *Microsomal MFO activities in liver and lung*

Activity	Lung	Liver	Lung/liver
Aniline	0.18	0.53	0.34
Benzphetamine	10.1	8.2	1.23
Biphenyl	3.99	3.35	1.19
NADPH cytochrome			
c reductase	43.0	48.0	0.90
Cytochrome P-450	0.24	1.82	0.13

Activities are expressed as nmoles/mg protein/min. Cytochrome P-450 is expressed as nmoles/mg protein.

that of lung microsomes, the overall activity of the MFO electron-transfer chain, as measured by benzphetamine demethylase or biphenyl hydroxylase was about the same in the two organs.

General Enzymology of the Microsomal MFO Systems in Lung and Liver

A large amount of information has accrued concerning the nature of the hepatic MFO system such as its cofactor requirements, its electron transfer chain, and its response to inhibitors. However, no comparable data were available regarding the pulmonary system, so we deemed it essential to examine these parameters in the two systems (2). Since there were no marked differences among the three substrates studied (aniline, benzphetamine, biphenyl), only the data for benzphetamine are presented for the sake of brevity. Moreover, there were no marked differences between the hepatic and pulmonary systems for these parameters.

NADPH or an NADPH-generating system was required for maximum enzyme activity (Table 3). NADH substituted inefficiently for NADPH and there was no additive effect when NADPH and NADH were both added; NADP and NAD were ostensibly inactive as cofactors in MFO activity. Microsomal benzphetamine demethylase of both liver and lung required oxygen for maximum activity; incubation under N_2 or CO essentially abolished activity (Table 4). MFO activity in both organs was inhibited by cytochrome c and by SKF 525-A (Table 5).

These data, taken together, suggest that the following qualitative inferences may be made regarding the MFO systems in liver and lung:

(a) The combined requirements for NADPH and oxygen suggest that MFO mechanisms are operative.

(b) The inhibition produced by CO and cytochrome c imply the participation of cytochrome P-450 and NADPH cytochrome c reductase respectively as components of similar electron transfer chains in the two organs.

TABLE 3. *Cofactor requirements of microsomal benzphetamine N-demethylase in rabbit liver and lung*

	Relative activity (%)	
	Lung	Liver
NADPH	100	100
No cofactor	9	9
Boiled enzyme + NADPH	8	15
NADPH generating system	110	130
NADP	16	14
NADH	30	23
NAD	8	8
NADPH + NADH	95	93

The concentration of all cofactors produced maximum effects and was 3.5 mM.

TABLE 4. *Atmospheric requirements of microsomal benzphetamine N-demethylase in rabbit liver and lung*

	Relative activity (%)	
Atmosphere	Lung	Liver
Air	100	100
O_2	95	105
N_2	15	10
CO	3	0
CO:air 1:1	7	25
CO:air 9:1	2	7

TABLE 5. *Effect of certain inhibitors of MFO on microsomal benzphetamine demethylase activity*

		Relative activity (%)	
Additions		Lung	Liver
None		100	100
Cytochrome c	0.1 mM	55	71
''	0.3 mM	35	50
SKF 525-A	0.1 mM	74	61
''	0.3 mM	55	44

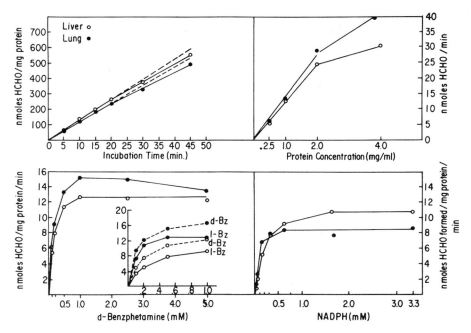

FIG. 1. *Some kinetic parameters of benzphetamine demethylase activity in microsomes from rabbit liver and lung.*

The general kinetic behavior of the microsomal MFO systems was remarkably similar in lung and liver preparations (Fig. 1). Optima of pH determined in three different buffers and temperature optima fell into the same ranges with both liver and lung (i.e., pH 7.0–7.8; temperature 35 to 45°C). Kinetic constants for the metabolism of three xenobiotics are given in Table 6. None of the apparent K_m values were significantly different between lung and liver although differences in V_{max} were observed.

TABLE 6. *Kinetic constants for the metabolism of xenobiotics by lung and liver microsomes*

	Apparent K_m (mM)		V_{max} (nmoles/mg protein/min)	
	Liver	Lung	Liver	Lung
Aniline	1.06	0.82	0.74^a	0.25^a
Benzphetamine	0.13	0.12	7.90^a	9.70^a
Biphenyl	0.42	0.48	2.94^a	3.50^a

$^a p < 0.05$, liver versus lung.

Cytochrome P-450 and Substrate Difference Spectra

Levels of cytochrome P-450 in lung microsomes were found to be only 10 to 20% those of liver (Table 2). However, the spectra obtained in the two organs were not different qualitatively and exhibited maxima at 450 nm. This contrasts with recent work performed with renal cortical microsomes in which the CO-binding pigment had an absorbance maximum at 454 nm (3). CO difference spectra revealed that lung microsomes bound hemoglobin much more avidly than did liver microsomes. This hemoglobin contamination of lung microsomes could not be abolished by several "washes" (resuspension and resedimentation) in dilute salt solutions but could be prevented by lung perfusion. Preliminary experiments suggested that the rates of reduction of cytochrome P-450 by NADPH in lung and liver microsomes were roughly comparable.

Type I substrate difference spectra obtained with benzphetamine were qualitatively similar in lung and liver microsomes (peak $\sim$ 385 nm, trough $\sim$ 423 nm). Moreover, K_s values obtained in the two organs did not differ significantly; ΔA_{max} was about 50% higher in liver microsomes. On the other hand, type II difference spectra obtained with aniline revealed some differences between lung and liver. Aniline interacted with liver microsomes to produce a typical type II difference spectrum (peak $\sim$ 426 nm, trough $\sim$ 388 nm). Interaction of aniline with lung microsomes, however, resulted in a somewhat atypical spectrum having a broad asymmetrical trough from about 390 to 410 nm and a peak at 430 to 435 nm. The ΔA_{max} obtained with lung microsomes was only about 15 to 20% that of liver and seemed to correlate roughly with levels of cytochrome P-450 (4). A similar anomalous aniline difference spectrum has been reported in liver microsomes from scorbutic guinea pigs (5).

Conjugation Reactions

In spite of their enormous importance in drug metabolism *in vivo* and in overall drug clearance, *in vitro* studies of the conjugation of foreign compounds in lung have been extremely limited. Transmethylation reactions involving amines (6) and phenols (7) have been documented, and a recent isolated report of glucuronide conjugation in lung (8) has appeared. Accordingly, we sought to investigate this question in greater detail.

Data presented in Table 7 indicate that the pulmonary N-acetyl transferase activity toward the substrate *p*-aminobenzoic acid is substantial and comparable to that of liver, whereas the activity in lung measured with sulfadiazine is very low.

UDP-glucuronyl transferase activity was detectable in lung microsomes with only one of three substrates investigated, namely, *o*-aminophenol. We

TABLE 7. *Conjugation reactions in lung and liver*

Parameter	Lung	Liver
Microsomal protein (mg/g)	9.1 ± 2.4 (10)	23.5 ± 2.7[a] (10)
Soluble (postmicrosomal) protein (mg/g)	44.1 ± 3.7 (10)	54.9 ± 8.9[a] (10)
N-acetyl transferase (nmoles/mg protein/min)		
PABA	0.86 ± 0.23 (9)	0.73 ± 0.24 (9)
sulfadiazine	0.02 ± 0.01 (8)	0.13 ± 0.07[a] (8)
UDP-glucuronyl transferase (nmoles/mg protein/min)		
o-aminophenol[b]	2.1 ± 1.4 (8)	7.5 ± 2.5[a] (8)
p-nitrophenol	0 (6)	4.1 ± 0.7[a] (6)
phenolphthalein	0 (10)	4.0 ± 0.6[a] (10)
Glutathione S-aryltransferase (nmoles/mg protein/min)	6.9 ± 1.4 (10)	32.6 ± 6.6[a] (10)

[a] $p < 0.05$, liver versus lung.
[b] $\Delta OD \times 10^{-4}$/mg protein/min.
Values represent mean ± standard deviation. The number of animals are in parenthesis.

were not able to demonstrate glucuronide synthesis by lung microsomes *in vitro* with *p*-nitrophenol or phenolphthalein. Glutathione S-aryltransferase activity in lung with 2,4-dichloronitrobenzene as substrate was about 20% that found in the soluble fraction of liver.

On teleological grounds, the comparatively low levels of transferase activity found in the lung are not difficult to understand in view of the increase in polarity and water solubility generally conferred by such conjugations. Whereas the liver secretes bile and thus has an aqueous excretory route for water-soluble conjugates such as glucuronides, the lung has no such clearance mechanism, and, hence, the formation of conjugates in lung would be energetically wasteful. The formation by liver of conjugates having greater water solubility than the parent drug, considered together with its aqueous biliary clearance mechanism, would appear to represent efficient integration of enzymatic or biochemical function and physiological function. The corollary of this, if the lung were to be important in detoxication, would be for the lung to possess the enzymatic capacity to catalyze the formation of metabolites with increased vapor pressure or volatility so that its remarkable gaseous excretory mechanism could be efficiently utilized.

REFERENCES

1. Hook, G. E., Bend, J. R., Hoel, D., Fouts, J. R., and Gram, T. E. (1972): *J. Pharmacol. Exp. Ther. 182*, 474.
2. Bend, J. R., Hook, G. E., Easterling, R. E., Gram, T. E., and Fouts, J. R. (1972): *J. Pharmacol. Exp. Ther. 183*, 206.

3. Ellin, A., Jakobsson, S. V., Schenkman, J. B., and Orrenius, S. (1972): *Arch. Biochem. Biophys. 150,* 64.
4. Gram, T. E. (1973): *Drug Metab. Rev. 2,* 1.
5. Zannoni, V. G., Flynn, E. J., and Lynch, M. (1966): *Biochem. Pharmacol. 15,* 599.
6. Dingell, J. V., and Sanders, E. (1966): *Biochem. Pharmacol. 15,* 599.
7. Axelrod, J., and Daly, J. (1968): *Biochim. Biophys. Acta 159,* 472.
8. Aitio, A. (1973): *Xenobiotica 3,* 13.

Drug Interactions, edited by P. L. Morselli,
S. Garattini, and S. N. Cohen. Raven Press,
New York © 1974

Fluorescence Spectroscopy as a Tool
for Monitoring Drug-Albumin Interactions

Colin F. Chignell

*National Heart and Lung Institute, National Institutes of Health, Bethesda, Maryland
20014*

INTRODUCTION

In recent years, spectroscopic techniques have played an important role
in studies of drug binding to proteins and other biologically important
macromolecules (1–3). When compared to the more classical methods available for studying drug binding, spectroscopic techniques have two distinct
advantages. Firstly, they are much more rapid than procedures such as
equilibrium dialysis. Secondly, they cannot only be used to measure the
amount of bound and free drug in a given system but can also yield additional information on the nature of the drug-protein interaction. For example,
changes in the ultraviolet or visible absorption spectrum of a drug may be
interpreted in terms of the polarity of a drug-binding site (4, 5). Nuclear
magnetic resonance spectroscopy often indicates which groups or parts of
a drug molecule are involved in the binding process (6), whereas circular
dichroism may yield information on the three-dimensional structure of the
drug-binding site (4, 7–11). Since fluorescence spectroscopy is one of the
most versatile of all the spectroscopic methods, this technique will be used
to illustrate the usefulness of a spectroscopic approach to drug-albumin
interactions.

The fluorescence of a drug molecule may be characterized by such parameters as the wavelengths of maximal activation and emission, quantum
yield, fluorescence lifetime, and degree of polarization (12). Since these
parameters are often exquisitely sensitive to changes in the microenviron-
ment of the fluorophore, it is perhaps not surprising that the fluorescence of
a drug molecule may be drastically altered when it binds to plasma albumin.
Similarly, the fluorescence characteristics of plasma albumin may be altered
by the binding of a drug. If neither the drug nor the protein has suitable
fluorescence properties, a drug-albumin interaction can often still be studied
by complexing (covalently or noncovalently) the protein with a fluorescent
label (13).

DRUGS THAT ALTER THE INTRINSIC FLUORESCENCE
OF PLASMA ALBUMIN

4-Butyl-1-(*p*-nitrophenyl)-2-phenyl-3,5-pyrazolidinedione

Human plasma albumin contains a single tryptophan residue which, when activated at 290 nm, emits fluorescence with a maximum at 335 nm. When 4-butyl-1-(*p*-nitrophenyl)-2-phenyl-3,5-pyrazolidinedione (II), an analogue of the anti-inflammatory drug phenylbutazone (I), binds to human plasma albumin, the tryptophan fluorescence of the protein is quenched (Fig. 1) (1). Förster has shown (14) that fluorescence quenching of this type is the result of nonresonance transfer of energy from the donor molecule

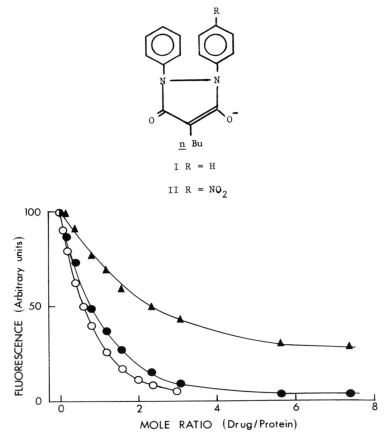

FIG. 1. The quenching of the fluorescence of human plasma albumin by the binding of 4-butyl-1-(*p*-nitrophenyl)-2-phenyl-3,5-pyrazolidinedione (II). The activation and emission wavelengths were 290 and 335 nm. Bandwidths were 12 nm. The concentrations of human plasma albumin were 6.44×10^{-7} M (——▲——▲——), 6.44×10^{-6} M (——●——●——), and 2.55×10^{-5} M (——○——○——). All solutions contained 0.1 M sodium phosphate (pH 7.4). Modified from ref. 3.

(i.e., the tryptophan of human plasma albumin) to the acceptor molecule (II). When the fluorescence of human plasma albumin is plotted as a function of the molar ratio between (II) and the protein, the degree of quenching is seen to be dependent upon protein concentration (Fig. 1). However, when the albumin concentration is 2.55×10^{-5} M or above, the drug is completely bound at all drug-protein ratios and the quenching curves are superimposable (Fig. 1). The amount of bound and free drug present during the titration of a low concentration of human plasma albumin (6.44×10^{-7} M) may be calculated with the aid of the curve obtained with the high protein concentration (2.55×10^{-5} M) (13). The Scatchard plot derived from these data indicates the presence of two binding sites with affinity constants of 3.1×10^5 M^{-1} (15). Equilibrium dialysis studies demonstrate the presence of two high-affinity sites ($K = 2.7 \times 10^5$ M^{-1}) and four lower affinity sites ($K = 2.9 \times 10^4$ M^{-1}) (15). The lower affinity sites cannot be detected by the fluorescence titration, since the binding of (II) to the two high-affinity sites results in the quenching of 95% of the albumin fluorescence (Fig. 1).

When a mixture containing human plasma albumin and (II) is titrated with lauric acid no change is observed in the tryptophan fluorescence of the protein until the concentration of lauric acid exceeds that of the drug. The intensity of albumin fluorescence then begins to increase (Fig. 2) until a lauric acid/drug ratio of 10 is reached and the fluorescence intensity is about 50% of that observed in the absence of added ligands. Since control experiments show that the binding of lauric acid to human plasma albumin does not alter the intrinsic fluorescence of the protein, the increase in fluorescence intensity (Fig. 2) must result from displacement of (II) by the fatty acid. The

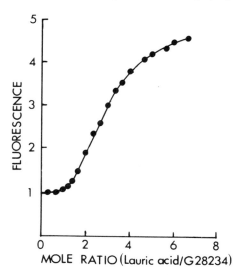

FIG. 2. The effect of lauric acid on the fluorescence of human plasma albumin (1×10^{-5} M) and II (G-28234) (3×10^{-5} M) in 0.1 M sodium phosphate (pH 7.4). The activation and emission wavelengths were 290 and 335 nm.

titration curve suggests that the sites initially occupied by lauric acid are not shared by (II). Furthermore, since, in the presence of a large excess of fatty acid, the intensity of albumin fluorescence is only 50% of that observed in the absence of (II) it would appear that lauric acid can only displace one of the bound drug molecules. It is of interest to compare these results with the equilibrium dialysis studies of Solomon and co-workers, who have found that lauric acid competitively displaces phenylbutazone (I) from its high-affinity site on human plasma albumin (16).

This fluorescence technique should be applicable to the measurement of drug-drug interactions at plasma-albumin binding sites provided that the binding of only one of the drug molecules quenches the intrinsic fluorescence of the protein.

DRUGS THAT CHANGE THEIR INTRINSIC FLUORESCENCE ON BINDING TO PLASMA ALBUMIN

Warfarin

III

When the anticoagulant drug warfarin (III) binds to human plasma albumin, the fluorescence quantum yield of the drug increases eightfold (Table 1) (8). The fluorescence quantum yield of warfarin also increases when the drug is dissolved in certain solvents, such as dimethylformamide and glycerol, but is relatively unaffected by other solvents, such as methanol and ethyl acetate (8) (Table 2). However, there is little correlation between the dielectric constant of the solvent and its effect on the fluorescence of warfarin. Whereas the organic solvents either have little effect on the fluorescence-emission maximum of warfarin or shift it to longer wavelengths (Table 2), the fluorescence-emission maximum of warfarin moves to shorter wavelengths when the drug binds to human serum albumin. Rat and canine plasma albumins induce even greater blue shifts in the fluorescence emission maximum of warfarin than does human plasma albumin (Table 1). Rat plasma albumin also causes the largest increase (13-fold) in the quantum yield of bound warfarin. Although it is not possible to interpret these changes in terms of the polarity of the warfarin binding site on the plasma albumins,

TABLE 1. *The quantum yield and fluorescence emission maximum of warfarin bound to different plasma albumins*

Plasma albumin	Fluorescence[a] quantum yield	Fluorescence[a] emission maximum (nm)
None	0.012	400
Human	0.090	390
Bovine	0.069	380
Rat	0.153	380
Porcine	0.080	385
Canine	0.083	380
Ovine	0.076	385
Equine	0.088	390
Rabbit	0.047	390

[a] Activation wavelength was 320 nm using 12-nm bandwidth.

the change in the fluorescence titration curve obtained by the addition of increments of warfarin to a fixed amount of rat plasma albumin (Fig. 3) can be replotted in terms of a Scatchard plot that shows that the protein has one binding site for the drug with an association constant of 8.2 × 10^5 M^{-1} (15).

Solomon and co-workers have reported that warfarin competitively displaces phenylbutazone from human plasma albumin (16). When phenylbutazone is added to a mixture of warfarin and human plasma albumin, the fluorescence intensity of the anticoagulant decreases (Fig. 4). However, even in the presence of a large excess of phenylbutazone, about 35% of the warfarin remains bound (Fig. 4). This suggests that although warfarin and phenylbutazone do share common binding sites on human plasma al-

TABLE 2. *Quantum yield of warfarin dissolved in various solvents*

Solvent dielectric constant (Debye units)	Solvent[a]	Quantum yield	Emission λ max (nm)
78.5	Water (0.05 M sodium phosphate, pH 7.4)	0.013	400
42.5	Glycerol	0.104	392
37.0	Ethylene glycol	0.047	400
36.7	Dimethylformamide	0.154	415
32.0	Propylene glycol	0.061	400
31.2	Methanol	0.016	400
25.8	Ethanol	0.033	400
19.2	1-Butanol	0.039	400
6.1	Ethyl acetate	0.010	400
3.0	Dioxane	0.022	412

[a] Solutions were made by adding 0.1 ml of a stock solution (made up in 0.01 N NaOH) to 9.9 ml of solvent. Fluorescence was excited at 320 nm.

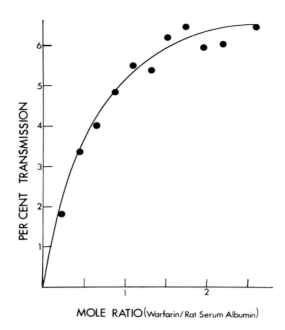

FIG. 3. Fluorometric titration of rat plasma albumin (1×10^{-5} M) with warfarin. The excitation and emission wavelengths were 320 and 390 nm respectively. The solution contained 0.1 M sodium phosphate buffer (pH 7.4). Adapted from ref. 15.

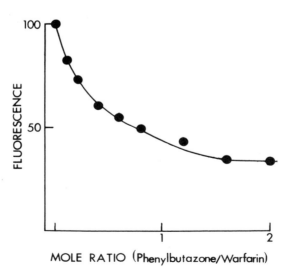

FIG. 4. The effect of phenylbutazone on the fluorescence of warfarin (4×10^{-5} M) and human plasma albumin (1×10^{-5} M) in 0.1 M sodium phosphate buffer (pH 7.4). The excitation and emission wavelengths were 320 and 390 nm, respectively.

bumin, the protein does have other sites which bind warfarin but not phenyl-butazone. This conclusion is in agreement with the recent equilibrium dialysis studies of Tillement and co-workers (17), who have found that the addition of a 30-fold excess of phenylbutazone (2.9×10^{-4} M) to a mixture containing warfarin (9.7×10^{-6} M) and human plasma albumin (2.9×10^{-4} M) causes a 58% reduction in the binding of the warfarin.

Camptothecin

Camptothecin (IV) is a cytotoxic alkaloid that is found in the stem wood of the oriental tree *Camptotheca accuminata*. In aqueous buffer solutions (pH 7.4), camptothecin is highly fluorescent with an emission maximum at 435 nm (18). When a fixed amount of camptothecin (1×10^{-6} M) is titrated

IV

with human plasma albumin, the fluorescence-emission maximum of the drug remains unchanged while its fluorescence intensity decreases to approximately 50% of the initial value (Fig. 5) (18). However, the fluorescence

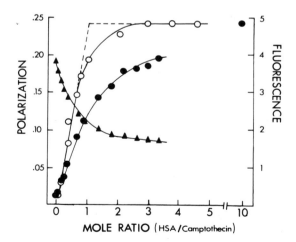

FIG. 5. The effect of human plasma albumin on the fluorescence intensity (—▲—▲—) and polarization (—●—●—) of camptothecin (2×10^{-6} M) and on the fluorescence polarization (—○—○—) of camptothecin (2×10^{-5} M). The wavelengths of activation and emission were 370 and 445 nm, respectively. All solutions contained 0.1 M sodium phosphate buffer (pH 7.4). Adapted from ref. 18.

polarization of camptothecin, which is 0.013 in the absence of plasma albumin, increases to 0.240 when the drug is completely bound to the protein
(Fig. 5). If the concentration of camptothecin is increased 20-fold, the titration curve approaches linearity and shows a distinct break at a protein/
drug ratio of 1.1 (Fig. 5). This indicates that human plasma albumin has a
single binding site for camptothecin. The binding of camptothecin to human
plasma albumin can be expressed in terms of the saturation fraction, $\bar{s}$,
which is the number of moles of ligand bound per mole of total ligand. The
value of $\bar{s}$ may be calculated from the data in Fig. 5 by means of the equation

$$\bar{s} = 1 - \frac{I}{I_0}\left(\frac{P_{max} - P}{P_{max} - P_{min}}\right) 0 \le s \le 1, \tag{1}$$

where P and I are the fluorescence polarization and intensity respectively
of the camptothecin human plasma albumin solution, P_{min} and I_0 are the
polarization and intensity of camptothecin in the absence of human plasma
albumin and P_{max} is the polarization of camptothecin in the presence of a
large excess of human plasma albumin (19). Since there is only one ligand
binding site per albumin molecule, the association constant, K, for the interaction can be obtained from the relationship

$$\frac{\bar{s}}{P} = K(1 - \bar{s}), \tag{2}$$

where P is the concentration of unbound protein. When the data of Fig. 5
are plotted according to Eq. 2 with $\bar{s}$ calculated from Eq. 1 an association
constant of 8×10^6 M^{-1} is obtained (18).

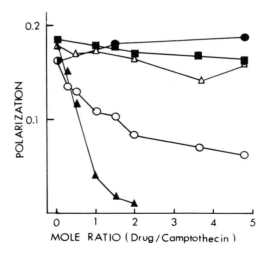

FIG. 6. The effect of stearic acid (——●——●——), α-(p-chlorophenoxy)-isobutyric acid
(——■——■——), warfarin (——△——△——), sulfaphenazole (——○——○——), and bilirubin
(——▲——▲——) on the fluorescence polarization of camptothecin (1 × 10^{-5} M). All solutions contained human plasma albumin (1 × 10^{-5} M) and 0.1 M sodium phosphate (pH
7.4). The wavelengths of activation and emission were 370 and 445 nm, respectively.

Fluorescence polarization provides a rapid and convenient method for monitoring drug-drug interactions that may occur at plasma-albumin binding sites. For example, when sulfaphenazole is added to a mixture of camptothecin and human plasma albumin, the fluorescence polarization of the drug decreases, reaching 38% of the initial value at a sulfaphenazole/camptothecin ratio of 5. The addition of an equimolar amount of bilirubin causes complete displacement of camptothecin from human plasma albumin. This finding is consistent with the high affinity of bilirubin for albumin (13). Other experiments have shown that dicoumarol also displaces camptothecin from human plasma albumin. In contrast, warfarin, α-(p-chlorophenoxy)-*iso*-butyric acid, stearic acid (Fig. 6), and phenylbutazone (18) do not alter the fluorescence polarization of albumin-bound camptothecin and hence do not displace the antitumor agent from its protein binding sites. One advantage of the fluorescence-polarization technique for studying drug-drug interactions at plasma-protein binding sites is that it can also be used to study drug displacement in plasma (18).

DRUGS THAT ALTER THE FLUORESCENCE OF COMPLEXES BETWEEN FLUORESCENT LABELS AND PLASMA ALBUMIN

Fluorescent labels are small molecules of known chemical structure which, after attachment (covalently or noncovalently) to a macromolecule, can be used to detect changes in the conformation of the macromolecule (20, 21). The most commonly employed labels for noncovalent attachment to proteins are 1-anilino-naphthalene-8-sulfonic acid (ANS), 2-p-toluidinyl-naphthalene-6-sulfonic acid (TNS) and 5-dimethylaminonaphthalene-1-sulfonyl (dansyl) derivatives of amino acids, such as glycine. These compounds all show a marked increase in their fluorescence quantum yields and a blue shift in their fluorescence emission maxima on going from a polar to a nonpolar environment (20, 21). Similar fluorescence changes are also observed when ANS, TNS, and the dansyl amino acids bind to certain proteins, such as plasma albumin. It has therefore been suggested that the dye binding sites on these proteins are nonpolar and that ANS, TNS, and the dansyl amino acids can be used as probes for the polarity of protein binding sites (20, 21).

When dansylglycine (V) binds to human serum albumin, the quantum yield of the ligand increases fivefold while its fluorescence emission maximum shifts from 580 to 480 nm (Table 3) (4). Fluorescence titration indicates that binding occurs at a single site for which dansylglycine has an association constant of 4.6×10^5 M^{-1} (Fig. 7). Phenylbutazone (I) competitively displaces dansylglycine from its binding site on human serum albumin (Fig. 7). The association constant of phenylbutazone for the dansylglycine binding site is 9×10^4 M^{-1} when calculated according to the procedure of Klotz et al. (22). Equilibrium dialysis studies have shown (4) that phenyl-

TABLE 3. *Quantum yields of dansylglycine, human plasma albumin,
and the dansylglycine-albumin complex*

Compound	Exciting wavelength (nm)	λ Max of emission (nm)	Quantum yield
Human plasma albumin	290	335	0.077
Dansylglycine	350	580	0.051
Dansylglycine-albumin	290	480	0.235
Dansylglycine-albumin	350	480	0.443
Dansylglycine-albumin	290	335	0.046

$N(CH_3)_2$

SO_2NHCH_2COOH

V

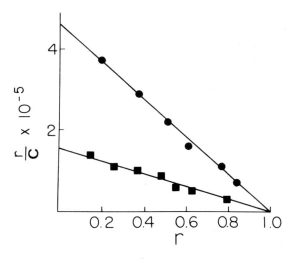

FIG. 7. Scatchard plot of the binding of dansylglycine to human plasma albumin in the presence of phenylbutazone. C = molar concentration of free dansylglycine, r = number of moles of dansylglycine bound per mole of HSA. Binding was measured by monitoring the increase in dansylglycine fluorescence at 480 nm while activating at 350 nm. Human plasma albumin alone (1×10^{-5} M) —●—●—; human plasma albumin (1×10^{-5} M) + phenylbutazone (2.5×10^{-5} M) —■—■—. All solutions contained 0.1 M sodium phosphate buffer (pH 7.4). Modified from ref. 4.

butazone has one high-affinity ($K = 1 \times 10^5$ M^{-1}) binding site and two others with a somewhat lower affinity ($K = 4 \times 10^4$ M^{-1}). Thus, it would appear that the human plasma-albumin high-affinity site for phenylbutazone is highly hydrophobic. This finding was confirmed by difference spectroscopy, which showed that when phenylbutazone is bound to human plasma albumin the drug chromophore is located in a nonpolar environment (4).

Several other drugs, such as flufenamic acid (7) and dicoumarol (8) also competitively displace dansylglycine from albumin whereas sulfaphenazole, α-(p-chlorophenoxy)-*iso*butyric acid do not affect the binding of the probe. Although the evidence is somewhat indirect, it seems reasonable to assume that those drugs that displace dansylglycine from albumin probably share at least one common binding site on the protein. Thus it seems probable that drug-drug interactions are to be expected with phenylbutazone, flufenamic acid, and dicoumarol.

PROGNOSIS

Fluorescence spectroscopy is undoubtedly one of the most versatile techniques that are currently available for the study of drug interactions with proteins. This technique is especially useful for measuring the binding of drugs to, and their displacement from, plasma proteins, since it is more rapid than equilibrium dialysis and is often more sensitive than other spectroscopic techniques, such as ultraviolet and visible absorption spectroscopy and nuclear magnetic resonance. In addition, fluorescence spectroscopy can also provide information on the structure of a drug binding site and the nature of the binding forces involved. Although fluorescence spectroscopy has been most frequently used as an analytical tool in pharmacology, the future should see a marked increase in the application of this technique to the study of drug interactions with biologically important macromolecules.

REFERENCES

1. Chignell, C. F. (1969): *Adv. Drug Res. 5*, 44.
2. Chignell, C. F. (1971): In: *Handbook of Experimental Pharmacology*, p. 187, Springer-Verlag, Berlin.
3. Chignell, C. F. (1972): *Crit. Rev. Toxic. 1*, 413.
4. Chignell, C. F. (1969): *Mol. Pharmacol. 5*, 244.
5. Baxter, J. H. (1964): *Arch. Biochem. Biophys. 108*, 375.
6. Jardetsky, O., and Wade-Jardetsky, N. (1965): *Mol. Pharmacol. 1*, 214.
7. Chignell, C. F. (1969): *Mol. Pharmacol. 5*, 455.
8. Chignell, C. F. (1970): *Mol. Pharmacol. 6*, 1.
9. Chignell, C. F., and Starkweather, D. K. (1971): *Mol. Pharmacol. 7*, 229.
10. Chignell, C. F. (1970): *Proc. Fourth Int. Cong. Pharmacol. 1*, 217.
11. Chignell, C. F. (1968): *Life Sci. 7*, 1181.
12. Chen, R. F. (1972): In: *Methods in Pharmacology*, Vol. 2, p. 1, Appleton-Century-Crofts, New York.

13. Chignell, C. F. (1972): In: *Methods in Pharmacology,* Vol. 2, p. 33, Appleton-Century-Crofts, New York.
14. Förster, T. (1951): In: *Fluoreszenz organischer Verbindungen,* p. 85, Vandenhoeck and Ruprecht.
15. Chignell, C. F. *(in press): Ann. New York Acad Sci.*
16. Solomon, H. M., Schrogie, J. J., and Williams, D. (1968): *Biochem. Pharmacol. 17,* 143.
17. Tillement, J. P, Zini, R., Mattei, C., and Singlas, E. (1973): *Eur. J. Clin. Pharmacol. 6,* 15.
18. Guarino, A. M., Call, J. B., Starkweather, D. K., and Chignell, C. F. (1973): *Cancer Chemother. Rep. 6,* 125.
19. Chien, Y., and Weber, G. (1973): *Biochem. Biophys. Res. Commun. 50,* 538.
20. Edelman, G. M., and McClure, W. O. (1968): *Accounts Chem. Res. 1,* 65.
21. Brand, L., and Gohlke, J. R. (1972): *Ann. Rev. Biochem. 41,* 843.
22. Klotz, I. M., Triwush, H., and Walker, F. M. (1948): *J. Am. Chem. Soc. 70,* 2935.

Drug Interactions, edited by P. L. Morselli,
S. Garattini, and S. N. Cohen. Raven Press,
New York © 1974

Redistributional Drug Interactions: A Critical Examination of Putative Clinical Examples

William M. Wardell

*Department of Pharmacology and Toxicology, University of Rochester Medical Center,
260 Crittenden Boulevard, Rochester, New York 14642*

INTRODUCTION

Competition between coadministered drugs for nonspecific binding sites in the body can result in displacement of one drug by another, with a resulting rise in the free and active fraction of a drug. It is widely believed that this displacement or redistribution phenomenon causes the enhanced clinical effects and toxicity seen when certain drugs and other substances interact in man (1–10). The object of this review is to examine critically the evidence underlying that belief.

The mechanisms of drug interactions can be broadly divided into those occurring at the receptor level or beyond, and those occurring by pharmacokinetic processes prior to the receptor. In the intact body, more than one mechanism may operate simultaneously. Therefore, before one can validly attribute a drug interaction to the process of redistribution, one must obtain positive evidence of redistribution, exclude or allow for other possible causes, and show that the result of the redistribution does indeed cause the pharmacological effect that one is attempting to explain.

In this chapter I shall set out the criteria needed to establish a redistributional cause for interactions involving the binding and displacement of drugs from plasma proteins. (A somewhat similar analysis could be applied to interactions involving displacement from tissue-binding sites, but for reasons of space the latter will not be dealt with here.) I shall then examine whether those clinically significant drug interactions popularly believed to be due to this redistributional mechanism actually satisfy the criteria.

CRITERIA FOR ANALYZING REDISTRIBUTIONAL INTERACTIONS INVOLVING PLASMA PROTEIN

Demonstration of Redistribution

A rudimentary first step is to demonstrate the displacement phenomenon with human plasma *in vitro,* using clinically relevant concentrations of both drugs.

Next, one should demonstrate qualitatively that the redistribution actually occurs in human subjects. One needs to show that there is a fall in the plasma total concentration of the displaced drug and that (on ultrafiltration of specimens taken from man) this fall consists of a fall in bound drug partially offset by a rise in the free concentration.

Finally, one needs to test quantitatively whether redistribution alone can wholly account for the pharmacokinetic changes, or whether other mechanisms need to be invoked. It is important to realize that redistribution, if it occurs, will tend to conceal any other (possibly more important) mechanisms that might occur simultaneously. Therefore the qualitative demonstration of redistribution is by itself insufficient proof of a causal role for this mechanism, and could even be a red herring. Only a quantitative approach can resolve this problem.

A balance sheet needs to be calculated for the whole body, comparing the loss in bound drug with the gain in free drug in all body compartments (not the plasma volume alone) in order to test whether the two quantities are equivalent (11, 12). If the whole body's gain in free drug is greater than the loss in plasma protein-bound drug (after due allowance for extravascular plasma protein), then obviously other sources of bound drug or other mechanisms of interaction must be sought. On the other hand, if the body's gain of free drug is equal to (or less than) the loss of bound drug, then displacement *could* be a sole cause of the observed pharmacokinetic changes.

A common fallacy is to postulate that if, for example, a drug is 99% bound in the plasma, then displacement of only 1% of the protein-bound drug will double the free concentration. This is true for plasma confined in a test tube, but in the whole body it would apply only in the unlikely event that both bound and free forms of the drug were wholly confined to the intravascular compartment. What will actually happen, of course, is that the liberated drug will distribute into other compartments, thus dissipating the rise in the concentration of free drug. If the latter distributed evenly into extracellular water, the rise would be only one-quarter of the postulated value, while if it distributed evenly into total body water, the rise would be only one-12th. Additional factors that must also be taken into account include the participation of binding sites on extravascular protein, and the effect of pH on the partitioning of free drug into various body compartments.

Thus for drugs with large volumes of distribution, where only a small fraction of the body load is present in the plasma, redistributional interactions involving plasma proteins can have only trivial direct effects on the concentration of free drug. Binding and displacement interactions involving tissues might have more direct significance for such drugs (12–15).

Indirect effects of redistribution might occur, however, and these could be important even for drugs with large volumes of distribution. For example, if the rate of a drug's metabolism or active excretion were limited by its rate of delivery to the site of this activity, and in turn by the drug's total plasma concentration, displacement from plasma proteins could diminish the rate of that drug's metabolism or excretion regardless of its volume of distribution. This effect would oppose any enhancement of metabolism or excretion caused by a rise in the concentration of free drug. Thus, the indirect effects of redistribution on a drug's pharmacokinetics could be complex.

Exclusion or Allowance for Other Pharmacokinetic Interactions

A fall in the concentration of plasma total drug, or a rise in free drug, could stem from processes other than displacement from plasma proteins. The very presence of a redistributional drug interaction makes it necessary — but at the same time difficult — to evaluate any other pharmacokinetic effects that might be occurring simultaneously.

The most important factors to exclude are other types of redistributional interaction (e.g., at the tissue level) and interactions at the other pharmacokinetic levels of absorption, metabolism, and excretion. The following considerations, in addition to the quantitative approach described above, would help to determine whether a given interaction was a purely redistributional one involving plasma proteins.

(a) The whole interaction should be mimicked by any drug with comparable displacing ability.

(b) Absorptive interactions should be excluded. For example, the interaction should be shown to occur when both drugs are administered parenterally or, alternatively, formal pharmacokinetic analyses of absorption should be undertaken.

(c) Metabolic and excretory rates should be measured. Any changes should be entirely predictable from changes in the concentrations of free (and, for the reasons discussed earlier, bound) drug.

If these conditions are not satisfied, some quantitative allowance must be made for the contributions of these other pharmacokinetic modes of interaction. If this is not done, it will be impossible to be certain of the ultimate contribution of the redistributional mechanism to the drug interaction observed.

Correlation with the Observed Effect

The change in drug effect resulting from a redistributional drug interaction should be entirely predictable from the changes in the concentration of free drug. This requires (a) that free-drug concentrations be measured, (b) that concentration-effect relationships be known for free-drug concentrations, and (c) that the influence of the displacing drug on the concentration-effect relationship of the first drug should be known in a dose-related fashion.

We have now arrived at the Achilles heel of redistributional explanations for drug interactions, and indeed of all mechanistic approaches, because hardly any of these factors are known. In only a few cases have the concentrations of free drug been measured; even fewer concentration-effect relationships are known for free-drug concentrations; and we are almost totally ignorant of the effect of other drugs on any such concentration-effect relationships in man. All this information is vitally necessary to exclude, for example, the very real possibility that the displacing drug alters the concentration-effect relationship of the first drug in some way such as sensitizing or antagonizing at the receptor level or altering processes beyond the receptor. Until such concentration-effect information becomes available, one will never be able to prove unequivocally that a given effect is caused by drug redistribution, no matter how plausible the rest of the evidence.

Nevertheless, helpful indirect evidence can be sought, for example, concerning the time course of the effect. With drug binding and displacements involving plasma proteins, the molecular events are for practical purposes instantaneous, whereas the biological processes render the redistribution well advanced within minutes (11, 12). Thus, at least at the pharmacokinetic level, the result of a displacement phenomenon should have a time course that parallels the concentration profile of the displacing agent. In other words, giving a dose of displacer drug should be tantamount to giving a dose of the drug that it is displacing.

Another characteristic is that (pharmacokinetically at least) the effect may be short lived. As Koch-Weser and Sellers (16) point out, a pulse of drug liberated by displacement will, in a first-order system, be metabolized faster until eventually the original free concentration is restored. A further reason for transience is that there is only a finite amount of bound drug available for displacement. With continued administration of displacer drug, the process will stop when the latter has accumulated to reach its plateau concentration. At that time, things will return more or less to their original condition, except that the original bound drug will be partially replaced by the displacer drug.

On the other hand, processes limited by the concentration of plasma total (rather than free) drug will not be transient in the manner just described. However, these indirect considerations, although valid, are peripheral to the main problem. No amount of pharmacokinetic argument can compensate for our ignorance of the pharmacodynamic aspects of drug interactions.

EXPERIMENTAL PHARMACOKINETIC STUDIES

Now we will examine how far the evidence actually available on redistributional drug interactions goes to satisfy the above criteria. I shall begin with an animal example that McQueen and I studied (11, 12), because this is one of the more detailed experimental analyses of the pharmacokinetics of a redistributional drug interaction.

We studied the displacement of the sulfonamide sulfadoxine (Fanasil) by phenylbutazone in live sheep (one needs to use a large animal in order to get large enough blood samples to ultrafilter).

We showed quite clearly the fall in total sulfonamide and the rise in free sulfonamide that occur when the displacing agent is injected (Fig. 1). We examined it quantitatively, paying particular attention to the distribution of free sulfadoxine into interstitial water and its pH-partitioning into intracellular water. We showed (Table 1A) that, if one allows for a modest contribution from drug bound to extravascular albumin, the body's gain in free drug is totally accounted for by the loss in bound drug. We excluded absorption, because both drugs were injected; we excluded metabolism and

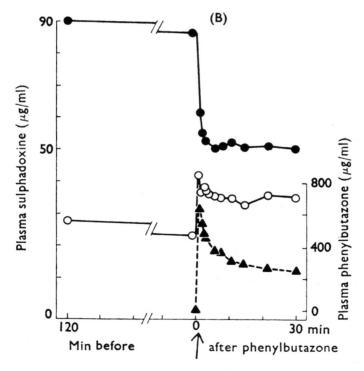

FIG. 1. Effect of 2.0 g intravenous phenylbutazone at zero time (arrow) on the total and free concentrations of sulfadoxine in plasma in one sheep. The three traces from above down are the concentrations of total sulfadoxine, free sulfadoxine, and total phenylbutazone. Abscissa: time in minutes before and after phenylbutazone. Left ordinate: sulfadoxine scale. Right ordinate: phenylbutazone scale. Reprinted from ref. 11 with permission.

TABLE 1.

	A	B
1. Demonstration		
(a) *In vitro*	+	+
(b) *In vivo* (qual.)		
↓ Plasma total	+	+
↓ Plasma bound	+	+
↑ Plasma free	+	+
(c) *In vivo* (quant.)		
Loss of bound	+	0
Gain of free	+	0
Equivalence?	+	0
2. Exclusion or allowance for:		
(a) Absorption	+	+
(b) Metabolism	+	+
(c) Excretion	+	+
3. Correlation of free level		
with effect	0	0

Criteria satisfied by two redistributional drug interactions. A — Sulfadoxine and phenylbutazone in live sheep (11, 12); B — penicillins and sulfonamides and aspirin in human volunteers (17).
  + Denotes evidence for redistribution.
  0 Denotes no evidence available.

excretion in a number of ways, including the very speed of the phenomenon, and by removing the kidneys and liver. Our conclusions were that in this particular example, the rise in the free sulfadoxine could be exclusively due to redistribution from plasma proteins.

This study was a pharmacokinetic analysis of the effects of single doses of the two drugs. We did not examine whether the phenomenon had any "therapeutic" significance. Presumably the temporarily increased free-sulfonamide concentration possessed enhanced antibacterial activity, but the wider effects of this are complex and would need to be studied under conditions of repetitive dosing.

In man, the evidence for redistributional interactions is rather less. The best demonstration I can find of the pharmacokinetics of redistribution in man is Kunin's study of penicillins in normal volunteers (17). Kunin studied the effects of three displacing agents (two sulfonamides and acetylsalicylic acid) on the distribution of a number of penicillins. The displacing agent was administered orally prior to the penicillin, and control studies with the penicillins alone were performed on separate days.

Experimentally, the evidence in this study was fairly extensive (Table 1B). The displacement was demonstrated *in vitro*. In man, a fall in plasma total and bound drug was demonstrated, together with a rise in the free concentration. Circumstantial evidence for a rise in volume of distribution was obtained by ruling out effects on metabolism and excretion (and, in most cases, absorption) by urinary measurements. However, since quantitative whole-body calculations were not made, it is not certain whether the gain in free drug could be totally ascribed to the loss of bound drug.

This again was a purely pharmacokinetic study, and, as in the previous example, there is no measure of clinical effect; Kunin pointed out that it would be hard to measure any such effect that might be produced. In any case, further data would be needed than are available here, since the pharmacokinetics were followed for only 2 hr after a single dose. The effect with chronic dosing is unknown and may be complex, since elimination of the penicillins would presumably be altered as a result of the displacement.

CLINICALLY SIGNIFICANT INTERACTIONS

When we turn to examine clinically significant drug interactions, the evidence for a redistributional mechanism becomes much less secure. There are three main interactions in which redistribution is thought to be the primary cause: these involve oral hypoglycemics, bilirubin, and oral anticoagulants.

Potentiation of Oral Hypoglycemics by Sulfaphenazole and Phenylbutazone

The hypoglycemic effect of tolbutamide has been shown to be potentiated in patients who are simultaneously given phenylbutazone (18) or sulfaphenazole (19) while the hypoglycemic effect of carbutamide was similarly potentiated by phenylbutazone (20). This has come to be very widely regarded as having a redistributional mechanism, although Christensen et al. (19) showed very elegantly that despite the occurrence of redistribution, this was definitely not the cause of the clinical effect. They showed that the mechanism was instead inhibition of tolbutamide's metabolism. It is ironic that this work has come to be misquoted, since it is the only clinical example in which redistribution has been convincingly ruled out as a cause by showing that the clinical potentiation does *not* occur with other equally potent displacing agents. In this example, as in some of the ones that follow, the attribution to a redistributional cause has been made not by the original authors but by subsequent reviewers.

Precipitation of Kernicterus by Sulfonamides (Table 2A)

In a well-designed prospective study in 1956, Silverman, Anderson, Blanc, and Crozier (21) showed that premature infants given prophylactic sulfisoxazole and penicillin had a high incidence of fatal kernicterus compared with a control group given oxytetracycline. Odell (22) proposed that

TABLE 2.

	A	B	C	D
1. Demonstration				
(a) *In vitro*	+	+	+	+
(b) In man (qual.)				
↓ Plasma total	+	+	−	+
↓ Plasma bound	0	0	0	0
↑ Plasma free	0	0	0	0
(c) In man (quant.)				
Loss of bound	0	0	0	0
Gain of free	0	0	0	0
Equivalence?	0	0	0	0
2. Exclusion or allowance for:				
(a) Absorption	(+)	0	0	0
(b) Metabolism	0	0	−	0
(c) Excretion	(+)	(+)	(+)	(+)
3. Correlation of free level with effect	0	0	0	0

Criteria satisfied by four clinical drug interactions. A —
Bilirubin and sulfonamides. Oral anticoagulents with B —
phenylbutazone; C — clofibrate; D — chloral hydrate.
+ Denotes evidence for redistribution.
− Denotes evidence against redistribution.
0 Denotes no evidence available.
( ) Denotes circumstantial evidence.

the mechanism of the increased kernicterus was displacement of bilirubin from plasma-binding by the sulfisoxazole.

The displacement was demonstrated qualitatively *in vitro* (22) and also in living animals (23). In the sulfonamide-treated infants, serum total bilirubin concentrations were substantially less than in the control group (24). However, serum-free (unbound) concentrations of bilirubin were not measured, and so no quantitative studies of the redistribution were possible.

Interactions at the levels of absorption and excretion do not apply in this situation, but the possibility that a metabolic interaction was occurring concealed by the changes in plasma concentrations has by no means been excluded.

Since serum-free levels of bilirubin were not measured, correlation with effect is not possible. However, the stronger bilirubin-staining of tissues in the sulfonamide-treated infants (24) despite their lower total serum concentrations supports the existence of redistribution, although not establishing a causal role for it.

In summary the evidence that exists, while incomplete in some crucial details, is consistent with a redistribution of bilirubin. It does not, however, exclude the possibility that other mechanisms (particularly at the metabolic level) are operating simultaneously, and it does not show the quantitative importance of redistribution as a cause of the kernicterus.

Potentiation of Oral Anticoagulants

By Phenylbutazone or Oxyphenbutazone (Table 2B)

It has often been suggested (1, 3–6, 25, 26) that the potentiation of oral-anticoagulant hypoprothrombinemia by phenylbutazone or oxyphenbutazone is due to displacement of the anticoagulant from binding sites on plasma protein.

This has been demonstrated *in vitro* (27, 28). In man, a fall in plasma total warfarin has been demonstrated (29, 30), but bound- and free-warfarin levels have not been measured. The loss of bound warfarin in the body has therefore not been calculated and neither has the gain, if any, of free warfarin. Consequently little is known about the redistribution in quantitative terms.

Alteration of the urinary excretion of warfarin can probably be ignored, but interaction at the level of absorption has by no means been ruled out. At first sight, a contribution from inhibition of metabolism seems to be excluded by O'Reilly and Aggeler's finding (30) that the half-life of warfarin is reduced by phenylbutazone. However, this finding is based solely on measurements of plasma total-warfarin levels, which have doubtful meaning in the presence of a displacing agent. The same objection applies to measurements of half-life in the two examples that are to follow. More sophisticated studies, including measurement of free-warfarin levels, are needed before a metabolic component can be excluded.

Another consequence of our ignorance of free-warfarin concentrations is that no correlation of these with effect is possible.

The fall in plasma total warfarin suggests that redistribution has occurred in man, and the clinical potentiation is consistent with a redistributional cause. However, no other unequivocal evidence exists to support this mechanism, other causes (31) have not been excluded, and the exact contribution of redistribution to the potentiation remains unknown.

By Clofibrate (Table 2C)

It has been reported that clofibrate increases the hypoprothrombinemic effect of bishydroxycoumarin (32) and, occasionally, warfarin (33, 34).

Although displacement of warfarin by clofibrate has been demonstrated *in vitro* (27, 28), what little *in vivo* evidence that exists seems to be at best nonsupporting. Instead of a fall in total bishydroxycoumarin, calculation from the data of Schrogie and Solomon's Table V (32) reveals no change or, if anything, a rise, whereas O'Reilly et al. (34a) found no significant fall of total-warfarin concentrations with clofibrate. Plasma-bound and free anticoagulant levels have not been measured, and neither has the volume of distribution of the anticoagulants in this situation. No quantitative examination of the redistribution has been made, nor is it possible with the data currently available.

The possibility of an absorptive interaction has not been excluded. Furthermore, an inhibition of the anticoagulant metabolism seems a distinct possibility: the half-life of bishydroxycoumarin (at least as reflected in measurements of plasma-total concentrations) did not fall; if anything [again calculating from Schrogie and Solomon's data (32)] it tended to increase.

Thus, in this interaction, little positive evidence exists to correlate the clinical effect with a redistributional cause and some of the evidence seems to be against it. Moreover, there is evidence for another mechanism, namely enhancement of the degradation rate of certain vitamin K–dependent clotting factors by clofibrate (34a).

By Chloral Hydrate (Table 2D)

Sellers and Koch-Weser (35) have shown elegantly and convincingly, in the most sophisticated analysis of its type, that chloral hydrate potentiates warfarin-induced hypoprothrombinemia in man. [There is some debate, however, about how troublesome the interaction actually is clinically (36–39).]

The displacement of warfarin by the chloral hydrate metabolite, trichloracetic acid, has been demonstrated *in vitro;* adequate concentrations of trichloracetic acid have been shown to accumulate in man (35), and a concomitant fall in plasma-total warfarin has been shown. It may be inferred, from the fact that peak warfarin levels after single doses were lower during chloral-hydrate therapy, that the volume of distribution of warfarin rose.

As in the previous examples, plasma-free anticoagulant levels have not been measured, so that neither qualitative nor quantitative evaluation of the magnitude of the redistribution is possible.

Whereas alteration of warfarin excretion can probably be ignored, an absorptive interaction has not been ruled out and neither has a metabolic one, although the presence of the overlying redistribution would make exclusion of the latter two possibilities difficult technically.

The authors' construction of warfarin concentration and dose indices is a sound way to demonstrate the fact of potentiation. The time course of the effect (onset and transience) is consistent with a redistributional cause, although again, because of the lack of free-warfarin levels, this proof must be regarded as circumstantial rather than direct. As in all the previous examples, the exact contribution of redistribution to the potentiation remains unknown.

DISCUSSION AND CONCLUSIONS

The concept of redistributional drug interactions is a plausible one and its feasibility, at least with binding involving plasma proteins, has been demonstrated many times *in vitro*. However, when we come to the question of its clinical significance, the picture is obscure.

The main defect is our lack of knowledge of plasma free-drug concentrations in all attempts to explain clinically significant interactions; since free-drug levels are the crucial point of the whole argument, this lack is a fatal one. Then there is failure to evaluate or exclude all other possible pharmacokinetic causes; and finally, we are in most cases ignorant of the effects of the displacer drug on the pharmacodynamics of the first drug and on the physiological or biochemical events under study. Whereas in most of the clinical interactions reviewed there is qualitative evidence that redistribution has occurred, we have no firm indication even of its significance in pharmacokinetic terms, let alone its contribution to the effect that is seen as an interaction.

Strong circumstantial evidence exists that the warfarin-phenylbutazone, warfarin–chloral hydrate, and bilirubin-sulfonamide interaction examples have at least some redistributional component. But it has not yet been rigorously shown that a redistributional drug interaction has ever, by itself, played an important part, or even a measurable part, in any of the clinically important drug interactions reviewed here. Much higher standards of proof are required before the redistributional mechanism can be accorded the position it currently holds in the literature.

One technical point that is often overlooked is that the displacement phenomenon, although not yet shown to produce clinical effects, does have a certain clinical significance. Any displacement that occurs during a drug interaction will always destroy the clinical meaning of plasma total levels of drugs, and thus invalidate any concentration-effect relationships based on these. In this respect, the situation resembles that in uremia, as discussed by Reidenberg, Odar-Cederlöf, Von Bahr, Borgà, and Sjöqvist (40). It is illogical to assume that plasma total concentrations of highly bound and displaceable drugs have the same meaning in the presence of displacing drugs as in the absence. Therefore, in both clinical and theoretical terms, if we really believe that it is the free level of drugs that is significant, it is high time we set about measuring this (by routinely ultrafiltering plasma specimens before measuring drug concentrations) and ignored the confusing and irrelevant protein-bound fraction.

ACKNOWLEDGMENTS

I am grateful to Drs. Olof Borgà, Paul Griner, and Michael Weintraub for making valuable suggestions.

REFERENCES

1. Brodie, B. (1965): *Proc. Roy. Soc. Med. 58,* 946.
2. Meyer, M., and Guttman, D. (1968): *J. Pharm. Sci. 57,* 895.

3. Thomas, J. (1969): *New Ethic. Med. Prog. March 1969, 64.*
4. Prescott, L. (1969): *Lancet 2,* 1239.
5. Deykin, D. (1970): *New Engl. J. Med. 283,* 801.
6. Melmon, K., and Morrelli, H. (1973): *Clinical Pharmacology: Basic Principles in Therapeutics,* Macmillan, New York.
7. Hansten, P. D. (1973): *Drug Interactions,* Lea and Febiger, Philadelphia.
8. Hartshorn, E. A. (1970): *Handbook of Drug Interactions,* Francke, Cincinnati.
9. Swidler, G. (1971): *Handbook of Drug Interactions,* Wiley-Interscience, New York.
10. Garb, S. (1971): *Clinical Guide to Undesirable Drug Interactions and Interferences,* Springer, New York.
11. McQueen, E., and Wardell, W. (1971): *Brit. J. Pharmac. 43,* 312.
12. Wardell, W. (1971): *Brit. J. Pharmac. 43,* 325.
13. Gillette, J. (1971): *Ann. N. Y. Acad. Sci. 179,* 43.
14. Yesair, D., Bullock, F., and Coffey, J. (1972): *Drug Metab. Revs. 1,* 35.
15. Weiner, M. (in press): In: *Symposium on Clinical Pharmacology Methods, Phase I-II,* New Orleans.
16. Koch-Weser, J., and Sellers, E. (1971): *New Engl. J. Med. 285,* 487.
17. Kunin, C. (1966): *Clin. Pharm. Therap. 7,* 180.
18. Gulbrandsen, R. (1959): *Tidsskrift Norske Laegeforen 79,* 1127.
19. Christensen, L., Hansen, J., and Kristensen, M. (1963): *Lancet 2,* 1298.
20. Kaindl, F., Kretschy, A., Puxkandl, H., and Wutte, J. (1961): *Wiener Klinische Wochenschrift 73,* 79.
21. Silverman, W., Anderson, D., Blanc, W., and Crozier, D. (1956): *Pediatrics 18,* 614.
22. Odell, G. (1959): *J. Clin. Invest. 38,* 823.
23. Johnson, L., Sarmiento, F., Blanc, W., and Day, R. (1959): *Dis. Children 97,* 591.
24. Harris, R., Lucey, J., and MacLean, R. (1958): *Pediatrics 21,* 875.
25. Sellers, E., and Koch-Weser, J. (1970): *New Engl. J. Med. 283,* 828.
26. Sellers, E., and Koch-Weser, J. (1971): *Ann. N. Y. Acad. Sci. 179,* 213.
27. Solomon, H., and Schrogie, J. (1967): *Biochem. Pharmacol. 16,* 1219.
28. Solomon, H., Schrogie, J., and Williams, D. (1968): *Biochem. Pharmacol. 17,* 143.
29. Aggeler, P., O'Reilly, R., Leong, L., and Kowitz, E. (1967): *New Engl. J. Med. 276,* 496.
30. O'Reilly, R., and Aggeler, P. (1968): *Proc. Soc. Exp. Biol. Med. 128,* 1080.
31. O'Reilly, R., and Aggeler, P. (1970): *Pharmacol. Revs. 22,* 35.
32. Schrogie, J., and Solomon, H. (1967): *Clin. Pharm. Therap. 8,* 70.
33. Hellman, L., Zumoff, B., Kessler, G., Kara, E., Rubin, I., and Rosenfeld, R. (1963): *Ann. Int. Med. 59,* 477.
34. Udall, J. (1969): *Clin. Res. 17,* 104.
34a. O'Reilly, R., Sahud, M., and Robinson, A. (1972): *Thromb. Diath. Haem. 27,* 309.
35. Sellers, E. Koch-Weser, J. (1970): *New Engl. J. Med. 283,* 827.
36. Griner, P., Raisz, L., Rickles, F., Wiesner, P., and Odoroff, C. (1971): *Ann. Int. Med. 74,* 540.
37. Griner, P., and Rickles, F. (1971): *Ann. Int. Med. 75,* 142.
38. Udall, J. (1971): *Ann. Int. Med. 75,* 141.
39. Boston Collaborative Drug Surveillance Program (1972): *New Engl. J. Med. 286,* 53.
40. Reidenberg, M., Odar-Cederlöf, I., Von Bahr, C., Borgå, O., and Sjöqvist, F. (1971): *New Engl. J. Med. 285,* 264.

Drug Interactions, edited by P. L. Morselli,
S. Garattini, and S. N. Cohen. Raven Press,
New York © 1974

Reserpine Measurements as a Model to Study the Complexity of Drug Interactions

L. Manara, S. R. Bareggi, C. Cerletti, F. Luzzani, and T. Mennini

Istituto di Ricerche Farmacologiche "Mario Negri", Via Eritrea, 62—20157 Milano, Italy

INTRODUCTION

A particular kind of interaction between drugs consists, partially if not entirely, in a different amount of one of the interacting agents being delivered to the sites of action. This is the ultimate reason for this type of altered drug response, no matter whether the corresponding drug interaction takes place at the level of absorption, excretion, metabolism, protein binding, or sites of action.

In this connection our laboratory has been interested in obtaining direct evidence by *in vivo* measurements of whether differences in drug levels can be demonstrated that are consistent with the altered drug response. For approaching this problem we have used an animal model system consisting in measurements of reserpine and of its depleting action on tissue catecholamine stores. These end points are evaluated in conditions of drug interactions, i.e., when the animals are treated with both reserpine and an agent interacting with it.

The short review that follows, based primarily on work performed in our laboratory, describes some of the most significant results obtained through such an approach.

RESERPINE MEASUREMENTS AS AN INDEX OF THE ACTION OF THE DRUG ON CATECHOLAMINE STORES

Reserpine presents several advantages as a model drug for studying the relationship between drug concentrations and drug effect *in vivo*. These advantages are mainly that reserpine acts by itself rather than through active biotransformation products (Plummer, Sheppard, and Schulert, 1957) and that reserpine measurements, even if performed on a gross specimen such as a whole organ, may reflect its concentrations at the sites of action. This is especially true in the case of reserpine levels measured in peripheral sympathetically innervated organs, such as the heart. Alpers and Shore (1969) maintain that, when different doses of this drug are administered to rats, by plotting the different amounts of reserpine found in the heart against the corresponding different concentrations of norepinephrine remaining in the same tissue, a highly significant linear regression is obtained, one molecule of reserpine present corresponding to about 500 of the missing catecholamine. Their data thus imply that the levels of reserpine measured upon assay of the heart are actually confined only to its adrenergic nerve endings.

Indeed, a similar conclusion may be drawn from the results of our study based on the use of 6-hydroxydopamine, a drug producing selective degeneration of the sympathetic terminals: when the latter in the heart were reduced by 6-hydroxydopamine to approximately 30% of normal, the administration of reserpine resulted in cardiac drug levels which were only about one-third of those of appropriate controls (Manara, Mennini, and Carminati, 1972). It is pointed out that this finding was apparent only 24 hr and not 30 min after the administration of reserpine. In fact, only at delayed intervals after reserpine administration do tissue concentrations in the target organs reflect those at the sites of action; they are, therefore, of functional significance.

THE TETRABENAZINE-RESERPINE INTERACTION

The functional significance of the nanogram amounts of reserpine persisting in tissues throughout the action of this agent (Plummer et al., 1957) which had been previously regarded as drug residues bound to nonspecific structures (Hess, Shore, and Brodie, 1956) was first established while studying the interaction between tetrabenazine and reserpine (Manara and Garattini, 1967).

Tetrabenazine is a reserpine-like drug, but its effects are much shorter-lasting than those of reserpine (Pletscher, 1957) so that, after tetrabenazine pretreatment, a prevention of the slowly reversible action of reserpine can be demonstrated (Quinn, Shore, and Brodie, 1959; Carlsson and Lindqvist, 1966). Such prevention is ascribed to reduced availability of the sites of action common to reserpine and tetrabenazine, to the former because of their occupancy by the latter (Sulser and Bass, 1968).

In order to obtain direct evidence that this is indeed the case, by means of reserpine measurements demonstrating lower reserpine levels in the target organs of tetrabenazine-pretreated animals, we had to measure the long-lasting nanogram amounts of reserpine (Manara and Garattini, 1967). The much higher concentrations that can be found early after the injection of this drug are in fact mostly nonspecific. They mask the small levels reflecting the concentrations of reserpine at the sites of action, so that even considerable differences in the latter fail to be detected by measuring the drug early after administration (Manara and Garattini, 1967, 1972).

Table 1 summarizes some of our data on the tetrabenazine-reserpine interaction in rats at the level of central and peripheral catecholamine stores. As to the brain, it should be pointed out that its reserpine content, unlike what was discussed for the heart in the previous section, cannot be regarded only as connected with the drug action on norepinephrine; no simple correlations exist between the amount of reserpine present and its action on the catecholamine (Manara and Garattini, 1972). Yet in Table 1, the data on brain reserpine content are consistent with those relative to the catecholamine concentrations and suggest that tetrabenazine prevents the depletion of norepinephrine induced by reserpine through a reduction of the levels of the latter. Also, for the heart, there is consistency between the results of reserpine measurements and those of norepinephrine analyses (i.e., only when tetrabenazine pretreatment is effective in reducing the levels of reserpine in the heart is a less extensive depletion of the cardiac catecholamine apparent).

However, in order to disclose that basically the same type of interaction between tetrabenazine and reserpine observed in the brain occurred also in the heart, appropriate adjustment of the doses of the two interacting agents was required. Reserpine in fact acts preferentially on heart norepinephrine stores as compared to tetrabenazine, which conversely is more active on the brain. Failure to consider similar factors may be misleading when studying drug interactions at the level of different tissues.

Since a similar prevention by tetrabenazine of the effects of reserpine on norepinephrine stores, as well as on those of other biogenic amines, was described also in mice and rabbits (Carlsson and Lindqvist, 1966), the discussed interaction between tetrabenazine and reserpine does not seem to be species-dependent.

THE COMPLEXITY OF THE PRENYLAMINE-RESERPINE INTERACTION

The choice of the animal species is important for the development of a given pattern of interaction between prenylamine and reserpine. In mice, pretreatment with prenylamine affects the action of reserpine in a way quite similar to that described for tetrabenazine in the previous section: the results are comparable to those shown in Table 1, and the same interpretations apply (Manara and Garattini, 1972).

Conversely, in order to obtain similar findings in rats, namely to show that also in this species pretreatment with prenylamine could prevent to some

TABLE 1. *Tetrabenazine-reserpine interaction on rat tissues: Norepinephrine depletion and reserpine concentrations*

Treatment		Assays			
		Brain		Heart	
Tetrabenazine (mg/kg i.p.)	Reserpine (mg/kg i.p.)	Norepinephrine (percent of normal ± SD)	Reserpine (ng/g ± SD)	Norepinephrine (percent of normal ± SD)	Reserpine (ng/g ± SD)
—	2.50	2.0 ± 0.6 (4)	15.5 ± 1.6 (4)	5.2 ± 2.7 (4)	4.5 ± 0.7 (4)
20	2.50	35.0 ± 15.7[b] (3)	7.9 ± 2.2[b] (5)	4.5 ± 1.6 (3)	5.4 ± 1.6 (5)
—	0.25			3.5 ± 1.9 (4)	4.4 ± 1.4 (3)[a]
60	0.25			23.0 ± 0.7[b] (4)	2.2 ± 0.3[b] (3)[a]

Male Sprague-Dawley rats of 180 to 220 g were treated as indicated in the table, tetrabenazine was given 30' prior to reserpine and animals sacrificed 12 hr after receiving reserpine. Norepinephrine assay was performed as described by Manara and Bareggi (1969). The animals used for reserpine assays were injected with tritium-labeled reserpine (Manara, 1967). The results of the assays are mean values based on the number of individually assayed specimens indicated in parentheses.

[a] The figures refer to the number of pools of three organs each.

[b] The mean is significantly different from that of the corresponding controls (Student's *t* test $p < 0.01$).

TABLE 2. *Prenylamine-reserpine interaction on norepinephrine stores in rats*

| Treatment | | Assays
Norepinephrine (μg/g $\pm$ SD) | | |
Prenylamine (mg/kg i.v.)	Reserpine (mg/kg i.v.)	Brain	Heart	Vas deferens
—	—	0.30 $\pm$ 0.02	0.61 $\pm$ 0.08	8.92 $\pm$ 0.76
5 $\times$ 2	—	0.33 $\pm$ 0.02	0.49 $\pm$ 0.11	6.40 $\pm$ 0.81
—	0.5	0.08 $\pm$ 0.01	0.04 $\pm$ 0.01	0.75 $\pm$ 0.23
5 $\times$ 2	0.5	0.15 $\pm$ 0.01[b]	<0.02	0.40 $\pm$ 0.08[a]

Prenylamine was repeated twice, 30 and 5 min before reserpine or its solvent (Manara and Bareggi, 1969). Norepinephrine assays were performed as indicated in Table 1. The results of the analyses are mean values, each based on four individually assayed specimens. (For the vasa deferentia, the 2 from the same animal represented one specimen.) Animals were sacrificed 24 hr after reserpine or at corresponding intervals.

[a] Significantly different from corresponding controls receiving reserpine alone (Student's *t* test, $p < 0.05$).

[b] Significantly different from corresponding controls receiving reserpine alone (Student's *t* test, $p < 0.01$).

extent the depleting action of reserpine on catecholamine stores, it was necessary to try a number of dosage schedules. Eventually we could determine the experimental condition described in Table 2, which is the only one resulting in a significant and reproducible reduction by prenylamine of the depleting action of reserpine on norepinephrine stores in the brain. In the other tissues (heart and vas deferens, see Table 2) taken from the same animals, prenylamine did not prevent reserpine-depleting action on catecholamine stores; the combination of these two drugs resulted rather in more extensive norepinephrine depletion than when reserpine alone was given. This is indeed an almost constant finding, irrespective of whether central (brain) or peripheral (heart and vas deferens) catecholamine stores are considered, when the effects of the combination of prenylamine and reserpine are studied in rats with different dosage schedules, some of which are illustrated in Table 3.

Species differences in the metabolism of prenylamine may possibly give a reason for the different aspects of the prenylamine-reserpine interaction when rats rather than mice are used (Manara and Garattini, 1972).

Measurements of reserpine (Table 4) show that in rats also prenylamine-pretreatment may result in some reduction of reserpine levels in tissues. In the brain, such a reduction (Table 4 and Fig. 2) is consistent with the antagonism by prenylamine of the norepinephrine-depleting action of reserpine (Table 2 and Manara and Garattini, 1972) and may be at the origin of this antagonism. However, the lack of a clear correlation between brain

TABLE 3. *Prenylamine-reserpine interaction on norepinephrine stores in rats*

Treatment		Assays Norepinephrine (percent of normal and SD or range)		
Prenylamine (mg/kg i.p.)	Reserpine (mg/kg i.v.)	Brain	Heart	Vas deferens
Experiment 1				
20 × 2	—	86 (82–90) (2)	86 (79–92) (2)	54 (50–58) (2)
—	1.25	10 ± 2.9 (5)	4.6 ± 1.3 (5)	6.9 ± 3.6 (5)
20 × 2	1.25	4.5 ± 1.8[a] (5)	0.8 ± 0.7[a] (5)	0.9 ± 0.7[a] (4)
Experiment 2				
20 × 2	—	78 (78–78) (2)	79 (93–65) (2)	58 (45–71) (2)
—	0.5	16 ± 1.5 (4)	7.2 ± 0.8 (4)	5.3 ± 0.6 (4)
20 × 2	0.5	15 ± 3.0 (3)	3.1 ± 1.4[a] (4)	0.9 ± 0.1[a] (3)
Experiment 3				
20 × 2	—	96 (102–90) (2)	87 (97–76) (2)	59 (46–72) (2)
—	0.25	50 ± 8.3 (4)	9.3 ± 2.4 (4)	14 ± 5.5 (4)
20 × 2	0.25	68 ± 13.0 (4)	3.9 ± 0.5[a] (4)	10 ± 3.6 (4)

Animals were treated with prenylamine 2 hr and 30′ before reserpine or its solvent and sacrified 24.5 hr after the second dose of prenylamine and/or 24 hr after reserpine. Norepinephrine assays were performed as indicated in Table 1.

The results of the assays are mean values, each based on the number of individually assayed specimens given in parentheses (for the vasa deferentia, the two from the same animal represented one specimen).

[a] Significantly different from corresponding controls receiving reserpine alone (Student's *t* test $p < 0.01$).

reserpine content and effect of this drug on the brain catecholamine (see the section "The Tetrabenazine-Reserpine Interaction") prevents the drawing of precise conclusions. In addition, the measurements of reserpine in Table 4 seem to exclude that the enhanced effects on catecholamine stores observed in the heart and vas deferens with the combination of prenylamine and reserpine, as compared with reserpine alone (Table 2), are due to changes in the metabolism of the latter drug. In fact the concentrations of reserpine found in the heart and vas deferens of prenylamine-pretreated animals do not exceed those of the appropriate controls.

TABLE 4. *Effect of prenylamine pretreatment on reserpine levels in rat tissues 24 hr after injection of 0.5 mg/kg i.v.*

Treatment	Assays Reserpine (ng/g ± SD)		
	Brain	Heart	Vas deferens
Controls	11.1 ± 0.9 (6)	4.2 ± 0.2 (3)[a]	7.1 ± 1.5 (3)[a]
Prenylamine-pretreated	8.6 ± 0.8[b] (6)	3.6 ± 0.1[b] (3)[a]	8.0 ± 0.7 (3)[a]

All the animals were injected with tritium-labeled reserpine (Manara, 1967), whereas those receiving prenylamine were treated according to the same dose and schedule as in Table 2.

The figures in the table are mean values, each based on the number of individually assayed specimens given in parentheses.

[a] The figures refer to the number of pools, consisting of two specimens each. For the vasa deferentia, the two from the same animal represented one specimen.

[b] Significantly different from corresponding controls receiving ^{3}H-reserpine alone (Student's *t* test, $p < 0.01$).

DRUGS INTERACTING WITH RESERPINE WITHOUT AFFECTING ITS TISSUE LEVELS

Reserpine has been employed frequently as a research tool in combination with agents capable of modifying its action. The functional significance of reserpine measurements discussed so far applies also to the possibility of verifying the specificity of such interactions on this ground: the finding of unchanged reserpine levels is required in order to support the concept that the observed interaction is based on a mechanism other than an alteration of the amount of reserpine reaching its sites of action.

In Table 5, several drugs are listed that, for the experimental conditions given, do not alter reserpine tissue levels when administered in combination with the latter. As an example metaraminol may be quoted.

In our laboratory, metaraminol was found to modify the depleting action of reserpine on cardiac norepinephrine (Manara and Bareggi, 1969). Since this finding could not be ascribed to a reduction by metaraminol of the amount of reserpine reaching the heart, the possible mechanism whereby metaraminol interacts with reserpine at the level of norepinephrine stores was investigated. The data collected led to the conclusion that metaraminol may act as a "functional" monoamine oxidase inhibitor, an action that also provides an alternative interpretation for the mechanism of the long-lasting pressor effect of this drug, which is of interest at the clinical level (Bareggi, Carminati, and Manara, 1971; Manara and Carminati, 1972; Manara and Garattini, 1972).

Another example of a drug interacting with reserpine without affecting its tissue levels refers to desipramine. This tricyclic antidepressant has been used extensively, as an antagonist of several pharmacological effects of reserpine, in animal studies aimed at the elucidation of the mechanism underlying "experimental depression" (Manara, Algeri, and Sestini, 1967). Our laboratory showed that desipramine and reserpine have a combined action on norepinephrine stores, thus providing a biochemical correlate for the interaction between these two drugs (Manara, Sestini, Algeri, and Garattini, 1966). We also confirmed the specificity of this interaction by showing no changes in reserpine levels by desipramine in any experimental condition among several tested (Table 5).

THE Ca^{++}-RESERPINE INTERACTION

As an example of an interaction with reserpine whose specificity could not be confirmed on the ground of reserpine measurements, reference is made to the proposed Ca^{++}-reserpine interaction at the level of brain monoamine stores (Radouco-Thomas, Tessier, Lajeunesse, and Garcin, 1971).

In Fig. 1, it can be seen that $CaCl_2$ pretreatment prevents brain norepinephrine depletion induced by subcutaneous administration of reserpine, in agreement with the findings of Radouco-Thomas et al. (1971). However, if reserpine is administered intravenously, the antagonism by the calcium salt is no longer apparent (Fig. 1).

Reserpine measurements in the same experimental conditions clearly indicate that a decreased delivery to the brain of reserpine administered subcutaneously may well account for the reduced action of this drug in the $CaCl_2$-pretreated animals. Conversely, the intravenous administration of reserpine results in comparable brain levels irrespective of whether the animals have been pretreated with the calcium salt (Table 6).

It is of interest to notice that, following subcutaneous administration of reserpine to $CaCl_2$-pretreated rats, as compared to controls receiving only distilled water in addition to reserpine, reduced brain levels of reserpine are already apparent 1 hr after its injection (Table 6). Since, as discussed in previous sections, only reserpine levels measured at delayed intervals reflect the concentration of the drug at the sites of action, such an early detectable difference in its whole-brain levels may be taken as an indication that the interaction between calcium and reserpine takes place far away from the sites of action.

Indeed in additional experiments we could show that $CaCl_2$ antagonizes the brain-norepinephrine depletion by reserpine only if both $CaCl_2$ and reserpine are administered subcutaneously in the same site of injection (this laboratory, *in preparation*). Consistently, an altered absorption from the injection site appears to be the most likely explanation for the reduced action on brain norepinephrine of subcutaneously administered **reserpine**

TABLE 5. *Drugs that do not alter tissue levels of reserpine when administered concurrently with it*

Drug	Dose and route	Interval	Dose of reserpine	Observation time	Tissue assayed Heart	Tissue assayed Brain
Amantadine HCl	100 i.p.	1 hr	0.50	24 hr		+
Bretylium tosylate	15 i.p.	30'	0.25	24 hr	+	
	20 i.p.	1 hr	0.25	6 hr	+	
p-Chloroamphetamine HCl	20 i.p.	1 hr	0.50	24 hr	+	+
Chlorpromazine HCl	20 i.p.	1 hr	0.25	6 and 24 hr	+	
Desipramine HCl	15 i.p.	6 hr (after reserpine)	2.50	1 and 12 hr	+	+
	15 i.p.	1 hr	2.50	5'; 1, 2, 6 and 12 hr	+	+
	15 i.p.	3 hr	0.25	24 hr	+	+
Guanethidine sulfate	20 i.p.	1 hr	0.25	5'	+	+
	20 i.p.	1 hr	0.25	1 hr	+	
	20 i.p.	1 hr	2.50	5'	+	+
	20 i.p.	1 hr	2.50	1 hr	+	
	20 i.p.	2 hr	0.25	24 hr	+	
Harmaline HCl	30 i.p.	30'	1.56	6 hr	+	+
	30 i.p.	1 hr	0.25	5'	+	+
	30 i.p.	1 hr	0.25	6 hr	+	
	30 i.p.	1 hr	2.50	5'	+	
Levo metaraminol	0.5 i.v.	1 hr	0.25	12 and 24 hr	+	
DL-metaraminol	1 i.v.	30'	0.25	24 hr	+	
Pheniprazine HCl	10 i.p.	12 hr	1.56	6 hr	+	+
	10 i.p.	2 hr	1.56	6 hr	+	+
	10 i.p.	24 hr	0.25	24 hr	+	
	10 i.p.	3 hr	0.25	24 hr	+	

Doses are in mg/kg; the interval is that between the administration of the drug and the intravenous injection of tritium-labeled reserpine (which was given always after, if not otherwise specified); the observation time is the interval after the administration of reserpine at which the animals were sacrificed; experiments were performed in rats and labeled reserpine assayed as indicated in Table 1.

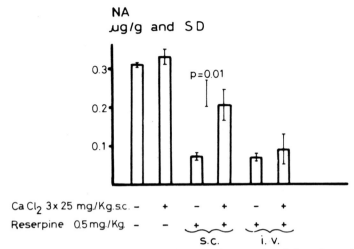

FIG. 1. Effect of CaCl$_2$ on the depletion of rat brain norepinephrine stores induced by reserpine. The doses of the drugs are those reported in the figure. CaCl$_2$ (or distilled water for the appropriate controls) was injected subcutaneously in the inguinal regions 45, 30, and 15 min before reserpine or its solvent: the first and the third injections were made in the right and the second in the left inguinal region. When administered subcutaneously, reserpine (or its solvent) was always injected in the left inguinal region. Animals were sacrificed 24 hr after the injection of reserpine or its solvent. The data on norepinephrine (NA) assays (Manara and Bareggi, 1969) are mean values, each based on three individually assayed brains: the vertical line below the probability level (p) represents the minimum significant difference (at $p = 0.01$) based on analysis of variance.

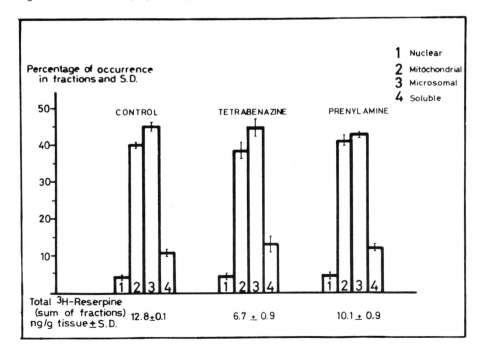

TABLE 6. *Reserpine brain levels after injection of 0.5 mg/kg to control and CaCl₂-pre-treated rats*

| | Assays Reserpine, ng/g and SD or range | | | |
| | 1 hr | | 24 hr | |
Treatment	Control	CaCl₂	Control	CaCl₂
Reserpine injected subcutaneously	13.6 ± 2.9 (3)	3.0 ± 1.2^a (4)	11.4 ± 1.9 (4)	6.2 ± 0.7^a (3)
Reserpine injected intravenously	28.8 (31.4–26.2) (2)	25.5 (23.8–27.3) (2)	12.5 ± 1.3 (3)	14.0 ± 1.0 (3)

Except for the use of tritium-labeled reserpine (Manara, 1967) which was used for all of the animals in this study, the doses of the drugs and the administration schedules were the same as in Fig. 1.

The results of the analyses are mean values based on the number of individually assayed specimens indicated in parentheses.

^{a} Significantly different from corresponding control (Student's *t* test *p* < 0.01).

in combination with calcium. Thus, in interpreting our data (Fig. 1 and Table 6), we do not favor the suggestion "that the calcium-reserpine antagonism is probably located at the level of the presynaptic axonal membrane" (Radouco-Thomas et al., 1971). In addition, we believe that our findings in Fig. 1 and Table 6 should be taken into account in a critical evaluation of the antagonism by calcium of the biochemical and behavioral effects following subcutaneous administration of reserpine (Radouco-Thomas et al., 1971; Boyaner and Radouco-Thomas, 1971*a, b*).

RESERPINE MEASUREMENTS IN SELECTED PARTS OF THE BRAIN

Enna and Shore (1971) have studied the regional distribution of reserpine in the rat brain and found no clear correlation between the concentration of the drug and that of any single endogenous monoamine.

FIG. 2. Subcellular distribution of reserpine in the rat brain and effect of tetrabenazine or prenylamine pretreatment. The doses and treatment schedules for reserpine and prenylamine were the same as in Table 7. Tetrabenazine, 5 mg/kg, i.p., was administered 1 hr prior to reserpine. Assays were performed on brains from animals sacrificed 24 hr after the injection of tritium-labeled reserpine (Manara, 1967) as described by Manara, Carminati, and Mennini (1972). The bars are mean percent values (the sum of ³H-reserpine activities of the four fractions derived from the same brain was made equal to 100%), each based on four individually assayed fractions, each obtained from a different and separately analyzed brain. The data on the total ³H-reserpine concentration in brain were derived from the sums of the amounts of reserpine in each different fraction from the same brain: the averages of the brains, from either tetrabenazine- or prenylamine-pretreated rats, are significantly different (*p* < 0.01, Student's *t* test) from that of control brains.

In our study, presented in Table 7, we have focused on the interaction between reserpine and either prenylamine or tetrabenazine at the level of three main brain regions. The results of our study suggest the widespread existence of sites of interaction with the binding of reserpine apparently unrelated to the relative distribution of the storage sites of the putative neurotransmitter monoamines. By using three different doses of tetrabenazine (Table 7), in fact, it can be shown that, within the same dose of the latter, the percent decrease in reserpine levels is of the same order for any of the three brain regions considered. This seems also to support the concept that the sites of interaction of tetrabenazine with the binding of reserpine in the different parts of the brain may have similar characteristics.

For prenylamine, the information is limited to one dose schedule, i.e., that which was found to antagonize brain norepinephrine depletion by reserpine (Table 2). At such a dose regimen, prenylamine pretreatment results only in a slight reduction (20 to 25%) of brain reserpine levels as compared to controls receiving reserpine alone. Yet this reduction is significant if the whole-brain concentrations of reserpine are considered (Table 4 and Fig. 2). However, in our study of the regional distribution of reserpine in the brain (Table 7), the percent decrease in reserpine content is not significant for all of the three regions studied, either when prenylamine or the lowest dose of tetrabenazine (which appears as effective as prenylamine in reducing brain reserpine levels) is used. Therefore, no safe conclusion can be drawn on the ground of the evidence presented as to whether saturable binding sites for the interaction with reserpine are common to prenylamine and tetrabenazine throughout the brain.

That our findings (Table 7) suggesting the existence of such sites of interaction in the brain are specific (independent of the aforementioned question, comparing the interaction by tetrabenazine with that by prenylamine, which remains an open one), is somehow confirmed by measurements of reserpine levels performed on the epididymal adipose tissues of the same animals whose brains were used for the assays reported in Table 7. In fact, tetrabenazine showed no consistent effect on the concentration of reserpine in the adipose tissue (which presumably reflects only the high lipid solubility of the latter), while a severalfold increase of reserpine levels was caused by prenylamine (this laboratory, *unpublished*). We do not yet have a satisfactory explanation for this finding with prenylamine. It is unlikely that the considerably higher amount of reserpine found in the adipose tissue of prenylamine-pretreated rats may simply derive from redistribution from other organs, since pretreatment with tetrabenazine had no such effect.

An additional aspect to be considered for a critical evaluation of the interactions by prenylamine and tetrabenazine with the binding of reserpine to specific sites is that the two former agents may act to an extent still to be determined through biotransformation products (Manara and Garattini, 1972).

TABLE 7. *Regional distribution of reserpine in the rat brain 24 hr after intravenous injection of 0.5 mg/kg and effect of prenylamine or tetrabenazine pretreatment*

Region	Control ng/g	Prenylamine (5 × 2 mg/kg i.v., 30' and 5' before reserpine)		Tetrabenazine (mg/kg i.p. 1 hr before reserpine)					
		ng/g	Percent of control	1		5		20	
				ng/g	Percent of control	ng/g	Percent of control	ng/g	Percent of control
Hemispheres	12.6 ± 0.5	10.8 ± 0.4	86	10.6 ± 0.5	84	7.2 ± 1.1	57	3.9 ± 1.1	31
Brainstem	13.7 ± 1.7	10.7 ± 3.1	78	10.7 ± 1.1	78	8.6 ± 0.2	63	5.3 ± 0.6	39
Cerebellum	1.7 (1.5–2.0)	1.2 (1.2–1.3)	71	1.3 (1.2–1.5)	77	1.2 (1.2–1.3)	71	0.8 (0.7–0.8)	44

Tritium-labeled reserpine (Manara, 1967) was used in this study. The concentrations of reserpine reported in the table are mean values and standard deviations (or range), each based on the results of three separately assayed pools, each consisting of two specimens. For the cerebellum the means refer to the results of the assays of two pools (given in parentheses) of three specimens each.

RESERPINE MEASUREMENTS AT THE SUBCELLULAR LEVEL

The results of studies on the subcellular distribution of drugs based on cell fractionation techniques are difficult to interpret because of artifacts of redistribution occurring in the course of such procedures. These difficulties apply also to reserpine (Alpers and Shore, 1969; Manara, Carminati, and Mennini, 1972; Wagner and Stitzel, 1972).

Our laboratory has used cell-fractionation methods as an approach to the isolation of specific sites of binding for reserpine in the rat brain. We found that the profile of subcellular distribution of reserpine in the brains of rats injected with this drug 24 hr previously differs from both patterns of distribution obtained either 1 hr after the administration of reserpine, or by its addition to brain homogenates from untreated rats. The two latter profiles closely parallel each other and derive primarily from the artifactual redistribution of "labile" bound reserpine, whereas the profile at 24 hr is more specific, suggesting the occurrence of a "persistent" binding of reserpine in the microsomal and possibly in the mitochondrial fractions (Manara et al., 1972). This interpretation is supported by recent data showing that the "labile" bound reserpine, resulting from the addition of the drug to the brain *in vitro* or from injection into animals 1 hr before, is removed by extraction into peanut oil, whereas such an extraction is slightly effective in removing reserpine "persistently" bound to the mitochondrial and microsomal fraction from brains of rats injected 24 hr before (Manara, Mennini, and Cerletti, 1974).

The interactions by prenylamine and tetrabenazine with the *in vivo* binding of reserpine to brain subcellular components were investigated quite recently. The corresponding results are reported in Fig. 2 and show that the profile of the relative distribution of reserpine in the different fractions at 24 hr is not altered by either prenylamine or tetrabenazine (which both reduce the total amount of bound reserpine).

As far as tetrabenazine is concerned, these findings appear somehow consistent with those obtained in the studies on the regional distribution of reserpine in the brain (see the previous section). They suggest, in fact, that different subcellular components, not necessarily associated with the monoamine storage organelles, may contain similar sites of interaction with the binding of reserpine. However, the difficulties in interpreting the results of this type of study, which have already been indicated at the beginning of this section, dictate caution in drawing conclusions from data such as those presented in Fig. 2.

As to the evaluation of the findings relative to prenylamine (Fig. 2), the same limitations apply. Moreover, although it may be tempting to speculate on the apparent similarities of the results obtained with tetrabenazine and prenylamine (Fig. 2), additional limitations refer in this case to the lack of more adequate supporting evidence for such a comparison from the data of the brain regional distribution studies (see the previous section).

Thus it is pointed out once more that, at the current status of these studies on the subcellular distribution of reserpine, only provisional indications should be cautiously derived from their results. Nonetheless, in our opinion the latter have been so far encouraging enough to support the concept that reserpine may be regarded as an interesting model also for the study of the significance of drug measurements at the subcellular level. Progress in this area appears highly desirable for a better understanding of the mechanism of drug action as well as of the interactions between drugs.

SUMMARY

Measurements of reserpine in several tissues give some indication of the action of the drug therein. Thus, it is possible to verify whether a given drug interacting with reserpine alters its action by affecting the levels of reserpine reaching the target sites.

Both tetrabenazine and prenylamine may prevent the binding of reserpine to specific sites; for prenylamine, however, different patterns of interaction with reserpine result depending on the animal species and on the target organ considered. Calcium salts, injected concomitantly, may antagonize the effects of subcutaneously administered reserpine by limiting its absorption.

Other drugs interact with reserpine without affecting its tissue levels. Since reserpine has been extensively used as a research tool, often in combination with agents capable of modifying its action, measurements of reserpine are also important for an appropriate evaluation of the nature of such interactions.

In view of their functional significance, reserpine measurements at the level of several organs are referred to as the main parameter considered for illustrating some general aspects of drug interactions by means of data derived from an animal model system.

Reserpine is further indicated as a model drug for approaching the difficult problem of interpreting the significance of drug measurements performed on subcellular components, also in connection with the interaction of different agents at such levels.

ACKNOWLEDGMENTS

The authors gratefully acknowledge Professor S. Garattini's advice and helpful discussion in the preparation of this chapter. The original work presented here was supported by U.S. Public Health Service Grant 1 P01 GM 18376–01, 02, 03, and 04 PTR from the National Institutes of Health.

REFERENCES

Alpers, H. S., and Shore, P. A. (1969): Specific binding of reserpine. Association with norepinephrine depletion. *Biochem. Pharmacol. 18,* 1363–1372.

Bareggi, S. R., Carminati, P., and Manara, L. (1971): Metaraminol and monoamine oxidase activity in the rat heart. *Res. Commun. Chem. Pathol. Pharmacol. 2,* 347–354.

Boyaner, H. G., and Radouco-Thomas, S. (1971a): Partial antagonism by exogenous calcium of the depressant effect of reserpine in rat shuttlebox behaviour. *Brain Res. 33,* 589–591.

Boyaner, H. G., and Radouco-Thomas, S. (1971b): Effect of calcium on reserpine-induced catalepsy. *J. Pharm. Pharmacol. 23,* 974–975.

Carlsson, A., and Lindqvist, M. (1966): The interference of tetrabenazine, benzquinamide, and prenylamine with the action of reserpine. *Acta Pharmacol. Toxicol. 24,* 112–120.

Enna, S. J., and Shore, P. A. (1971): Regional distribution of persistently bound reserpine in rat brain. *Biochem. Pharmacol. 20,* 2910–2912.

Hess, S. M., Shore, P. A., and Brodie, B. B. (1956): Persistence of reserpine action after the disappearance of drug from brain: Effect of serotonin. *J. Pharmacol. Exp. Ther. 118,* 84–89.

Manara, L. (1967): Identification and estimation of tritium-labeled reserpine in biological material by a combination of thin-layer chromatography and liquid-scintillation radioassay. *Eur. J. Pharmacol. 2,* 136–138.

Manara, L., Algeri, S., and Sestini, M. G. (1967): Some modifications of the adrenergic mechanism induced by DMI-reserpine interactions. In: *Antidepressant Drugs,* ed. S. Garattini and M. N. G. Dukes, pp. 51–60, Excerpta Medica, Amsterdam.

Manara, L., and Bareggi, S. R. (1969): Modification by metaraminol of reserpine action on noradrenaline stores in the rat heart. *Eur. J. Pharmacol. 7,* 115–117.

Manara, L., and Carminati, P. (1972): Is metaraminol a selective monoamine oxidase inhibitor? In: *Monoamine Oxidase: New Vistas,* ed. E. Costa and M. Sandler, pp. 421–422, Raven Press, New York.

Manara, L., Carminati, P., and Mennini, T. (1972): "*In vivo*" persistent binding of 3H-reserpine to rat brain subcellular components. *Eur. J. Pharmacol. 20,* 109–113.

Manara, L., and Garattini, S. (1967): Time course of 3H-reserpine levels in brains of normal and tetrabenazine-pretreated rats. *Eur. J. Pharmacol. 2,* 139–141.

Manara, L., and Garattini, S. (1972): Actions and interactions of reserpine, reserpine-like and other catecholamine releasing agents. In: *Le Catecolamine,* Atti Convegno Farmitalia, pp. 21–45, Minerva Medica, Torino.

Manara, L., Mennini, T., and Carminati, P. (1972): Reduced binding of 3H-reserpine to the hearts of 6-hydroxydopamine-pretreated rats. *Eur. J. Pharmacol. 17,* 183–185.

Manara, L., Mennini, T., and Cerletti, C. (1974): 3H-reserpine persistently bound "in vivo" to rat brain subcellular components: limited removal by peanut oil extraction. *Life Sci. in press.*

Manara, L., Sestini, M. G., Algeri, S., and Garattini, S. (1966): On the ability of desipramine to interfere with reserpine induced noradrenaline release. *J. Pharm. Pharmacol. 18,* 194–195.

Pletscher, A. (1957): Release of 5-hydroxytryptamine by benzoquinolizine derivatives with sedative action. *Science 126,* 507.

Plummer, A. J., Sheppard, H., and Schulert, A. R. (1957): The metabolism of reserpine. In: *Psychotropic Drugs,* ed. S. Garattini and V. Ghetti, pp. 350–362. Elsevier, Amsterdam.

Quinn, G. P., Shore, P. A., and Brodie, B. B. (1959): Biochemical and pharmacological studies of Ro-1-9569 (tetrabenazine), a non-indole tranquilizing agent with reserpine-like effects. *J. Pharmacol. Exp. Ther. 127,* 103–109.

Radouco-Thomas, S., Tessier, L., Lajeunesse, N., and Garcin, F. (1971): Role of calcium in the reserpine-induced cerebral monoamines depletion. *Int. J. Clin. Pharmacol. 5,* 5–12.

Sulser, F., and Bass, A. D. (1968): Pharmacodynamic and biochemical considerations on the mode of action of reserpine-like drugs. In: *Psychopharmacology. A Review of Progress,* Proc. 6th Annual Meeting American College of Neuropsychopharmacology, San Juan, Puerto Rico, 1967, ed. D. H. Efron, pp. 1065–1075, Government Printing Office, Washington, D.C.

Wagner, L. A., and Stitzel, R. E. (1972): The relation between the subcellular distribution of 3H reserpine and its proposed site of action. *J. Pharm. Pharmacol. 24,* 396–402.

Drug Interactions, edited by P. L. Morselli, S. Garattini, and S. N. Cohen. Raven Press, New York © 1974

Estrogen Interactions at the Hypothalamic Subcellular Level

Jean-Pierre Raynaud

Centre de Recherches Roussel-Uclaf, 93230 Romainville, France

INTRODUCTION

Previous studies have established that, in the immature rat, estradiol is bound by a specific plasma binding protein, EBP (1), the concentration of which is very high in the fetus (80 μM) and decreases linearly from birth with a half life of 4 days, the level falling to zero at weaning and remaining at zero in normal and castrated adults (2). Binding to this protein affects biological response (2), since the highly potent synthetic estrogen R 2858 (11β-methoxy-17-ethynyl-1,3,5(10)-estratriene-3,17β-diol), which is not bound by EBP, is more uterotrophic than estradiol, although its affinity for the uterine cytosol receptor is less (3). In any study on mechanism at a cellular, and *a fortiori* subcellular, level in the immature rat, R 2858 is therefore a more sensitive tool than the natural hormone for tracking down possible estrogen target organs.

Autoradiographic studies on the hypothalamus have located the regions of maximum estrogen concentration as the medial preoptic area, the periventricular nuclei of the anterior region, and the arcuate and ventral medial nuclei (4, 5). *In vitro* sucrose-gradient studies on whole hypothalami have demonstrated that an estradiol receptor is already present at 14 days (6). The concentration of binding sites in the nuclear fraction and the dissociation constant of the receptor-estradiol complex have been measured at 4 weeks by an *in vitro* uptake method (7). The most recent gradient studies by Kato (8) on the adult castrated rat have confirmed that this receptor is indeed primarily located in the anterior hypothalamus as suggested by autoradiographic studies. *In vivo* studies have shown that the uptake by the anterior hypothalamus and median eminence of the adult castrated rat follows a pattern similar to that shown by the uterus and vagina (9) and that the onset of preferential uptake appears to be at approximately 3 weeks (10).

If the estrogen receptor in the anterior hypothalamus cytosol is translocated to the nucleus to trigger off the biological response, as described for the uterus (11–13), then the *in vivo* nuclear uptake following injection of a physiological dose of steroid should be both saturable and hormone specific. The *in vivo* nuclear radioactivity uptake by the anterior, middle, and posterior hypothalamus of immature 2- and 5-week-old rats following intravenous injection of labeled estradiol and R 2858 was therefore investigated in order to take into account in a single study all the parameters so far considered in the literature as well as the influence of plasma binding.

MATERIALS AND METHODS

Animals

Immature female Wistar rats bred by Charles River were used. The animals were given food and water *ad libitum* and maintained in air-conditioned surroundings under controlled lighting conditions.

Steroids

6,7 ^{3}H-estradiol-17β (58 C/mmole) and 6,7 ^{3}H 11β-methoxy-17-ethynyl-1,3,5(10)-estratriene-3,17β-diol (R 2858) (44 C/mmole) were synthesized by Roussel-Uclaf and tested for purity (>98%) by thin-layer chromatography in benzene:ethyl acetate (7:3, v/v). The corresponding nonradioactive compounds and 11α-methoxy-17-ethynyl-1,3,5(10-estratriene-3, 17β-diol (RU 16117) were also used.[1]

Radioactivity Measurements

Following dissolution of samples in methoxy ethanol:toluene (2:3, v/v) containing naphthalene (8%, w/v) and butyl PBD (0.4%, w/v), radioactivity was counted in a Tricarb Packard liquid scintillation spectrometer (model 3320) with a standard error of counting of less than 1%. All counts were corrected to 100% efficiency by the channel ratio method or external standardization.

Sucrose Gradient Studies. Fetal Plasma

One milliliter of $^1/_{100}$ dilute plasma from 20-day fetuses was incubated for 2 hr at 0°C with the radioactive steroid (0.4 nM) in 0.05 M Tris-HCl, 0.15 M NaCl buffer (pH 7.4) and then layered (0.2 ml) on a 5 to 20% sucrose gradient. The gradients were centrifuged at 42,000 rpm for 17 hr at 4°C in a Spinco ultracentrifuge (model $L_2$65B) using an SW 50.1 rotor. The radioactivity of 2-drop fractions, collected from the bottom of the tubes, was counted.

---

[1] For the sake of simplicity, the following abbreviations have been used in the tables: E, 11βMEE, 11αMEE. RU 16117 has been prepared by A. Pierdet in our Research Center.

Sucrose Gradient Studies. Hypothalamic Tissue

The anterior hypothalamus, middle hypothalamus, and cortex from 5-week-old rats were homogenized in 1 ml of 0.01 M Tris-HCl, 1.5 mM EDTA, 12 mM thioglycerol buffer (pH 7.4) in a Teflon-glass homogenizer at 4°C (~660 mg of tissue per ml of buffer) and centrifuged at 105,000 g for 1 hr in a Spinco $L_2$65B centrifuge using a 50 Ti rotor. The supernatant or 1 ml of $\frac{1}{5}$ dilute plasma was incubated for 30 min at 4°C with 0.2 nM labeled estradiol in the presence or absence of nonradioactive competitor (20 nM) and then layered (0.3 ml) on a linear sucrose gradient containing 10% glycerol [6.5 to 20% (w/v) sucrose in solution in buffer]. The gradients were centrifuged at 47,000 rpm for 16 hr at 4°C in a Spinco $L_2$65B centrifuge using an SW 50.1 rotor. The radioactivity of 2-drop fractions was counted.

Determination of *in vivo* Radioactivity Uptake by the Hypothalamus.

In the Fetus

Groups of three 22-day-old female rat fetuses were injected intravenously into the umbilical vein with 0.05 μC of labeled compound in 0.1 ml of a 10% solution of ethanol in physiological saline. The fetuses were killed by decapitation 30 min later and the radioactivity of the plasma, cortex, and hypothalamus was determined by liquid scintillation following combustion in an Oximat auto-oxidizer.

In the Immature Rat

Groups of three rats were injected intravenously with 10 or 44 μC of radioactive compound in 0.5 ml (5-week-old rats) or 0.25 ml (2-week-old rats) of physiological saline. In competition studies they received 2.5 μg radioinert steroid 30 min prior to the injection of radioactivity. They were killed by decapitation 15 min, 30 min, or 2 hr after injection. Blood samples were collected in heparinized tubes and centrifuged at 6,000 rpm for 10 min at 4°C. The entire hypothalamus was cut out as a block, limited anteriorly by a cut through the center of the optic chiasma, laterally by the hypothalamic fissures, and posteriorly by the anterior border of the mammillary bodies (4). The depth from the basal surface of the hypothalamus was 2 to 3 mm. The excised area was then divided into three parts: anterior, middle, and posterior. Tissue was homogenized in 1 ml of 0.32 M sucrose and then treated as shown in Fig. 1. Samples from the cerebral cortex served as control tissue for total radioactivity determination.

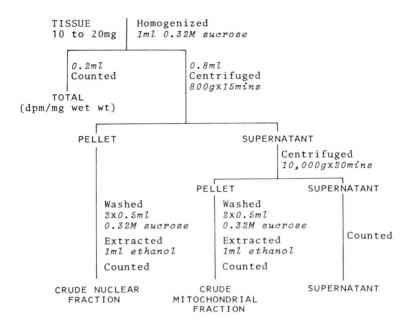

FIG. 1. Scheme for the preparation of subcellular fractions.

RESULTS

Specific Plasma Binding

As shown in the sucrose gradients in Fig. 2, an estradiol-plasma binding protein complex is formed, which sediments in the "4S" region. The steroid, 11β-methoxy-ethynyl-estradiol (R 2858), on the other hand, remains unbound and is recovered at the top of the gradient.

Saturability and Specificity of Total Radioactivity Uptake

The total radioactivity incorporated by the anterior, middle, and posterior regions of the hypothalamus, by the cerebral cortex and plasma 30 min and 2 hr after intravenous injection of labeled estradiol to 5-week-old female rats has been entered in Table 1. After 30 min, the highest radioactivity levels are recorded in the plasma and anterior hypothalamus, the level in the middle hypothalamus being somewhat lower and in the posterior hypothalamus and cortex very much lower. The radioactivity disappearance, as indicated by the change in concentration from 30 min to 2 hr, is fairly rapid in the case of the cortex and posterior and middle hypothalamus, slower in the case of the plasma and anterior hypothalamus. These results

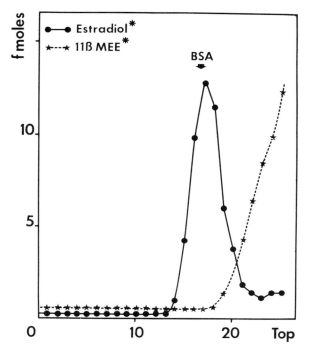

FIG. 2. Specific plasma binding in the 22-day-old fetus.

TABLE 1. *Saturability and specificity of radioactivity uptake by various regions of the rat brain*

Tissue	Time (hr)	*E dpm/mg	t/c	t/p	*E+E dpm/mg	*E+11βMEE dpm/mg	*E+11αMEE dpm/mg
Anterior	0.5	325 ± 35	2.4	0.9	214 ± 6	192 ± 34	298 ± 15
hypothalamus	2.0	162 ± 38	5.6	1.1	40 ± 4	27 ± 6	98 ± 4
Middle	0.5	256 ± 30	1.9	0.7	172 ± 26	189 ± 9	266 ± 28
hypothalamus	2.0	74 ± 4	2.6	0.5	33 ± 1	33 ± 7	64 ± 8
Posterior	0.5	159 ± 13	1.2	0.4	170 ± 34	197 ± 6	209 ± 35
hypothalamus	2.0	44 ± 8	1.5	0.3	25 ± 3	23 ± 5	38 ± 7
Cerebral	0.5	137 ± 12	1.0	0.4	136 ± 31	167 ± 21	172 ± 39
cortex	2.0	29 ± 3	1.0	0.2	28 ± 2	26 ± 4	35 ± 4
Plasma	0.5	364 ± 38		1.0	409 ± 64	430 ± 44	472 ± 27
	2.0	148 ± 9		1.0	138 ± 25	182 ± 31	225 ± 40

Uptake was measured following i.v. injection of 44 μC of labeled estradiol (0.2 μg) alone or after injection 30 min before with 2.5 μg of radioinert competitor to the 5-week-old female rat. Results are expressed as the mean uptake (±SEM) calculated from measurements on three rats and as the ratio of the concentrations between tissue and cerebral cortex *(t/c)* or tissue and plasma *(t/p)*.

imply specific retention in the anterior hypothalamus. The only true reflection of the power of tissular retention is however the value of the ratio of the concentrations between target tissue and nontarget tissue of similar cellular structure (in this case cerebral cortex). The tissue/cortex ratios at 2 hr reveal marked retention in the anterior hypothalamus (t/c = 5.6), moderate retention in the middle hypothalamus (t/c = 2.6), and virtually negligible retention in the posterior hypothalamus (t/c = 1.5), whereas the tissue/plasma ratios just indicate that slight retention occurs in the anterior hypothalamus only (t/p = 1.1). It is interesting to note for the purposes of comparison that in the immature 3-week-old rat the estradiol uterus/plasma ratio is 3.2 at 30 min and 5.3 at 2 hr (3).

The injection of 2.5 μg of radioinert steroid 30 min prior to the injection of radioactive estradiol has the following effect on uptake by the anterior hypothalamus (Table 1): the highly estrogenic compound 11β-methoxy-ethynyl-estradiol (R 2858) gives rise to the greatest decrease in bound radioactive steroid, this decrease being much more marked 2 hr than 30 min after injection. Since at 2 hr the amount of nonspecific binding has diminished faster than specific binding, competition with the specifically retained labeled steroid is consequently more apparent; estradiol itself has an effect that is nearly as marked, whereas the only very slightly estrogenic derivative 11α-methoxy-ethynyl-estradiol is much less effective. Somewhat parallel results are observed in the case of the middle and posterior hypothalamus: the radioactivity disappearance from these regions is however faster and the competitive effect less marked, implying that nonspecific binding exceeds by far specific binding. No competitive effect is observed in the cerebral cortex.

The picture as regards competition in the plasma is completely different since, as shown in Table 1, the addition of radioinert competitor has no effect on the level of circulating labeled estradiol. An increase is even observed and may be explained by the saturation of specific tissular binding sites since the competitor is injected 30 min prior to administration of the labeled compound.

Subcellular Total Radioactivity Uptake

The radioactivity taken up by the various regions of the hypothalamus after injection of labeled estradiol is distributed subcellularly as shown in Fig. 3. The major part of the radioactivity in the anterior hypothalamus is found in the supernatant fraction after 30 min but in the nuclear pellet at 2 hr, thus demonstrating retention at the nuclear level. Uptake in the crude mitochondrial fraction is insignificant in comparison. In the middle hypothalamus, uptake is marked, but less pronounced than in the anterior region. In this case also, disappearance from the nuclear fraction is less rapid than from the cytosol. On the other hand, no specific retention of radioactivity

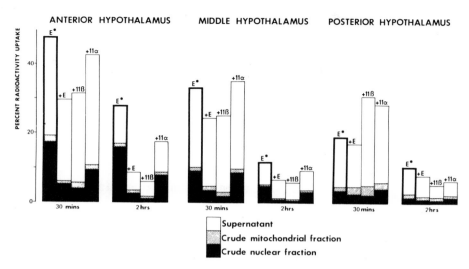

FIG. 3. Subcellular radioactivity uptake by the anterior, middle, and posterior regions of the rat hypothalamus. Uptake was measured 30 min and 2 hr following i.v. injection of 44 μC of labeled estradiol (0.2 μg) either alone or 30 min after the injection of 2.5 μg of radioinert compound to the 5-week-old immature female rat. Results are expressed as a percentage of the total radioactivity incorporated by the whole hypothalamus at 30 min.

has been recorded in the posterior hypothalamus. Competition by radio-inert steroid confirms the estrogen specificity of the uptake and reveals that for each hypothalamic region, excluding the posterior hypothalamus, competition is most apparent at the nuclear level. Nuclear radioactivity is therefore the most sensitive indicator of specific *in vivo* estrogen uptake.

Uptake as a Function of Age

The above experiments have all been carried out in 5-week-old animals after the disappearance of EBP; in 2-week-old animals, somewhat different results are recorded as shown in Table 2. Once again, a higher radioactivity level is found in the anterior hypothalamus ($t/c = 1.3$) as compared to the other regions, but in this instance an extremely high concentration is detected in the plasma on account of the presence of EBP. Whereas the cortex/plasma ratio was 0.2 in 5-week-old animals for estradiol (Table 1), it is 0.06 in 2-week-old animals. The distribution pattern obtained with the highly active synthetic estrogen 11β-methoxy-ethynyl-estradiol (R 2858) is different, much less radioactivity being retained in the plasma ($c/p = 0.4$) and correspondingly more radioactivity being associated with the anterior hypothalamus ($t/c = 2.1$). The subcellular distribution of radioactivity as a function of age is given in Table 3. More radioactivity is incorporated in the nuclear fraction of all target tissues, and in particular of the anterior hypo-

TABLE 2. *Radioactivity uptake in the 2-week-old immature rat and in the 22-day-old fetus*

| | 2-week-old immature rat | | | | | | 22-day-old fetus | | | | | |
| | E* | | | 11βMEE* | | | E* | | | 11βMEE* | | |
	dpm/mg	t/c	t/p	dpm/mg	t/c	t/p	dpm/mg	t/c	t/p	dpm/mg	t/c	t/p
Anterior hypothalamus	112 ± 8	1.3	0.07	401 ± 29	2.1	0.9						
Middle hypothalamus	84 ± 13	1.0	0.06	251 ± 2	1.3	0.6	8 ± 1	0.8	0.1	16 ± 1	0.8	1.0
Posterior hypothalamus	73 ± 6	0.9	0.05	175 ± 5	0.9	0.4						
Cerebral cortex	86 ± 10	1.0	0.06	191 ± 9	1.0	0.4	10 ± 2	1.0	0.2	21 ± 2	1.0	1.2
Plasma	1522 ± 134		1.0	426 ± 40		1.0	63 ± 10		1.0	17 ± 1		1.0

In the 2-week-old female rat, uptake was measured 2 hr following i.v. injection of 10 μC of either labeled estradiol (0.05 μg) or 11βMEE (0.07 μg). In the fetus, uptake was measured 30 min following i.v. injection via the umbilical vein of 0.05 μC of either labeled estradiol (0.25 ng) or 11βMEE (0.35 ng). Results are expressed as the mean uptake (±SEM) calculated from measurements on three rats and as the ratio of the concentrations between tissue and cerebral cortex *(t/c)* or tissue and plasma *(t/p)*.

thalamus, on administration of R 2858 at 2 weeks than on administration of estradiol, which tends to be retained in the plasma owing to the presence of EBP.

Restricted access to the tissues in the case of estradiol, but not R 2858, is further demonstrated by the results obtained for the 22-day-old fetus, which

TABLE 3. *Subcellular distribution of radioactivity as a function of age*

Tissue	Crude fractions	2 weeks E*	11βMEE*	5 weeks *E
Anterior hypothalamus	Nucleus	7	14	57
	Mitochondria	6	7	3
	Supernatant	87	79	40
Middle hypothalamus	Nucleus	7	12	41
	Mitochondria	6	4	3
	Supernatant	87	84	56
Posterior hypothalamus	Nucleus	4	4	15
	Mitochondria	6	5	10
	Supernatant	90	91	75
Cerebral cortex	Nucleus	3	5	
	Mitochondria	5	5	
	Supernatant	92	90	

Radioactivity distribution was determined 2 hr following i.v. injection of 10 μC of either labeled estradiol or 11βMEE. Results are expressed as percentages.

has a very high EBP concentration (2). Since in the fetus it is not possible to divide the hypothalamus accurately into its various parts, radioactivity determinations were carried out on the whole organ. No specific radioactivity uptake was observed, the values being lower than those for the cortex even on administration of R 2858 (Table 2). Whether the 22-day-old fetus or the 2-week-old immature rat is concerned, the 11βMEE/E ratio as determined from the tissue/plasma values is of the order of 10, implying that the EBP concentration is high enough, at least up to 2 weeks, to effectively control the bioavailability of estradiol.

In Vitro Binding

Following *in vitro* incubation of labeled estradiol in the presence or absence of radioinert steroid with cytosol from the hypothalamus or cerebral cortex or with plasma, the sucrose density patterns illustrated in Fig. 4 were obtained. An "8S" peak is observed with estradiol and anterior hypothalamic tissue which is completely suppressed on addition of radioinert estradiol. The middle hypothalamus gives a similar but much lower peak with the same sedimentation coefficient; this peak is also completely suppressed by the addition of radioinert compound. The cerebral cortex does not specifi-

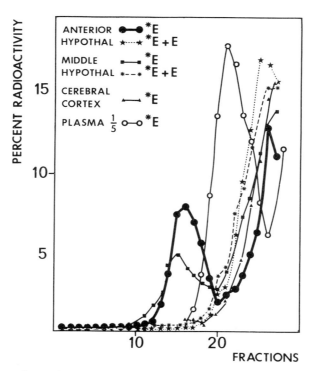

FIG. 4. Binding of estradiol to hypothalamus and cerebral cortex cytosol and to plasma in the 5-week-old rat. (For details, refer to Materials and Methods).

cally bind estradiol and all the radioactivity is recovered at the top of the gradient. Binding of estradiol to plasma ("4S") was taken as a reference for the determination of the sedimentation coefficient.

Uptake as a Function of Time

Figure 5 illustrates the *in vivo* radioactivity uptake of the crude nuclear, mitochondrial, and supernatant fractions of anterior, middle, and posterior hypothalamic cells as a function of time. Over the period 15 min to 2 hr, the percentage radioactivity uptake increases most markedly in the case of the crude nuclear fraction of the anterior hypothalamus. A similar but less pronounced increase is recorded for the middle hypothalamus, whereas the level for the posterior hypothalamus decreases. In the case of the super-

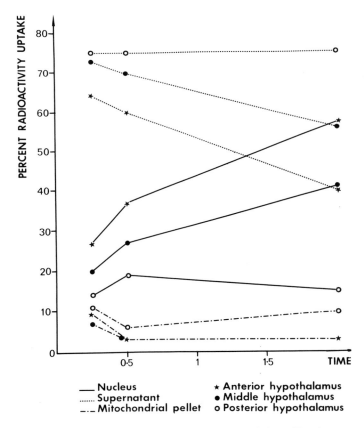

FIG. 5. Subcellular radioactivity uptake as a function of time. Uptake was measured following i.v. injection of 44 μC of labeled estradiol (0.2 μg) to the 5-week-old immature female rat. Results are expressed as a percentage of the total radioactivity taken up by each region of the hypothalamus.

natant, a decrease, which parallels the increase observed for the crude nuclear fraction, is recorded. No change is observed for the crude mitochondrial fraction. These results confirm those for total radioactivity uptake and clearly demonstrate translocation from supernatant to nucleus.

DISCUSSION

If a target organ cytosol receptor is translocated to the nucleus after binding to the biologically active ligand, *in vitro* sucrose-gradient studies on cytosol and *in vivo* nuclear uptake studies (7) should alone be able to establish the presence of specific binding eliciting a response. *In vivo* gradient studies are superfluous. In the present investigation, it has in fact been shown that estradiol and its highly potent 11β-methoxy-ethynyl derivative are taken up preferentially by the nuclear fraction of the anterior region of the hypothalamus, this uptake being saturable at a physiological dose and hormone specific. A similar but much less marked retention is observed for the middle hypothalamus. Uptake by the posterior hypothalamus and cerebral cortex is nonspecific. These results were followed up by the confirmation of the existence of a specific receptor protein in the anterior and middle hypothalamus cytosol by sucrose-gradient studies. The peaks obtained corroborated the *in vivo* nuclear uptake results, since the amplitude of the peak was considerably lower for the middle than the anterior hypothalamus.

Detection of *in vivo* specific nuclear uptake is however only valid if all factors affecting the plasma concentration of free, i.e., active, steroid are taken into consideration, in particular the effect of metabolism and binding to plasma proteins. For this reason a highly potent estradiol derivative which, on the one hand, is not bound by EBP and, on the other, is known to be active per se and not as a result of metabolic degradation was chosen in these experiments. A comparison was carried out with the 11α-isomer which as a result of a change in the configuration of the 11-methoxy bond is only weakly estrogenic. Immature animals were preferred to castrated animals, since although there is no EBP in castrated animals, the concentration of target tissue receptor protein is diminished (15), and consequently a loss in sensitivity occurs. The age of the immature animals was also of importance: up to 4 weeks, EBP still persists in the plasma, and as from 5 weeks endogenous estrogen is secreted in appreciable amounts. It was therefore preferable to use animals of 4 to 5 weeks.

The above experiments clearly demonstrate that certain physiological conditions preclude the use of natural hormones and that consequently to obtain detailed and reliable information on mechanisms of action, in particular at a subcellular level, the use of highly potent synthetic derivatives is essential. R 2858 has enabled the detection of a specific receptor in the anterior hypothalamus of the 2-week-old rat and established the probable absence of such a receptor in the 22-day-old rat fetus.

SUMMARY

Interactions at the subcellular level are a fundamental aspect of the mechanism of action of a drug, but their study is only meaningful insofar as the results may be integrated into a general scheme covering all facets of the mechanism from administration to the triggering of the biological response. For example, the uterine cell response to estrogen in the immature rat is partly governed by the presence of a specific plasma binding protein, EBP, which limits cellular uptake by controlling the plasma free-steroid concentration. The free steroid interacts with a cytosolic macromolecule, which may be considered a hormonal receptor, if it is saturable at a physiological dose and hormone specific. This receptor is then translocated with the hormone to the nucleus in order to elicit the response. If the mechanism of estrogen action is one and the same for all target tissues, it should be possible to observe hormone specific nuclear uptake and to identify a specific cytosol binding protein for each tissue, as in the present studies on rat anterior hypothalamus with estradiol and R 2858, a highly potent synthetic estrogen not bound by EBP, which enables the influence of plasma binding on interactions at the subcellular level to be correctly determined.

ACKNOWLEDGMENTS

The technical assistance of Mrs. Joelle Humbert and Mrs. Dominique Gofflo is gratefully acknowledged.

REFERENCES

1. Raynaud, J. P., Mercier-Bodard, C., and Baulieu, E. E. (1971): *Steroids 18*, 767.
2. Raynaud, J. P. (1973): *Steroids 21*, 249.
3. Raynaud, J. P., Bouton, M. M., Gallet-Bourquin, D., Philibert, D., Tournemine, C., and Azadian-Boulanger, G. (1973): *Mol. Pharmacol. 9*, 520.
4. Stumpf, W. E. (1968): *Science 162*, 1001.
5. Anderson, C. H., and Greenwald, G. S. (1969): *Endocrinology 85*, 1160.
6. Kato, J., Atsumi, Y., and Inaba, M. (1971): *J. Biochem. (Tokyo) 70*, 1051.
7. Clark, J. H., Campbell, P. S., and Peck, E. J. (1972): *Neuroendocrinology 10*, 218.
8. Kato, J. (1973): *Acta Endo. 72*, 663.
9. Kato, J., and Villee, C. A. (1967): *Endocrinology 80*, 567.
10. Presl, J., Röhling, S., Horsky, J., and Herzmann, J. (1970): *Endocrinology 86*, 899.
11. Jensen, E. V., Suzuki, T., Kawashima, T., Stumpf, W. E., Jungblut, P. W., and Desombre, E. R. (1968): *Proc. Nat. Acad. Sci. 59*, 632.
12. Gorski, J., Toft, D., Shyamala, G., Smith, D., and Notides, A. (1968): *Rec. Progr. Hormone Res. 24*, 45.
13. Baulieu, E. E., Alberga, A., Jung, I., Lebeau, M. C., Mercier-Bodard, C., Milgrom, E., Raynaud, J. P., Raynaud-Jammet, C., Rochefort, H., Truong, H., and Robel, P. (1971): *Rec. Progr. Hormone Res. 27*, 351.
14. McGuire, J. L., and Lisk, R. D. (1968): *Proc. Nat. Acad. Sci. 61*, 497.
15. Steggles, A. W., and King, R. J. B. (1970): *Biochem. J. 118*, 695.

Drug Interactions, edited by P. L. Morselli,
S. Garattini, and S. N. Cohen. Raven Press,
New York © 1974

The Role of Calcium in Drug Action

Ronald P. Rubin

*Department of Pharmacology, State University of New York, Downstate Medical Center,
Brooklyn, New York 11203*

INTRODUCTION

Presenting an overview of drug-calcium interaction in a somewhat abridged form represents a Herculean task. One can adopt a narrow and limited scope, and review one's own already published findings, or, by contrast, one can attempt to cover the entire diverse field of calcium-drug interaction in a very cursory way. I have attempted a middle course by first reviewing the biological significance of calcium and its cellular distribution and metabolism. Then, by using the adrenal medulla as the prototype tissue, examples will be given to illustrate how pharmacologic agents may influence this calcium-dependent secretory process. On the basis of these data, a model will be presented to explain the facilitatory and inhibitory actions of drugs on calcium metabolism in the medulla. Finally, this model will be extended to other biological systems to establish certain general concepts concerning calcium-drug interactions.

BIOLOGICAL IMPORTANCE OF CALCIUM

The biological importance of calcium is a well-established fact. Not only does calcium aid in providing the structural framework of the organism by comprising one of the basic constituents of bone, but its presence in the extra- and intracellular environment allows it to control a myriad of other biological functions (Table 1). For example, calcium regulates cohesiveness and permeability of cells by actions at the cell surface. The importance of calcium in maintaining the normal permeability properties of the cell membrane deserves special consideration here, because agents that alter membrane function could do so directly or indirectly by affecting calcium binding to the cell membrane. Thus certain agents, by displacing membrane calcium, could produce effects that mimic those of calcium deprivation, leading to increases in membrane permeability. Conversely, other agents may produce membrane effects that resemble those of high calcium, resulting in membrane stabilization with a decrease in permeability.

TABLE 1. *Biologic importance of calcium*

Blood coagulation
Cellular adhesion — intercellular binding
Permeability properties of cell membrane
  "stabilizing" effect of calcium
Protoplasmic motility
Muscle contraction ("excitation-contraction coupling")
Secretion ("stimulus-secretion coupling")
Effects on enzyme systems (e.g., control of glycogenolysis)

Calcium also exerts actions within the cell by affecting metabolic processes (1–3) and by altering the physicochemical properties of the cytoplasm (4). Heilbrunn originally suggested that the prominent role that calcium plays in the chemical reactions involved with blood coagulation could be extended to its coagulative effects on protoplasmic processes. This effect of calcium may underlie a fundamental mechanism in most cells concerned with protoplasmic motility. It seems to involve an actomyosin-like protein complex that splits high-energy phosphates and is triggered by calcium (5). Examples of this phenomenon may include muscle contractility, amoeboid movements, secretory phenomena, and neuronal transport of substances from the soma to the nerve terminal. The microtubular-microfilamentous systems found in many cells may serve to modulate the function of these processes. Agents such as colchicine, vinblastine, and cytochalasin, which are thought to exert their primary pharmacologic actions on the microtubular-microfilamentous systems, block these processes, perhaps by competing with calcium at some critical cellular site.

CALCIUM REDISTRIBUTION DURING STIMULATION

In many types of cells, most notably those of excitable tissue, stimulation is associated with an increase in membrane permeability with a transmembrane flux of calcium. For example, acetylcholine causes the adrenal medulla to secrete by facilitating the entry of extracellular calcium into the chromaffin cell (6, 7) (Fig. 1). A variety of other agents, including nicotine, histamine, serotonin, polypeptides, ouabain, and sympathomimetic amines, also stimulate the adrenal medulla to secrete by a calcium-dependent mechanism (8). Amphetamine is an especially potent amine-releasing agent, both from the medulla (9) and from brain (10), and this releasing activity also proceeds through a calcium-dependent mechanism. Thus, at least certain pharmacologic actions of amphetamine clearly involve calcium, and its interaction with other central nervous system (CNS) active agents may also be somehow related to calcium metabolism.

Pharmacologic agents inhibit the sequence of events concerned with medullary secretion not only by interfering with agonist-receptor interac-

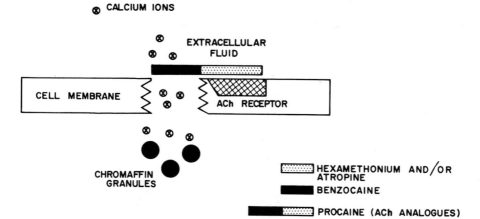

FIG. 1. Schematic representation of the action of acetylcholine (ACh) on the adrenal medulla. In the resting gland—because of the low permeability to calcium ions—there is no appreciable influx of extracellular calcium, despite the large concentration gradient between extra- and intracellular ionized calcium. ACh triggers an increase in the permeability of the membrane to calcium ions, causing the level of free calcium to rise within the cell. This event causes the catecholamine-containing chromaffin granules to release their contents to the extracellular fluid. Inhibition of this sequence can occur either by an action on ACh-sensitive receptor sites, or by a blockade of the calcium channel. Certain local anesthetics, because of their structural resemblance to ACh, inhibit medullary catecholamine release by (a) interfering with the response to ACh by an action on or near ACh-sensitive sites, and (b) blocking the influx of calcium that follows chromaffin cell stimulation. Local anesthetics that do not have a tertiary amino group, such as benzocaine, produce their inhibitory activity solely by an action on calcium flux.

tions, but also by inhibiting the resultant transmembrane calcium flux resulting from membrane recognition of stimulus-receptor interaction (Fig. 1). The latter effect can be demonstrated by employing excess potassium as a secretogogue, which circumvents drug-receptor interaction by directly depolarizing the cell (cf. 8).

The ability of certain pharmacologic agents to block calcium-evoked release (Fig. 2) by antagonizing calcium movement (Fig. 3) was first demonstrated with the use of the local anesthetic tetracaine (11), and was therefore ascribed to a "local anesthetic" action; however, it was subsequently ascertained that this property is shared by a variety of diverse agents, which may or may not have local-anesthetic activity. Guanethidine, desmethylimipramine, propranolol, and diphenhydramine are only a few of the diverse agents that are able to inhibit the calcium flux and resultant catecholamine release associated with potassium depolarization (12, 13).

The demonstration of this "local anesthetic" activity on secretory systems is not confined to the adrenal medulla. In the β cell of the pancreas, glucose is the essential physiological signal for insulin secretion. Although some have attempted to explain its secretory activity in strictly biochemical

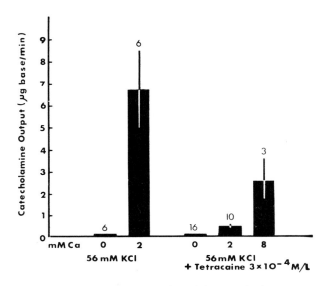

FIG. 2. The inhibitory effect of tetracaine on the calcium-evoked secretory response of the cat adrenal medulla and its reversal by excess calcium. Glands were perfused with calcium-free, high K⁺ (56 mM) Locke's solution with and without tetracaine for 10 min. Calcium (2 mM or 8 mM) was then added to the perfusion fluid. The perfusate was collected and analyzed for total catecholamine (epinephrine plus norepinephrine). The vertical bars represent the mean ($\pm$SE) catecholamine outputs obtained during a 2-min collection period, and the number of glands is indicated by the figure at the top of each bar (taken from ref. 11).

terms, others have drawn attention to the action of glucose to produce changes in membrane permeability, resulting in the redistribution of cations, including calcium (14, 15). It is of interest to our present discussion that in this tissue propranolol as well as tetracaine is able to block glucose-induced insulin release, presumably by interfering with the redistribution of calcium (16).

There is additional evidence that warrants carrying this generalization over to at least one other system. Adrenergic blocking agents that appear to produce inhibition by presynaptic rather than postsynaptic blockade also interfere directly or indirectly with calcium participation in stimulus-secretion coupling. Burn and Welsh (17) found that inhibition of the rabbit ileum to sympathetic nerve stimulation by guanethidine could be restored by increasing the external calcium concentration. These observations were extended by Kirpekar and co-workers (18), who suggested that adrenergic neuronal blockade by guanethidine was due to the prevention of the access of calcium to its site of action in the sympathetic nerve ending. Moreover, the blockade of amine release produced by bretylium and lithium is also reversed by excess calcium, suggesting that the inhibitory effects of these

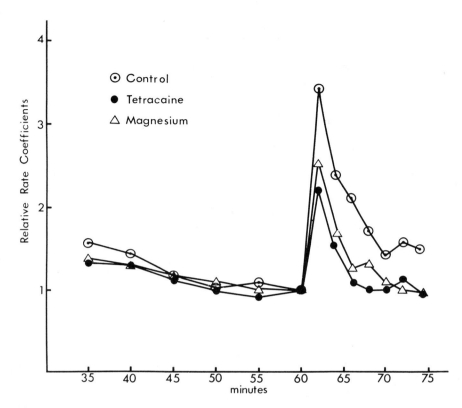

FIG. 3. The effect of tetracaine on the exchange of nonradioactive calcium in perfusate with ^{45}Ca in the perfused cat adrenal gland. Adrenal glands were initially perfused with Locke's solution plus ^{45}Ca and ACh to stimulate calcium uptake, and then washed out for 60 min with calcium-free Locke's solution. Calcium (2 mM) was added to the perfusion fluid between the 65th and 75th min of perfusion. Some glands were perfused with solutions containing tetracaine (3×10^{-4} M), commencing at 50 min. The inhibitory effect of magnesium (5 mM) is also shown, for comparison. Each point represents the mean relative rate coefficient for ^{45}Ca in six glands. The relative rate coefficient gives an indication of the rate of radiocalcium efflux relative to the amount of radioactivity in the gland during the same interval (taken from ref. 11).

therapeutic agents are mediated through some calcium-mediated process (19, 20).

REGULATION OF CELL CALCIUM

One should not infer that in all calcium-dependent secretory systems stimulation results in an enhanced influx of extracellular calcium. There is evidence that suggests that in certain secretory systems, such as the adrenal cortex (21) and the thyroid (22), stimulation causes a redistribution of

TABLE 2. *Regulation of cell calcium*

Binding and sequestration
(a) Membranes
(b) Microsomes — (incl. sarcoplasmic reticulum)
(c) Mitochondria
Cation exchange
(a) Ca^{+2}-Ca^{+2} exchange
(b) Na^{+1}-Ca^{+2} exchange
Calcium pump
(a) Ca^{+2}-activated ATPase in red cells

---

cellular calcium rather than an entry of extracellular calcium. Drugs may alter cell function in such systems by affecting the mechanisms that exist to maintain the low free-calcium concentrations characteristic of most cells. These mechanisms are summarized in Table 2.

Binding and Sequestration

The avid binding of calcium to membrane systems provides an efficient mechanism for sequestering free calcium. Although membranes act as cation exchangers, the affinity of calcium for these membrane sites is orders of magnitude greater than sodium or potassium, which helps to explain the fact that calcium is a basic component of natural membrane systems (23).

Calcium not only binds to the plasma membrane but also to cellular membrane systems such as the endoplasmic reticulum. The sarcoplasmic reticulum of muscle is a specialized form of reticulum, and the calcium-sequestering activity of this organelle has been studied extensively (24). Many pharmacologic agents exert effects on the sarcoplasmic reticulum — including the methylxanthines, such as caffeine (25), which cause muscle contractures by releasing calcium from these vesicular structures.

The mitochondria also avidly take up calcium; the avidity with which calcium is transported into mitochondria is exemplified by the fact that calcium is taken up in preference to ADP (26). Thus, calcium uptake appears to have primacy over the phosphorylation of ADP, which has been generally thought to be the primary function of mitochondria. Diverse agents, in addition to classical metabolic inhibitors, affect calcium accumulation by mitochondria *in vitro*. Studies concerned with the effects of local anesthetics have shown both inhibition (27) and stimulation of calcium uptake (28). Chlorpromazine, a psychoactive agent with local anesthetic properties, also inhibits calcium transport by mitochondria isolated from liver (29) and nerve tissue (30) and by sarcoplasmic reticulum of skeletal muscle (31). Such findings further extend the relationship between local anesthetic activity and effects on calcium metabolism; in view of the importance of calcium in neuronal excitability, transmitter release, and muscle contraction, the action of chlorpromazine on calcium transport processes may have important implications for its pharmacologic effects *in vivo*.

Cation Exchange

Not only is calcium inactivated by binding to intracellular structures, but it is also removed from cells by exchanging with extracellular cations. Cat adrenal glands that have been labeled with radiocalcium show a marked increase in calcium efflux when "cold" calcium is returned to the perfusion medium (11) (Fig. 3). The calcium-calcium exchange does little to bring about a lowering of intracellular calcium, but it does succeed in preventing the cell calcium levels from rising to toxic concentrations.

Evidence for a linking of calcium and sodium exchange has been demonstrated in a number of excitable tissues (32). This type of exchange is not directly linked to a coupled sodium-potassium pump but involves sodium-calcium exchange. Under physiologic conditions the enhancement of sodium entry that follows stimulation results in a loss of intracellular calcium. However, conditions that decrease the electrochemical gradient for sodium, as for example, an increase in internal sodium, will decrease the sodium-dependent calcium efflux and increase calcium uptake. This exchange provides a basis for explaining the cardiotonic activity of cardiac glycosides. These agents, by inhibiting Na-K-ATPase, bring about an increase in cell sodium, which, in turn, increases calcium and enhances contractility. A similar mechanism may be invoked to explain the well-known secretory activity of ouabain (see ref. 8).

Active Transport

The sodium-calcium exchange diffusion process is distinct from the calcium-activated ATPase system, which exists in erythrocytes and is responsible for maintaining an extremely low level of intracellular calcium by an active transport mechanism (33). This latter process is similar to the calcium uptake system in the endoplasmic reticulum, which also involves a calcium-activated ATPase and ATP hydrolysis. Both systems are not affected by cardiac glycosides but are inhibited by mersalyl and ethacrynic acid (34).

CALCIUM-DRUG INTERACTION *IN VITRO*

The intracellular accumulation and translocation of ionized calcium in cells reflect the existence of a mechanism for the transport of calcium from an extracellular aqueous phase through the lipid-containing membranes. Woolley (35) was the first to show that lipids extracted from excitable tissues promote the transport of calcium from an aqueous through a lipid-solvent phase *in vitro*. Feinstein (36) later demonstrated that local anesthetics, including procaine, interact with lipids in such a way as to inhibit or depress their ability to transport ionized calcium from an aqueous to a lipid-solvent phase.

However, the displacement of calcium from lipid molecules by drugs is not restricted to the classical local-anesthetic agents. Propranolol, quinidine, and various CNS-active drugs, including morphine and other opiate analgesics, also inhibit the facilitation of calcium transport *in vitro* (37, 38). The ability of local-anesthetic agents, including propranolol and quinidine, to inhibit calcium transport *in vitro*, as well as in secretory systems, allows one to consider the possibility that their antifibrillatory activity is based upon an interference with calcium distribution in cardiac muscle cells.

The importance of calcium in modulating neuronal excitability and in "stimulus-secretion coupling" also suggests an action for the morphine-like drugs at the level of calcium metabolism. Indeed, morphine is able to obtund synaptic transmission by inhibiting peripheral neurosecretory mechanisms (39), and a similar effect on synaptic transmission in the CNS would almost certainly interfere with brain function. Such speculation attains added significance when it is realized that calcium has been implicated in the action of CNS-active drugs *in vivo* by a group of Japanese workers who showed that the intracisternal administration of calcium to rats markedly suppressed the analgesic effects of morphine (40). On the basis of their data, they suggested that calcium does indeed play a very important role in the mechanism of opiate analgesia at the level of synaptic transmission.

SUMMARY

It seems clear that the ubiquity of calcium action makes this cation a prime target for pharmacologic agents. Calcium and drug interaction may occur at the cell membrane or intracellularly with molecular events that follow membrane stimulation. Drug effects on the membrane may be stimulatory and produce activation and/or depolarization, or they may be inhibitory. In systems where recognition of agonist-receptor interaction results in a transmembrane flux or a cellular translocation of calcium, pharmacologic agents can directly affect the receptor response or the subsequent redistribution of calcium.

Inhibition mediated through a depression of calcium influx, as opposed to a drug-receptor interaction, has been ascribed to a "local anesthetic" action, which is shared by a variety of agents including the classical local anesthetics. Drugs can not only control cell calcium levels by actions on transmembrane calcium fluxes but also by intracellular actions on calcium-binding structures. Since the free intracellular calcium concentration is controlled by binding to the endoplasmic reticulum and mitochondria and by extrusion to the extracellular fluid through cation exchange and active transport, pharmacologic agents can readily modulate ionized calcium levels by exerting effects on these systems.

Although this discussion has covered a variety of biological systems and many important points have been all too briefly considered, its overall purpose was to emphasize the scope of calcium influence; for the ubiquitous effects of calcium militate that this cation should always be considered as a potential site of drug action. It is hoped that this general point has been definitively made.

REFERENCES

1. Lehninger, A. L., Carafoli, E., and Ross, C. S. (1967): *Adv. Enzymol. 29,* 259.
2. Rasmussen, H., and Nagata, N. (1970): In: *Calcium and Cellular Function,* p. 198, MacMillan, London.
3. Landowne, D., and Ritchie, J. M. (1971): *J. Physiol. 212,* 503.
4. Heilbrunn, L. V. (1956): *The Dynamics of Living Protoplasm.* Academic Press, New York.
5. Jahn, T. L., and Bovee, E. C. (1969): *Physiol. Rev. 49,* 793.
6. Douglas, W. W., and Rubin, R. P. (1961): *J. Physiol. 159,* 40.
7. Douglas, W. W., and Rubin, R. P. (1963): *J. Physiol. 167,* 288.
8. Rubin, R. P. (1970): *Pharmacol. Rev. 22,* 389.
9. Rubin, R. P., and Jaanus, S. D. (1966): *Naun. Schmied. Arch. Pharmacol. 254,* 125.
10. Ziance, R. J., Azzaro, A. J., and Rutledge, C. O. (1972): *J. Pharmacol. Exp. Ther. 182,* 284.
11. Rubin, R. P., Feinstein, M. B., Jaanus, S. D., and Paimre, M. (1967): *J. Pharmacol. Exp. Ther. 155,* 463.
12. Jaanus, S. D., Miele, E., and Rubin, R. P. (1968): *Brit. J. Pharmacol. 33,* 560.
13. Rubin, R. P., and Miele, E. (1968): *Naun. Schmied. Arch. Pharmacol. 260,* 298.
14. Dean, P. M., and Matthews, E. K. (1970): *J. Physiol. 210,* 265.
15. Randle, P. J., and Hales, C. N. (1972): In: *Handbook of Physiology,* Sec. 7, Endocrinology, p. 219, American Physiological Society, Washington, D.C.
16. Bressler, R., and Brendel, K. (1971): *Diabetes 20,* 721.
17. Burn, J. H., and Welsh, F. (1967): *Brit. J. Pharmacol. 31,* 74.
18. Kirpekar, S. M., Wakade, A. R., Dixon, W., and Prat, J. C. (1969): *J. Pharmacol. Exp. Ther. 165,* 166.
19. Katz, R. I., and Kopin, I. J. (1969): *J. Pharmacol. Exp. Ther. 169,* 229.
20. Katz, R. I., and Kopin, I. J. (1969): *Biochem. Pharmacol. 18,* 1935.
21. Jaanus, S. D., and Rubin, R. P. (1971): *J. Physiol. 213,* 581.
22. Williams, J. A. (1972): *Endocrinology 90,* 1459.
23. Dawson, R. M. C., and Hauser, H. (1970): In: *Calcium and Cellular Function,* p. 17, MacMillan, London.
24. Weber, A., Herz, R., and Reiss, I. (1966): *Biochem. Zeit. 345,* 329.
25. Bianchi, C. P. (1968): *Cell Calcium,* p. 58, Appleton-Century-Crofts, New York.
26. Lehninger, A. L. (1970): *Biochem. J. 119,* 129.
27. Azzi, A., and Scarpa, A. (1967): *Biochim. Biophys. Acta 135,* 1087.
28. Mela, L. (1968): *Arch. Biochem. Biophys. 123,* 286.
29. Dawkins, M. J. R., Judah, J. D., and Rees, K. R. (1960): *Biochem. J. 76,* 200.
30. Tjioe, S., Haugaard, N., and Bianchi, C. P. (1971): *J. Neurochem. 18,* 2171.
31. Balzer, H., Makinose, M., Fiehn, W., and Hasselbach, W. (1968): *Naun. Schmied. Arch. Pharmacol. 260,* 456.
32. Baker, P. F. (1972): *Progr. Biophys. Mol. Biol. 24,* 177.
33. Schatzmann, H. J. (1970): In: *Calcium and Cellular Function,* p. 85, MacMillan, London.
34. Schatzmann, H. J., and Vincenzi, F. (1969): *J. Physiol. 201,* 369.
35. Woolley, D. W. (1963): In: *The Transfer of Calcium and Strontium Across Biological Membranes,* p. 375, Academic Press, New York.

36. Feinstein, M. B. (1964): *J. Gen. Physiol. 48,* 357.
37. Nayler, W. (1966): *J. Pharmacol. Exp. Ther. 153,* 479.
38. Mulé, S. J. (1969): *Biochem. Pharmacol. 18,* 339.
39. Kennedy, B. L., and West, T. C. (1967): *J. Pharmacol. Exp. Ther. 157,* 149.
40. Kakunaga, T. K., Kaneto, H., and Kotobuki, H. (1966): *J. Pharmacol. Exp. Ther. 153,* 134.

Drug Interactions, edited by P. L. Morselli,
S. Garattini, and S. N. Cohen. Raven Press,
New York © 1974

Covalent Binding of Chloramphenicol as a Biochemical Basis for Chloramphenicol-Induced Bone Marrow Damage

G. Krishna and L. Bonanomi*

Laboratory of Chemical Pharmacology, National Heart and Lung Institute, National Institutes of Health, Bethesda, Maryland 20014

Drug-induced tissue damage as exemplified by pulmonary, hepatic, and renal necrosis, bone marrow depression and aplasia, and certain types of hypersensitive reactions, is a major obstacle in the development of new and useful therapeutic agents. Moreover, many of the drugs developed in the past have become of limited usefulness because of their toxicity. A clear understanding of the biochemical events leading to the toxicity of drugs may help in the development of new drugs or in the modification of old ones.

Chloramphenicol was developed in the mid 1940s as an effective broad spectrum antibiotic. It has become of limited usefulness mainly because it produces occasionally aplastic anemia in certain susceptible individuals (1). An understanding of the mechanism of this toxicity would greatly help in the development of new analogues of chloramphenicol that have the therapeutic efficacy of this drug, without its serious side effects. But the biochemical mechanism by which chloramphenicol produces bone marrow damage leading to aplastic anemia remains poorly understood (2–6).

During the past few years, we have been investigating the possibility proposed by Brodie a number of years ago (7), that chemically inert therapeutic agents may produce tissue damage by being metabolized in the body to highly reactive intermediates that combine covalently with tissue macromolecules. A similar mechanism has also been proposed for the carcinogenicity of various chemicals (8). In these studies, we have developed a simple *in vitro* method in our laboratory for the study of the covalent binding of drugs to tissue macromolecules (9–11). This method consists of incubating the radiolabeled drug with rat liver microsomes and a NADPH-generating system. The incubation is terminated at various periods of time by precipitating the protein with trichloroacetic acid. The protein is washed repeatedly with solvents and finally dissolved in sodium hydroxide. Aliquots are taken for determinations of protein and of radioactivity associated with the pro-

* Supported by a fellowship from Zambon Research Labs, Via Del Duca 12 Bresso, Milan, Italy.

tein. In order to understand the enzyme system involved in the activation of the drug, we used phenobarbital as well as 3-methylcholanthrene-induced microsomes in these studies. Moreover, various inhibitors of the cytochrome P-450 system are used in order to delineate the enzyme system involved in the activation.

In some of our studies we have established that the binding of drugs to microsomes and other macromolecules is covalent by isolating the proteins containing the labeled drug, hydrolyzing them by pronase to amino acid derivatives of the reactive metabolites and separating these amino-acid derivatives in an amino acid analyzer. The covalent binding of drugs that we have established so far appeared to be bound to one or two amino acids. The exact structure of the amino acid drug derivatives, however, is being investigated using mass spectrometry.

It occurred to us that chloramphenicol may be metabolized to chemically reactive metabolites since it contains both the nitro group and chlorine in the molecule. Previously, various authors have implicated the involvement of the nitro group in the toxicity of chloramphenicol, but none of these studies have considered the possible involvement of the chlorine group (3–6). We, and several others, have shown that compounds such as carbon tetrachloride (CCl_4), chloroform ($CHCl_3$), and trichlorobromomethane (CCl_3Br) produce various liver and other tissue damage by being converted into highly reactive intermediates that combine covalently with various tissue macromolecules (10–14). We have been able to show from both *in vivo* and *in vitro* studies that a cytochrome P-450 system is involved in the reductive cleavage of the carbon chlorine bond of carbon tetrachloride leading to the formation of CCl_3 free radical which combines covalently with tissue macromolecules (15). In order to determine whether chloramphenicol could be converted to chemically reactive metabolites, we studied its covalent binding to liver microsomes and to bone marrow cells. We have also performed *in vivo* studies on rats in order to test the possibility that covalent binding to various tissues, especially bone marrow cells, also occurs *in vivo*.

Thiamphenicol is a synthetic analogue obtained by replacement of the nitro group of chloramphenicol by a methylsulfonyl group and has been used widely in Europe and Japan. Although thiamphenicol has not been used to the same extent as chloramphenicol, it has been used by 15 to 20 million people and not a single case of aplastic anemia has been reported (16). By contrast chloramphenicol has been shown to cause aplastic anemia with the incidence of 1/50,000 to 1/500,000 (1). Thus, it was of interest to compare the covalent binding of thiamphenicol to tissue macromolecules and bone marrow cells with that of chloramphenicol.

Figure 1 shows that ^{14}C-chloramphenicol binds covalently to rat liver microsomes when incubated in the presence of oxygen and NADPH. The rate of covalent binding of chloramphenicol is 12 times greater than that of

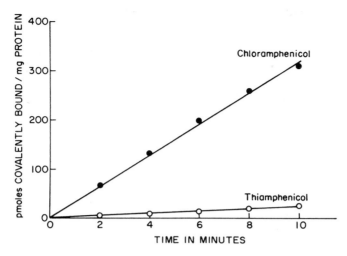

FIG. 1. Covalent binding of ^{14}C-chloramphenicol and ^{14}C-thiamphenicol to rat liver micro-somes *in vitro*. Rat liver microsomes (1 mg protein) isolated from phenobarbital-pre-treated rats were incubated for various periods of time either with ^{14}C-chloramphenicol or ^{14}C-thiamphenicol as described in the footnote to Table 1. Proteins containing the covalently bound materials were isolated as described earlier (11).

thiamphenicol. The covalent binding of both compounds was linear for 10 min. The apparent K_m for the conversion of chloramphenicol to its reactive metabolite was 50 μM and the apparent V_{max} was 50 pmoles/mg protein/min. When microsomes from phenobarbital-treated rats were used, the covalent binding of chloramphenicol and thiamphenicol was increased 10-fold and threefold, respectively (17). As shown in Table 1, the enzyme catalyzing the formation of the reactive metabolites required both NADPH and oxygen and was inhibited by carbon monoxide and SKF 525-A. These findings thus suggest that the formation of the reactive metabolites is catalyzed by a cytochrome P-450 system in liver microsomes.

In order to understand whether similar mechanisms exist for the covalent binding of chloramphenicol to bone marrow cells, rat bone marrow cells were isolated and incubated with chloramphenicol and thiamphenicol. Table 2 shows that chloramphenicol binds to a greater extent than does thiamphenicol to rat bone marrow cells *in vitro*. In these experiments we also used an analogue of CCl_4, namely CCl_3Br, which is 30 times more potent than CCl_4 in causing liver necrosis as a result of extensive covalent binding (18, 19). In bone marrow cells CCl_3Br is also capable of binding covalently to these cells.

The mechanism by which chloramphenicol binds covalently is not yet clearly understood. At first it seemed possible that the hydroxylamine derivative of chloramphenicol, formed during the reduction of the nitro

TABLE 1. *Inhibition of covalent binding of chloramphenicol and thiamphenicol by inhibitors of cytochrome P-450 system*

Inhibitors	Chloramphenicol covalently bound (pmoles/mg protein/min)	Thiamphenicol covalently bound (pmoles/mg protein/min)
None	20.4	3.9
SKF 525-A (1 mM)	5.6	3.0
CO:O₂ (8:2)	10.4	1.8
N₂	2.4	2.8
GSH (3 mM)	7.5	1.1
Minus NADPH	0.8	0.9

Rat liver microsomes (1 mg protein) isolated from phenobarbital-treated rats were incubated under an atmosphere of air for 10 min with 0.5 μC of 1,2-^{14}C-chloramphenicol or 1-^{14}C-thiamphenicol (10^{-4} M) in 1 ml of Tris-KCl buffer (20 mM Tris 1.15% KCl pH 7.4) containing NADPH (0.2 mM)–NADH (0.125 mM) nicotinamide (2 mM) and NADPH-generating system consisting of glucose-6-phosphate (2 mM) and glucose-6-phosphate dehydrogenase (1 unit/ml). Protein-containing covalently bound materials were isolated and quantitated as described earlier (11). Drugs were dissolved in Tris-KCl buffer and added to the incubation mixture. Air was replaced by a mixture of CO:O₂ or N₂. ^{14}C-Chloramphenicol or ^{14}C-thiamphenicol dissolved in 10 μl of dimethylformamide were added to the incubation mixture.

group, might be the reactive intermediate. But the finding that the covalent binding of chloramphenicol was decreased by 80 to 90% when liver microsomes were incubated under anaerobic conditions is inconsistent with this view. Other plausible mechanisms for covalent binding of chloramphenicol are illustrated in Fig. 2. These are based on previous studies with bromobenzene, CCl_4, and $CHCl_3$ (15, 20, 21). For example, we had postulated an

TABLE 2. *Covalent binding of chloramphenicol and thiamphenicol to rat bone marrow cells in vitro*

	Picomoles covalently bound per milligram protein at		
	10 min	20 min	30 min
^{14}C-Chloramphenicol	48	80	100
^{14}C-Thiamphenicol	3	5	6
^{14}C-CCl₃Br	227	334	336

Bone marrow cells of rats were isolated from the tibia of five rats and were suspended in 50 ml of Krebs ringer phosphate buffer (pH 7.4) containing one-third of normal calcium concentration. Bone marrow cell suspensions (1 ml aliquots) were incubated with ^{14}C-chloramphenicol (0.8 mM S.A. 30 cpm/pmole) or ^{14}C-thiamphenicol (0.1 mM S. A. 15 cpm/pmole) or ^{14}C-CCl₃Br (1 mM S. A. 2 cpm/pmole). The incubations were terminated with 1 ml of 10% trichloroacetic acid and the protein-containing covalently bound materials were isolated as described earlier.

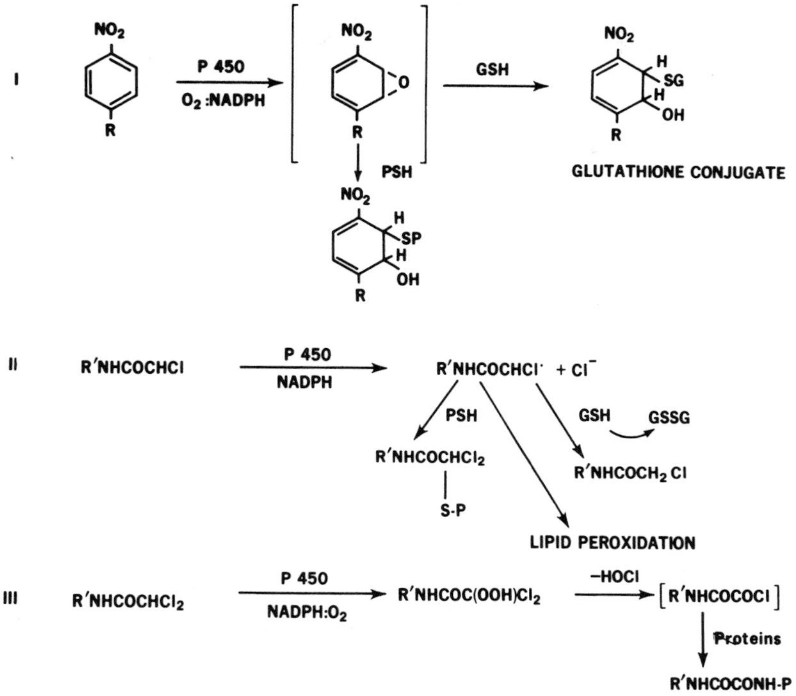
I
P 450
O2 :NADPH
GSH
PSH
GLUTATHIONE CONJUGATE
II
R'NHCOCHCl
P 450
NADPH
R'NHCOCHCl· + Cl⁻
PSH
GSH GSSG
R'NHCOCHCl2
S-P
R'NHCOCH2 Cl
LIPID PEROXIDATION
III
R'NHCOCHCl2
P 450
NADPH:O2
R'NHCOC(OOH)Cl2
-HOCl
[R'NHCOCOCl]
Proteins
R'NHCOCONH-P

FIG. 2. Proposed mechanisms for covalent binding of chloramphenicol.

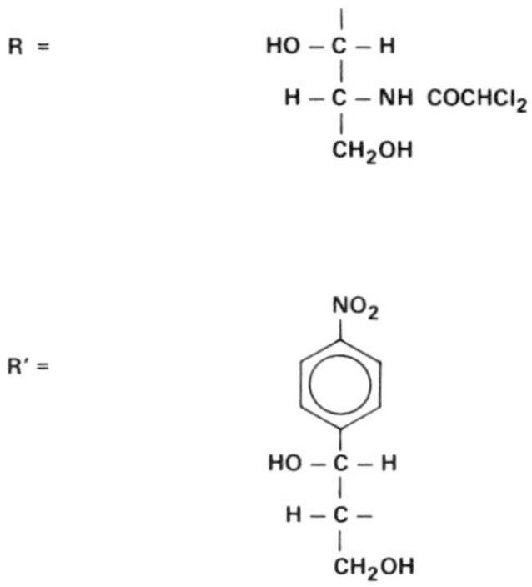
R =
HO – C – H
H – C – NH COCHCl2
CH2OH
R' =
NO2
HO – C – H
H – C –
CH2OH

PSH Protein Sulfhydryl group

P-450 Cytochrome P-450

arene oxide intermediate in the covalent binding of bromobenzene (20). By a similar mechanism, an arene oxide of the nitrobenzene ring of chloramphenicol might be formed by the cytochrome P-450 system and NADPH and oxygen. Once formed, the arene oxide might react covalently with tissue macromolecules or with glutathione to form a glutathione conjugate or with water to form a dihydrodiol. A second mechanism may be also proposed which involves the formation of a free radical in a fashion similar to the formation of the free radical of CCl_4 (15) by cytochrome P-450 and NADPH. The free radical of chloramphenicol might react covalently with tissue macromolecules or glutathione to give rise to monochloro derivative of chloramphenicol. A third mechanism which might be proposed involves a hydroxylation of the dichloroacetamide group followed by elimination of HOCl which gives rise to a phosgene analogue of chloramphenicol that then can react covalently with tissue macromolecules (17).

Whatever the mechanism of activation may be, the electronegativity of the nitro group in chloramphenicol appears to influence its capacity to be activated and bound covalently to tissue macromolecules. More experiments are needed to understand the reason for the lower extent of covalent binding of thiamphenicol in comparison to chloramphenicol. In order to evaluate the validity of the *in vitro* covalent-binding studies, we have studied the covalent binding of the drugs to tissue macromolecules in untreated rats and in rats that had the pretreatment with phenobarbital. The results of these studies are summarized in Table 3. The highest covalent binding of chloramphenicol occurred to proteins of plasma, liver, and bone marrow. The covalent binding was markedly increased by phenobarbital pretreatment of the animals. More than half of the covalent binding of chloramphenicol occurred within 2 hr after the administration of the drug (17). By contrast the covalent binding of thiamphenicol to these tissues was lower than that of chloramphenicol. Moreover, phenobarbital pretreatment did not greatly increase the covalent binding of thiamphenicol (Table 3).

At 24 hr after administration of ^{14}C-chloramphenicol all of the radioactivity found in plasma is bound covalently to plasma proteins. In phenobarbital-pretreated animals at this time, as much as 60 μg of chloramphenicol or its metabolite is covalently bound to plasma protein per milliliter of plasma. This binding has been found to be covalent by a variety of methods including solvent extraction, Sephadex gel filtration, and agarose gel electrophoresis. Most of the covalently bound chloramphenicol is associated with a protein that has a molecular weight similar to that of albumin but has a mobility lower than albumin as measured by agarose gel electrophoresis.

These studies thus demonstrate that chloramphenicol in rats is converted to a chemically reactive metabolite that reacts covalently with macromolecules in various tissues including bone marrow cells. They further show that thiamphenicol, which apparently does not cause aplastic anemia (16), becomes covalently bound to a much smaller extent. But whether any of the toxicities including aplastic anemia caused by chloramphenicol are mediated by the chemically reactive metabolites remains to be determined. It would be of obvious importance to determine whether the magnitude of the covalent binding of chloramphenicol is related to the incidence and

TABLE 3. *In vivo covalent binding of ^{14}C-chloramphenicol and ^{14}C-thiamphenicol to various tissue macromolecules of rat*

Tissues	Chloramphenicol covalent binding (pmoles/mg protein)		Thiamphenicol covalent binding (pmoles/mg protein)	
	Normal rats	Phenobarbital-induced rats	Normal rats	Phenobarbital-induced rats
Plasma	698	3205	150	229
Liver	423	1646	159	305
Bone marrow	324	1398	110	178
Adrenal	316	680	75	142
Fat pad (epididymal)	273	834	87	73
Kidney	212	782	85	126
Lung	155	602	75	119
Spleen	95	742	83	126
Testis	76	339	37	37
Heart	69	273	38	45
Brain	38	191	17	23
Erythrocytes	36	60	43	40
Muscle	23	113	23	19

100 mg/kg ^{14}C-chloramphenicol (100 μC_1/kg) or 100 mg/kg ^{14}C-thiamphenicol (150 μC_1/kg) were injected i.p. into normal or phenobarbital-pretreated rats. The animals were killed 24 hr later and various tissues were removed for analysis of covalent binding of drugs (10).

severity of bone marrow damage including aplastic anemia. But various attempts to produce aplastic anemia in animals by treatment with chloramphenicol have not been successful. In one long-term study lasting up to 6 months, we were not able to show any aplastic anemia by examination of bone marrow sections even though the animals showed a 25% depression of circulatory leukocytes after treatment with chloramphenicol. Presently, we are attempting to produce aplastic anemia with chloramphenicol in other animal species. We are also at present studying other analogues of chloramphenicol that are as effective as chloramphenicol but that may not cause serious side effects on the bone marrow. It has been shown recently that the trifluoro acetamide analogue of chloramphenicol is more effective as an antibiotic than chloramphenicol (22). We are currently examining whether this analogue binds covalently to macromolecules and whether it produces bone marrow damage in animals.

ACKNOWLEDGMENTS

We wish to thank Dr. James R. Gillette for critical reviewing of this manuscript and Miss E. Boykins for expert technical assistance. We also wish to thank Prof. Davide Della Bella for the gift of ^{14}C-thiamphenicol used in these studies.

REFERENCES

1. California Medical Association Report (1967).
2. Woodward, T. C., and Wisseman, C. L., Jr. (1955): In: *Chlormycetin (Chloramphenicol), Antibiotic Monographs*, no. 8, p. 28, Medical Encyclopedia, New York.
3. Yunis, A. A., and Bloomberg, G. R. (1964): *Progr. Hematol. 4*, 138.
4. Yunis, A. A. (1969): *Adv. Intern. Med. 15*, 357.
5. Pisciotta, A. V. (1971): *Clinical Pharmacol. Therap. 12*, 13.
6. Polak, B. C. P., Wesseling, H., Schut-Diew, Herxheimer, A., and Meyler, L. (1972): *Acta Med. Sci. 192*, 409.
7. Brodie, B. B. (1967): In: *Ciba Foundation Symposium on Drug Response in Man*, p. 188. Churchill, London.
8. Miller, E. C., and Miller, J. R. (1966): *Pharmacol Rev. 18*, 805.
9. Corsini, G. U., Sipes, I. G., Krishna, G., and Brodie, B. B. (1972): *Fed. Proc. 31*, 548.
10. Reid, W. D., and Krishna, G. (1973): *Exp. Mol. Pathol. 18*, 80.
11. Sipes, I. G., Stripp, B., Krishna, G., Maling, H. M., and Gillette, J. R. (1973): *Proc. Soc. Exp. Biol. Med. 142*, 237.
12. Ilett, K. F., Reid, W. D., Sipes, G., and Krishna, G. (1973): *Exp. Mol. Pathol. 19*, 215.
13. Reynolds, E. S. (1967): *J. Pharmacol. Exp. Therap. 155*, 117.
14. Sipes, I. G., Corsini, G. U., Krishna, G., and Gillette, J. R. (1972): *Fifth Int. Congr. Pharmacology*, San Francisco, Karger, Basel, p. 215.
15. Krishna, G., Sipes, I. G., and Gillette, J. R. (1973): *Pharmacologist 15*, 260.
16. Zambon Research Laboratories (1968): *Thiamphenicol: Experimental and Clinical Basis of New Antibiotic*, English edition, p. 105, Zambon, S. P. A. Milan-Vicenza.
17. Krishna, G. *(in press):* Postgrad. Med. J. (1974).
18. Slater, T. F., *Free Radical Mechanisms in Tissue Injury*, p. 165, Pion Ltd., London.
19. Sipes, I. G., Docks, E., Asghar, K., Boykins, E., and Krishna, G. (1973): *Fed. Proc. 32*, 319.
20. Brodie, B. B., Reid, W. D., Cho, A. K., Sipes, G., Krishna, G., and Gillette, J. R. (1971): *Proc. Nat. Acad. Sci. 68*, 1960.
21. Gillette, J. R. (1973): In: *Pharmacology and the Future of Man*, Proc. 5th Int. Congr. Pharmacology, San Francisco, Vol. 2, p. 187, Karger, Basel.
22. Hansch, C. R., Heman-Ackah, S. M., and Won, C. H. (1973): *J. Med. Chem. 6*, 917.

Drug Interactions, edited by P. L. Morselli,
S. Garattini, and S. N. Cohen. Raven Press,
New York © 1974

The Role of Genetic Factors in Drug Interactions

Elliot S. Vesell

*Department of Pharmacology, Milton S. Hershey Medical Center, Pennsylvania State
University College of Medicine, Hershey, Pennsylvania 17033*

Drug interactions refer to effects of one or more therapeutic agents on the absorption, distribution, biotransformation, binding at receptor sites, and/or excretion of other drugs. This definition reveals why major emphasis in discussions and studies of drug interactions has generally focused on environmental rather than genetic factors. However, in certain drug interactions genetic characteristics of the host significantly influence the nature and magnitude of the interaction, thereby determining whether adverse side effects will ensue. Thus, it should be stressed that individuals with particular genotypes are more liable than others to develop adverse reactions based on drug interactions when they receive certain drugs. Table 1 lists 13 of these monogenically transmitted conditions which, in man, predispose to adverse reactions when certain classes of drugs are administered. These conditions have been described in detail elsewhere (1–4), but three of them are reviewed here in the context of drug interactions.

Diphenylhydantoin (DPH) toxicity is more common in slow than in rapid acetylators of isoniazid when both drugs are administered simultaneously. The mechanism for this interaction appears to be DPH accumulation due to competition for metabolism (5).

A second, much more common interaction is hemolysis resulting from administration alone or in combination of drugs listed in Table 1 to individuals deficient in glucose-6-phosphate dehydrogenase (G-6-PD). Hemolysis is generally more severe when two or more of these drugs are administered simultaneously. More than 100,000,000 people suffer from this condition. Approximately 80 distinct mutations at the sex-linked locus controlling G-6-PD synthesis have been identified through physicochemical studies of the G-6-PD molecule (6). Several of these different alleles are associated with clinically distinguishable courses of hemolysis even with administration of the same dose of drug.

The third example is warfarin resistance, an apparently rare condition transmitted as an autosomal dominant trait thus far described in only two pedigrees (7). In affected individuals a structural alteration in the hepatic receptor site at which warfarin and vitamin K compete for binding probably is responsible for increased binding of vitamin K but appreciably re-

TABLE 1. *Pharmacogenetic conditions with putative aberrant enzyme, mode of inheritance, frequency, and drugs that can elicit the signs and symptoms of the disorder*

Name of condition	Aberrant enzyme and location	Mode of inheritance	Frequency	Drugs that produce the abnormal response
Genetic conditions probably transmitted as single factors altering the way the body acts on drugs (altered drug metabolism)				
1. Acatalasia	Catalase in erythrocytes	Autosomal recessive	Mainly in Japan and Switzerland, reaching 1% in certain small areas of Japan	Hydrogen peroxide
2. Slow inactivation of isoniazid	Isoniazid acetylase in liver	Autosomal recessive	Approximately 50% of U.S.A. population	Isoniazid, sulfamethazine, sulfamaprine, phenelzine, dapsone, hydralazine
3. Suxamethonium sensitivity or atypical pseudocholinesterase	Pseudocholinesterase in plasma	Autosomal recessive	Several aberrant alleles; most common disorder occurs one in 2500	Suxamethonium or succinylcholine
4. Diphenylhydantoin toxicity due to deficient parahydroxylation	? Mixed-function oxidase in liver microsomes that parahydroxylates diphenylhydantoin	Autosomal or X-linked dominant	Only one small pedigree	Diphenylhydantoin
5. Bishydroxycoumarin sensitivity	? Mixed-function oxidase in liver microsomes that hydroxylates bishydroxycoumarin	Unknown	Only one small pedigree	Bishydroxycoumarin
6. Acetophenetidin-induced methemoglobinemia	? Mixed-function oxidase in liver microsomes that deethylates acetophenetidin	Autosomal recessive	Only one small pedigree	Acetophenetidin
Genetic conditions probably transmitted as single factors altering the way drugs act on the body				
1. Warfarin resistance	? Altered receptor or enzyme in liver with increased affinity for vitamin K	Autosomal dominant	Two large pedigrees	Warfarin

Condition	Defect	Inheritance	Frequency	Drugs/Agents
2. Glucose-6-phosphate dehydrogenase deficiency, favism or drug-induced hemolytic anemia	Glucose-6-phosphate dehydrogenase	X-linked incomplete codominant	Approximately 100,000,000 affected in world; occurs in high frequency where malaria is endemic; 80 biochemically distinct mutations	A variety of analgesics [acetanilide, acetylsalicylic acid, acetophenetidin (phenacetin), antipyrine, aminopyrine (Pyramidon)], sulfonamides and sulfones [sulfanilamide, sulfapyridine, N_2-acetylsulfanilamide, sulfacetamide, sulfisoxazole (Gantrisin), thiazolsulfone, salicylazosulfapyridine (Azulfadine), sulfoxone, sulfamethoxypyridazine (Kynex)], antimalarials [primaquine, pamaquine, pentaquine, quinacrine (Atabrine)], nonsulfonamide antibacterial agents [furazolidone, nitrofurantoin (Furadantin), chloramphenicol, p-aminosalicyl acid], and miscellaneous drugs [naphthalene, vitamin K, probenecid, trinitrotoluene, methylene blue, dimercaprol (BAL), phenylhydrazine, quinine, quinidine]
3. Drug-sensitive hemoglobins a) Hemoglobin Zurich	Arginine substitution for histidine at the 63rd position of the β-chain of hemoglobin	Autosomal dominant	Two small pedigrees	Sulfonamides
b) Hemoglobin H	Hemoglobin composed of four β-chains	Autosomal recessive	Approximately one in 300 births in Bangkok	Same drugs as listed above for G6PD deficiency
4. Inability to taste phenylthiourea or phenylthiocarbamide	Unknown	Autosomal recessive	Approximately 30% of Caucasians	Drugs containing the N-C-S group such as phenylthiourea methyl and propylthiouracil
5. Glaucoma due to abnormal response of intraocular pressure to steroids	Unknown	Autosomal recessive	Approximately 5% of U.S.A. population	Corticosteroids
6. Malignant hyperthermia with muscular rigidity	Unknown	Autosomal dominant	Approximately one in 20,000 anesthetized patients	Various anesthetics, especially halothane
7. Methemoglobin reductase deficiency	Methemoglobin reductase	Autosomal recessive heterozygous carriers affected	Approximately one in 100 are heterozygous carriers	Same drugs as listed above for G6PD deficiency

duced warfarin binding. Thus, several times higher than usual doses of warfarin must be administered to these patients to produce anticoagulation. When these patients who are hypersensitive to vitamin K receive even very small additional doses of vitamin K, anticoagulation achieved with very high doses of warfarin can be impaired.

The role of genetic factors in drug interactions extends well beyond the conditions listed in Table 1. In order to evaluate the role of genetic factors in drug interactions beyond those suggested in Table 1, it is desirable first to describe genetic control of large interindividual differences in response to a single drug. Such large interindividual differences in response to single drugs constitute a major medical problem in therapeutics and a basis for adverse drug reactions when compounds are administered alone or in combination.

During the past 9 years, we have attempted to assess the relative contributions of genetic and environmental factors to large interindividual differences in rates of clearance of commonly used drugs. Numerous environmental factors, such as exposure to inducing agents, degree of health or illness, and hormonal or nutritional status, are known to alter the rates at which humans metabolize certain drugs. Several drugs such as phenylbutazone enhance their own metabolism in certain species (8). In mice, responsiveness to a drug such as hexobarbital differs according to age, sex, liter, painful stimuli, ambient temperature, degree of crowding, time of day of drug administration, and type of bedding (9). Such experiments would imply that in man a large component in the causation of variations among individuals in drug metabolism would be environmental.

The environmental and heritable components of individual variations in rates of drug metabolism can be determined through the use of human twins. Galton developed and introduced this use of twins in 1875. The approach has the virtue of simplicity in experimental design and execution, although it contains some important, rarely examined assumptions about environmental equality among identical and fraternal twins. By applying the twin method, we could estimate to what extent individual variations in drug metabolism were genetically controlled, reproducible, and of predictive value in the determination of individually optimum doses of drugs. Should extensive individual variations in drug response be maintained by genetic factors, then the rates at which patients metabolize drugs could be employed therapeutically to adjust doses of drugs prior to chronic administration. On the other hand, if rates of drug elimination in a given individual or in groups were predominantly under environmental control, then they would be expected to fluctuate extensively, depending on environmental alterations, and therefore would not be anticipated to constitute sufficiently stable values upon which to base long-term dosage.

In a series of studies conducted over the past 9 years, normal, adult, Caucasian twins living in the Washington, D.C. area were given single oral doses of various drugs to quantitate the genetic and environmental components of large individual variations in rates of drug elimination from plasma (10–15).

The environments of the volunteer twins were ascertained and during the course of the investigation were maintained unchanged from their usual patterns. Although no therapeutic agents were administered for 1 month preceding the study, this single limitation, imposed because of our goal to determine in the uninduced state the extent of and mechanisms responsible for individual variations in rates of drug elimination, did not represent much of a change for these volunteers. None had been on chronic medication. Many commonly encountered therapeutic agents enhance rates of drug elimination by inducing hepatic microsomal drug-metabolizing enzymes (8), so that to accomplish our purpose the twins could not ingest such drugs either during or for a short period before our investigation.

Because the environments prevalent in many large American cities contain compounds capable of altering rates of drug metabolism (8), differential individual exposure to such compounds as chlorinated hydrocarbons and insecticides was expected to produce an appreciable environmental contribution to large interindividual differences in rates of drug elimination from plasma. To assess the full extent of this environmental component, subjects should not be hospitalized either preceding or during the study. Therefore, the twins were permitted their customary range of activity at home and at work. All twins spent their working day apart, and only two pairs of the identical and two pairs of the fraternal twins lived in the same house so that most ate their noon and evening meals in different places.

An important aspect of this investigation concerned selection of drugs and the methods of administering them. The drugs chosen were phenylbutazone, antipyrine, bishydroxycoumarin, and ethanol because in man these agents are handled almost exclusively by biotransformation rather than by excretion of the unaltered parent drug. Phenylbutazone (16) and bishydroxycoumarin (17) are avidly bound to plasma proteins; however, antipyrine and ethanol binding to albumin is negligible (18). Administration of multiple doses of phenylbutazone (8) and antipyrine (19) alters rates of drug metabolism, and bishydroxycoumarin is poorly absorbed from the gastrointestinal tract after multiple doses (17, 20) so that we were reluctant to employ the method of steady-state blood levels in our studies. Sjöqvist and his colleagues effectively used the steady-state method of repeated drug administration in studies in nortriptyline (21), which presents problems in gastrointestinal absorption and redistribution that make the steady-state method more suitable. However, we were obliged to measure plasma half-lives of the drugs we selected after only a single oral dose because chronic administration of these agents produces induction of the hepatic microsomal drug-metabolizing enzymes.

In our study, the volunteers were normal, adult, Caucasian twins who were typed for approximately 30 blood group antigens to document the nature of their twinship. At 9:00 A.M. each volunteer received a single oral dose of phenylbutazone tablets (6 mg/kg), several months later a single oral dose of antipyrine (in a solution of 18 mg/kg), and several months later a single oral dose of bishydroxycoumarin tablets (4 mg/kg). Blood specimens, drawn at regular intervals after drug ingestion, were analyzed for drug concentration in plasma and the values plotted as shown for phenylbutazone, antipyrine and bishydroxycoumarin in Figs. 1–3, respectively (10–12). These curves illustrate typical examples of rates of phenylbutazone, antipyrine, and bishydroxycoumarin elimination from plasma of identical and fraternal twins. Phenylbutazone and bishydroxycoumarin, which were administered in tablet form, exhibit considerable interindividual variations in gastrointestinal absorption, as indicated by interindividual differences in y-intercept (Figs. 1 and 3), whereas antipyrine given in a solution was almost entirely absorbed in each subject and shows only small interindividual variations in y-intercept (Fig. 2).

The half-life of ethanol was determined in the plasma of these twins after each twin received a single oral dose of 95% ethanol (1 ml/kg) at 9:00 A.M. (14). Plasma levels were estimated by gas chromatography (22).

For each of these four compounds intratwin differences in half-life are appreciably greater in fraternal than identical twins. Therefore, it can be concluded that genetic rather than environmental factors maintain large individual differences in rates of elimination of phenylbutazone, antipyrine, bishydroxycoumarin, and ethanol. Application of the following formula described by Neel and Schull (23) and Osborne and DeGeorge (24) allowed estimation of the contribution of heredity to large individual variations in the plasma half-lives of these drugs:

$$\frac{(\text{Variance within pairs of fraternal twins}) - (\text{Variance within pairs of identical twins})}{(\text{Variance within pairs of fraternal twins})}$$

This formula permits a range of values from 0, indicating negligible hereditary and complete environmental control, to 1, indicating virtually complete hereditary influence. The contribution of heredity to variations in the half-life of phenylbutazone, antipyrine, bishydroxycoumarin, and ethanol was calculated to be 0.99, 0.98, 0.97, and 0.99, respectively. In these investigations we obtained intraclass correlation coefficients not very far from theoretical expectation on the basis of complete genetic control, according to which fraternal twins, having in common approximately half their total number of genes, should exhibit a value of 0.5, whereas identical twins should have a value of 1. The intraclass correlation coefficients of identical twins for phenylbutazone, antipyrine, bishydroxycoumarin, and ethanol were 0.83, 0.85, 0.85, and 0.82, respectively, whereas in fraternal twins the values for these drugs were 0.33, 0.47, 0.66, and 0.38, respectively (10–12,

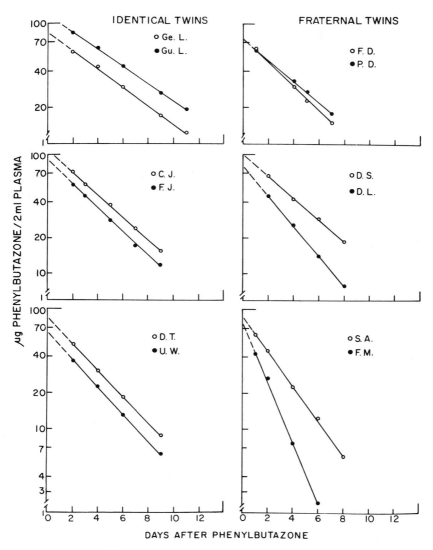

FIG. 1. Decline of phenylbutazone in the plasma of three sets of identical twins (left) and of three sets of fraternal twins (right) after a single oral dose of 6 mg/kg. Reproduced by permission from Vesell and Page (10).

14). Thus, in normal subjects not receiving other therapeutic agents large individual differences in rates of elimination of these drugs from plasma are surprisingly free of environmental influence. Repeated half-life determinations revealed that nonmedicated, normal subjects have very reproducible plasma half-lives for these drugs. Phenylbutazone (16) and bishydroxy-

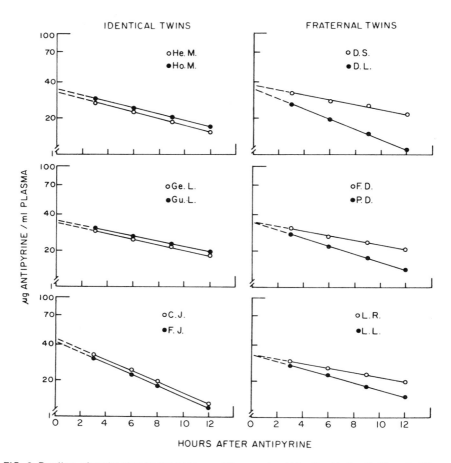

FIG. 2. Decline of antipyrine in the plasma of three sets of identical twins (left) and of three sets of fraternal twins (right) after a single oral dose of 18 mg/kg. Reproduced by permission from Vesell and Page (11).

coumarin (17) are 98% bound to plasma proteins, so that differences among individuals in rates of plasma clearance of these drugs might possibly involve binding to albumin. Antipyrine and ethanol, on the other hand, are not appreciably bound to plasma proteins (18). Therefore, for antipyrine and ethanol, if not also for phenylbutazone and bishydroxycoumarin, variations in plasma half-life arise from genetic differences that involve metabolism rather than distribution. The ranges for the plasma half-lives of ethanol, antipyrine, phenylbutazone, and bishydroxycoumarin of two-fold, three-fold, six-fold, and 10-fold, respectively, among the 28 individuals in our study indicate large variations among these individuals in rates of plasma clearance.

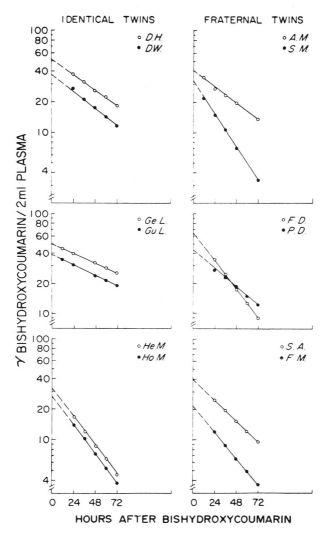

FIG. 3. Decline of bishydroxycoumarin in the plasma of three sets of identical twins (left) and of three sets of fraternal twins (right) after a single oral dose of 4 mg/kg. Reproduced by permission from Vesell and Page (12).

Another study of these same twins revealed almost fourfold variations in metabolism of a single intravenous dose of 3.4 mg of radioactive halothane (13). Large individual differences in halothane metabolism were demonstrated to be predominantly controlled by genetic factors (13), although the corrected value of 0.88 and the uncorrected value of 0.63 for the contribution of heredity to individual differences in rates of halothane metabolism indicate a larger environmental component for this drug than was observed for ethanol, phenylbutazone, antipyrine, or bishydroxycoumarin. Two reasons that could account for the greater environmental influence over variations in halothane than in phenylbutazone, antipyrine, or bishydroxycoumarin metabolism include the possibility of its control by a different enzyme system more susceptible to induction by commonly encountered environmental substances or alternatively the fact that halothane is metabolized to a much smaller extent than the other drugs we investigated. The percent of the administered dose of halothane metabolized ranges in these 20 subjects from only 2.7 to 11.4. When such a small fraction of an administered dose is metabolized, environmental contributions to variations in biotransformation could play a proportionately larger role. For halothane, the intraclass correlation coefficient for identical twins was 0.52 and for fraternal twins 0.36, respectively.

Table 2 shows heritability of variations in the metabolism of these drugs as calculated by several other methods. Other methods were employed because the technique utilized in the preceding estimates assumes that environmental differences between twinships are negligible, and, therefore, these calculations are too high to the extent that such differential environmental factors operate. Falconer (25) approached the problem by partitioning variance into several genetic and environmental components; although this approach can be utilized in the family studies (26), it cannot be applied to twin data. Halothane shows a very small genetic component of control by the Holzinger (27) index

$$\frac{r_I - r_F}{1 - r_F}$$

or by the method of Falconer (25), modified by using values of V_A/V_P, (variance due to additive gene effects and phenotypic factors, respectively) provided from the family study of Whittaker and Price Evans (28). The estimation of hereditary control of a trait, according to Falconer (25), is

TABLE 2. *Heritability of variations in drug metabolism of twins utilizing different methods of data analysis*

	Antipyrine	Phenylbutazone	Bishydroxycoumarin	Ethanol	Halothane
$\dfrac{V_F - V_I}{V_F}$	0.98	0.99	0.97	0.98	0.88
r_I	0.85	0.83	0.85	0.82	0.52
r_F	0.47	0.33	0.66	0.38	0.36
$\dfrac{r_I - r_F}{1 - r_F}$	0.72	0.75	0.56	0.71	0.25
$2(r_I - r_F)$	0.76	1.00	0.38	0.88	0.32

r = Intraclass correlation coefficient.

based on the proportion of the phenotypic variance contributed by the two genetic components of variance, the so-called addition and dominance components of variance:

$$H = 2(r_1 - r_F) = \frac{V_A + 1.5\, V_D}{V_P}.$$

A twin study performed in Stockholm on variations in steady-state blood concentrations of nortriptyline in otherwise nonmedicated, nonhospitalized twins showed appreciably smaller intratwin differences in identical than in fraternal twins (29). These marked differences between identical and fraternal twins in steady-state blood levels of nortriptyline confirmed our conclusions from twin studies with phenylbutazone, antipyrine, bishydroxycoumarin, ethanol, and halothane. A value of 0.98 for heritability of variations among individuals in nortriptyline metabolism was calculated from the twin data of Alexanderson et al. (29).

Recently, Whittaker and Price Evans (28) performed a family study to assess the genetic contribution to variability among individuals in phenylbutazone metabolism. They concluded that variability among individuals in phenylbutazone metabolism was under polygenic control. Previously, a similar conclusion was reached by Motulsky (30) from a family study on variability in the plasma half-lives of bishydroxycoumarin after a single oral dose. Whittaker and Price Evans (28) obtained a normal distribution of phenylbutazone half-lives in plasma after correcting for height and also after administering a 3-day course of phenobarbital to "render the environment more uniform." A significant regression of mean offspring value on midparent value indicated to Whittaker and Price Evans (28) that approximately 65% of the observed phenotypic variance was caused by the additive effects of genes. These results agree closely with those from our earlier study on phenylbutazone metabolism in twins (10) if V_D (variance due to the effect of dominance) is not neglected in the following formula derived from Falconer (25).

$$H = \frac{\frac{1}{2} V_A + \frac{3}{4} V_D}{\frac{1}{2} V_A + \frac{3}{4} V_D = V_E} = \frac{V_F - V_I}{V_F}$$

where V_A = the variance due to additive effects of genes controlling the trait, V_E = the variance due to environment, F = fraternal twins, and I = identical twins. Whittaker and Price Evans (28) state that V_D is too small to be significant, although they admit that V_{Ec} is probably large. ($V_E = V_{Ew} + V_{Ec}$, where V_{Ew} and V_{Ec} are the within-twin-pair variance and the common variance between twin pairs, respectively.) Neither V_D nor V_{Ec} was measured in their family study. In other studies of polygenically controlled traits in man, V_D is small but not negligible. For example, in their classic study of height and intelligence, Burt and Howard (26) reported a value of 0.16 and 0.17 for the contribution of V_D to height and intelligence, respectively. If their value for V_D of 0.16 is utilized as an estimate of V_D in calculating the family data of Whittaker and Price Evans (28) — and it seems more reasonable to use this hypothetical value than to disregard V_D completely — there is good agreement between the results of the family study of Whittaker and Price Evans ($H = 0.88$) and our twin data on phenylbutazone ($H = 0.75$ or 1.00) (Table 2). Since these values are close to the estimate (0.99) based on the formula for heritability that we employed

$$H = \frac{V_F - V_I}{V_F},$$

we may conclude that differential environmental factors operating between twinships in our investigation were quite small. Another recent study in two extensive Swedish pedigrees with high steady-state plasma concentrations of nortriptyline suggested that the appreciable individual differences in the steady-state plasma concentrations of this drug were polygenically controlled (31). Thus far both the family studies and the twin data have agreed in their conclusions that large differences among healthy, nonmedicated volunteers in rates of drug metabolism are primarily controlled by genetic factors.

The use of twins has lost favor in human genetics; although the defects inherent in twin studies have been repeatedly emphasized, their advantages in investigating variations among individuals in rates of drug metabolism have not previously been described. Even the assumption that "monozygotic human twins have identical inheritance" has been challenged by Storrs and Williams (32) on the basis of large differences in 20 parameters among newborn monozygotic quadruplet armadillos. The twin method does suffer from several disadvantages including its inability to establish conclusively the mode of inheritance of a genetically controlled trait and its assumption of an environmental equality in all subjects, identical as well as fraternal twins. It has been argued that in man this latter assumption is invalid because identical twins make more similar choices and have more similar tastes than fraternal twins in eating, drinking, and even toothpaste. However, in our studies the identical twins lived for the most part in different homes and ate different meals so that these environmental similarities that might possibly affect drug metabolism seemed superficially no greater among the identical than among the fraternal twins. Each of our subjects was over 21 years of age and had established for himself a life pattern relatively independent of and different from that of his twin.

Some reviewers maintain that "while twin studies can define the heritable nature of an unusual response to a drug, they are of little value in elucidating the genetics of a disorder further" (33). However, twin studies can provide important clues toward the elucidation of the mode of inheritance of pharmacogenetic variation. A trimodal distribution curve strongly suggests single-factor inheritance of variations among only 10 sets of twins in response to isoniazid (34). By way of contrast, another twin study, also of a very small number of twins, reveals a unimodal distribution of antipyrine half-lives (11), suggesting polygenic control of these variations. Thus, even for the very small number of twins, construction of a distribution curve clearly helps to suggest the mode of inheritance of genetically controlled variations in response to drugs.

Twin studies can be a particularly profitable initial step in identifying the relative genetic and environmental contributions to a new trait. Then, the construction of a distribution curve of these twins can provide a useful hint as to whether such variations are transmitted polygenically or as simple single factors. It should be emphasized here that for a rare autosomal recessive trait, a unimodal curve might be obtained if too few individuals were tested. This eventuality could lead to an erroneous interpretation of polygenic control. Twin studies alone cannot conclusively establish the mode of inheritance of a pharmacogenetic entity, but, through distribution curves of drug response, twin data can be utilized more than they have been previously. Family studies should, as the third step in the genetic delineation of a new trait, then be performed at the extremes of this distribution curve where pedigrees would be most likely to prove genetically informative.

In the evaluation of variations in drug metabolism, twin studies enjoy several distinct advantages over family studies and have been utilized on rare occasions as subjects for investigations of the genetic component of individual variations in drug metabolism (34, 35). Twins are by definition age corrected, and dizygotic twins of the same sex can easily be selected. As studies in rodents have shown (9) and as studies in man have suggested (36), rates of drug metabolism change with age and sex. Thus the genetic analysis of data on drug metabolism from family studies is complicated by incorporation of variations in rates of drug metabolism from differences in age and sex, two factors readily eliminated in twin studies. Furthermore, differences in the environment of children, parents, and grandparents with respect to exposure to certain environmental compounds capable of inducing or inhibiting the hepatic microsomal drug-metabolizing enzymes must be considered a source of possible variation in family studies. Such environmental influences on drug metabolism arising from common exposure in the same household to inducers or inhibitors of drug-metabolizing enzymes could explain why, in the family study of Whittaker and Price Evans, there was a correlation in phenylbutazone metabolism between husbands and wives before phenobarbital administration.

Compounds capable of shortening either their own duration of action or that of other drugs administered simultaneously (37, 38) have been utilized clinically, and, therefore, the magnitude of differences among individuals in responsiveness to such inducing agents becomes a therapeutically important problem. The simplest assumption would be that if comparable blood levels of an inducing agent were obtained, then the activity of the drug-metabolizing enzymes would rise to a similar extent. However, this was not the case; for phenobarbital, the inducing agent most commonly employed therapeutically in man, large, genetically determined differences exist in the inductive response, even in the face of similar blood concentrations of phenobarbital (39). In four sets of identical and four sets of fraternal twins, antipyrine half-lives were measured before and after 2 weeks of sodium phenobarbital administered in a daily dose of 2 mg/kg. Intrapair differences in the extent to which phenobarbital altered antipyrine half-lives were significantly greater in fraternal than in identical twins, as shown in Table 3 (39). The contribution of heredity to variations in the extent of pheno-barbital-induced reduction in plasma antipyrine half-life, and hence to variations in the induction of hepatic, microsomal drug-metabolizing enzymes by phenobarbital, was calculated to be 99% by the formula for H described above.

In these studies, phenobarbital decreased the standard deviation of the mean antipyrine half-life by more than twofold and the variation in anti-pyrine half-life from 2.8-fold to 1.8-fold (Table 3). These results suggest that if extensive interindividual differences in drug metabolism produce thera-peutic problems, relatively innocuous inducing agents might be adminis-tered to minimize such variability.

With respect to this suggestion, a direct relationship occurred between initial antipyrine half-life and the percent shortening of antipyrine half-life produced by phenobarbital administration; the longer the initial anti-pyrine half-life, the greater the reduction caused by phenobarbital treatment (Fig. 4) (39). This relationship permits prediction of the extent to which phenobarbital will reduce initial antipyrine half-life; since phenobarbital shortens the antipyrine half-life of slow metabolizers more than it shortens the antipyrine half-life of fast metabolizers, use of phenobarbital to reduce toxic blood levels of various drugs would appear to aid preferentially those individuals most in need of such therapy, namely, the slow metabolizers. Because the genes controlling variations among individuals in inducibility after phenobarbital may be different from the genes controlling variations among relatively uninduced individuals in the metabolism of drugs such as phenylbutazone and antipyrine, it is difficult to interpret results of a study that mixes these two phenomena by measuring variations among individ-uals in the metabolism of a drug such as phenylbutazone only after all the subjects have been induced by phenobarbital (28).

Recent studies (40, 41) on genetically controlled differences of the extent of induction of benzpyrene hydroxylase activity in human peripheral lymphocytes after methylcholanthrene administration are in harmony with the general results of the phenobarbital investigation (39). The mode of in-heritance of this control over induction was shown in family studies (40) to be autosomal codominant.

It is known that many commonly administered drugs enhance the activity

TABLE 3. *Response of plasma antipyrine half-life to phenobarbital administration with smoking, coffee, tea, and alcohol history in 16 twins*

Twin	Age, Sex	Plasma antipyrine half-life Before phenobarbital (hr)	After phenobarbital (hr)	Decrease in half-life produced by phenobarbital (percent)	Percentage difference between siblings in response to phenobarbital	Plasma phenobarbital levels at 156hr	212hr	Smoking (pack/ day)	Coffee (cup/ day)	Tea (cup/ day)	Beer (bottles/ day)	Wine (glasses/ day)	Hard liquor (oz/ day)
Identical twins													
Dan. E.	22, M	13.6	9.6	29.4	0	20.0	23.0	0	2	0	1/4	0	1/4
Dav. E.	22, M	13.6	9.6	29.4		20.0	23.2	1/4	0	2	1/4	0	1/4
A. M.	35, F	8.0	6.3	21.2	0	17.0	18.0	1/2	0	3	0	0	0
B. Z.	35, F	8.0	6.3	21.2		15.0	16.0	2	6–7	0	0	0	1
Bar. J.	23, F	18.2	8.4	53.8	0	16.8	17.1	0	0	0	0	0	0
Bev. J.	23, F	18.2	8.4	53.8		17.9	25.0	0	0	0	0	0	0
B. F.	26, F	10.8	7.3	32.4	2.6	16.0	23.4	0	0	0	0	0	0
B. J.	26, F	11.4	7.4	35.0		17.4	24.4	0	0	1	0	0	1/4
Fraternal twins													
F. D.	49, M	12.0	10.3	14.2	14.2	14.8	19.4	0	1	2	0	0	0
P. D.	49, M	9.3	9.3	0		15.2	18.3	1 1/2	5	0	0	0	1
C. K.	49, M	17.5	5.5	68.6	8.6	—	23.0	1 1/2	2	0	1	0	18
N. R.	49, F	14.5	5.8	60.0		—	19.0	1 1/2	4	0	0	0	0
H. H.	47, F	12.3	9.2	25.2	9.8	17.8	16.6	2	2	0	1/2	0	1/2
P. M.	47, F	6.5	5.5	15.4		16.0	20.8	1 1/2	2	0	1/2	0	0
E. W.	54, F	15.0	6.9	54.0	30.7	20.0	29.0	0	4	0	0	0	1/2
E. E.	54, F	9.0	6.9	23.3		20.0	30.0	1	2	2	0	0	1/4

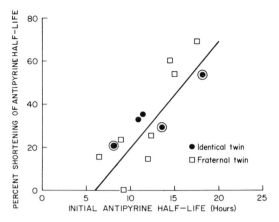

FIG. 4. Positive correlation (0.84) between the initial antipyrine half-life in plasma and the phenobarbital-induced shortening of antipyrine half-life. Reproduced by permission from Vesell and Page (39).

of hepatic microsomal drug-metabolizing enzymes. However, inhibition of drug metabolism in man is less well appreciated, although the clinical consequences of drug inhibition may be more severe than the sequelae of induction. Very few inhibitors of drug metabolism have been identified. Inhibition of drug metabolism would appear to be much less frequent an occurrence than induction, but sufficient studies have not been performed to establish this conclusively. Inhibition may occur for short periods after a drug is administered; most studies unfortunately examine only one or two time points so that inhibition may be missed (42).

A recent twin study compared identical and fraternal twins with respect to the extent to which phenylbutazone inhibited DPH metabolism (43). Although plasma DPH half-lives exhibited greater similarity among sets of identical than among sets of fraternal twins, DPH half-lives were prolonged by phenylbutazone to the same degree in identical and fraternal twinships (43). Thus the greater similarity among identical than among fraternal twins with respect to induction of drug-metabolizing enzymes after phenobarbital (39) was not observed in the case of inhibition of DPH metabolism by phenylbutazone (43). A consideration of the major differences in mechanism between induction and inhibition of drug metabolism reveals why this difference might have been predicted. Induction involves increased protein synthesis through effects on the primary genetic material, DNA and/or RNA, thereby being under genetic control, whereas many examples of inhibition of drug metabolism involve the presence of compounds that compete with substrate for enzymatic transformation in the endoplasmic reticulum. This process of competition for biotransformation would not appear as likely as induction to be under genetic control. Rather it would seem to be more subject to influence by various environmental circumstances affecting physicochemical conditions and concentrations of numerous compounds near the active sites of hepatic microsomal mixed-function oxidases. It must be noted, however, that several inhibitors of drug metabolism exist that exhibit noncompetitive kinetics (44).

CONCLUSION

Drug interactions can be significantly influenced by genetic factors, although this fact has been obscured by the essentially environmental nature of drug interactions and by the numerous studies on environmentally controlled conditions that can modify drug interactions. Both monogenically and polygenically transmitted traits predispose to adverse drug reactions occurring as a result of drug interactions. Some of these genetically transmitted conditions have been discussed in this chapter. Large interindividual differences in rates of elimination of many commonly used drugs occur, are under predominantly genetic control, as revealed by twin and family studies, and constitute a major source of drug toxicity from drug accumulation since these interindividual differences are not sufficiently taken into account in adjusting drug dosage.

Large differences in the extent of induction of drug-metabolizing enzymes also appear to be under predominantly genetic control, whereas large interindividual differences in the extent of inhibition of drug metabolism appear to be influenced more by environmental than genetic factors. Consideration of the markedly different mechanisms for induction and inhibition of drug metabolism renders these results compatible.

ACKNOWLEDGMENT

Support in part by U.S. Public Health Service Grant No. MH 21327 from the National Institutes of Health.

REFERENCES

1. Kalow, W. (1962): *Pharmacogenetics: Heredity and Response to Drugs*, Saunders, Philadelphia.
2. LaDu, B. N., and Kalow, W., eds. (1965): Pharmacogenetics, *Ann. N.Y. Acad. Sci. 151*, 691–1001.
3. Vesell, E. S., ed. (1971): Drug metabolism in man, *Ann. N.Y. Acad. Sci., 179*, 1–773 (1971).
4. Vesell, E. S. (1973): *Progr. Med. Genet. 9*, 291.
5. Brennan, R. W., Dehejia, H., Kutt, H., and McDowell, F. (1968): *Neurology 18*, 283.
6. Motulsky, A. G., Yoshida, A., and Stamatoyannopoulos, G. (1971): *Ann. N.Y. Acad. Sci. 179*, 636–644.
7. O'Reilly, R. A. (1970): *New Engl. J. Med. 282*, 1448–1451.
8. Conney, A. H. (1967): *Pharmacol. Rev. 19*, 317–366.
9. Vesell, E. S. (1968): *Pharmacology 1*, 81–97.

10. Vesell, E. S., and Page, J. G. (1968): *Science 159*, 1479–1480.
11. Vesell, E. S., and Page, J. G. (1968): *Science 161*, 72–73.
12. Vesell, E. S., and Page, J. G. (1968): *J. Clin. Invest. 47*, 2657–2663.
13. Cascorbi, H. F., Vesell, E. S., Blake, D. A., and Hebrich, M. (1971): *Clin. Pharmacol. Ther. 12*, 50–55.
14. Vesell, E. S., Page, J. G., and Passananti, G. T. (1971): *Clin. Pharmacol. Ther. 12*, 192–201.
15. Vesell, E. S., Passananti, G. T., Greene, F. E., and Page, J. G. (1971): *Ann. N.Y. Acad. Sci. 179*, 752–773.
16. Burns, C., Rose, R. K., Chenkin, T., Goldman, A., Schulert, A., and Brodie, B. B. (1953): *J. Pharmacol. Exp. Ther. 109*, 346–357.
17. Weiner, M., Shapiro, S., Axelrod, J., Cooper, J. R., and Brodie, B. B. (1950): *J. Pharmacol. Exp. Ther. 99*, 409–420.
18. Soberman, R., Brodie, B. B., Levy, B. B., Axelrod, J., Hollander, V., and Steele, J. M. (1949): *J. Biol. Chem. 179*, 31–42.
19. Breckenridge, A., and Orme, M. (1971): *Ann. N.Y. Acad. Sci. 179*, 421–431.
20. O'Reilly, R. A., and Aggler, P. M. (1965): *Pharmacol. Rev. 22*, 35–96.
21. Hammer, W., Martins, S., and Sjöqvist, F. (1969): *Clin. Pharmacol. Ther. 10*, 44–49.
22. Goldbaum, L. R., Domanski, T. J., and Schloegel, E. L. (1964): *J. Forensic Sci. 9*, 63–71.
23. Neel, J. V., and Schull, W. J. (1954): In: *Human Heredity*, p. 280, University of Chicago Press, Chicago.
24. Osborne, R. H., and DeGeorge, F. V. (1959): *Genetic Basis of Morphological Variation, an Evaluation and Application of the Twin Study Method*, Harvard University Press, Cambridge, Mass.
25. Falconer, D. S. (1960): *Introduction to Quantitative Genetics*, Ronald, New York.
26. Burt, C., and Howard, M. (1956): *Brit. J. Statist. Psychol. 8/2*, 95–131.
27. Holzinger, H. J. (1929): *J. Educ. Psychol. 20*, 241–248.
28. Whittaker, J. A., and Price Evans, D. A. (1970): *Brit. Med. J. 4*, 323–328.
29. Alexanderson, B., Price Evans, D. A., and Sjöqvist, F. (1969): *Brit. Med. J. 4*, 764–768.
30. Motulsky, A. (1964): *Progr. Med. Genet. 3*, 49–74.
31. Asberg, M., Price Evans, D. A., and Sjöqvist, F. (1971): *J. Med. Genet. 8*, 129–135.
32. Storrs, E. E., and Williams, R. J. (1968): *Proc. Nat. Acad. Sci. USA 60*, 910–914.
33. Cohen, S. N., and Weber, W. W. (1972): *Pediat. Clin. N. Amer. 19/1*, 21–36.
34. Bönicke, R., and Lisboa, B. P. (1957): *Naturwissenschaften 44*, 314.
35. Kappas, A., and Gallagher, T. F. (1960): *J. Clin. Invest. 39*, 620–625.
36. O'Malley, K., Crooks, J., Duke, E., and Stevenson, I. H. (1971): *Brit. Med. J. 3*, 607–609.
37. Yaffe, S. J., Levy, G., Matsuzawa, T., and Baliah, T. (1966): *New Engl. J. Med. 275*, 1461–1465.
38. Ramboer, C., Thompson, R. P. H., and Williams, R. (1969): *Lancet 1*, 966.
39. Vesell, E. S., and Page, J. G. (1969): *J. Clin. Invest. 48*, 2202–2209.
40. Kellerman, G., Luyten-Kellermann, J., and Shaw, C. R. (1973): *Amer. J. Human Genet. 25*, 327.
41. Cantrell, E. T., Warr, G. A., Busbee, D. L., and Martin, R. R. (1973): *J. Clin. Invest. 52*, 1881.
42. Vesell, E. S., Lee, C. J., Passananti, G. T., and Shively, C. A. (1972): *Pharmacology 8*, 217.
43. Andreasen, P. B., Froxland, A., Skovsted, L., Andersen, S. A., and Hauge, M. (1973): *Acta. Med. Scand. 193*, 561.
44. Hutson, D. H. (1970): In: *Foreign Compound Metabolism in Mammals*, Vol. 1, p. 390, The Chemical Society, London.

Drug Interactions, edited by P. L. Morselli,
S. Garattini, and S. N. Cohen. Raven Press,
New York © 1974

Kinetics of Tolbutamide Interactions

Malcolm Rowland, Shaik B. Matin, Jake Thiessen,* and John Karam**

*Department of Pharmacy, School of Pharmacy, University of California, San Francisco, California 94143, *Faculty of Pharmacy, University of Toronto, Toronto, Ontario, Canada, and **Department of Metabolic Diseases, School of Medicine, University of California, San Francisco, California 94143*

The coadministration of two or more drugs can result in an adverse reaction or ineffective therapy. Those concerned with drug therapy are increasingly aware of these phenomena, commonly known as drug interactions. Many review articles (1–5) and books (6–8) cover the whole array of drug interactions. Whereas many are useful, other sources lack critical evaluation regarding the clinical significance or mechanism of the cited interaction.

A common cause of the pharmacological sequelae following multiple-drug therapy is the alteration by one drug on the rate and extent of absorption, distribution, metabolism, and excretion of another. Prescott (9) has called these "pharmacokinetic interactions" to distinguish them from the numerous interactions between drugs at their sites of action (10), although this distinction is somewhat arbitrary as any or all possibilities can occur *in vivo*. Our knowledge of the pharmacokinetics of drugs in animals and man has increased substantially over the past few decades (11). Models have been developed that accurately describe the concentration-time profile of drugs and metabolites in various biological fluids following drug administration. Considerable success has also been gained in relating the kinetics of a graded pharmacologic response to a drug with its pharmacokinetics (12, 13). Since many pharmacokinetic drug interactions are dependent on the concentration of the interacting species, the degree of interaction should also be a graded phenomenon varying with drug (and metabolite) concentrations and, therefore, drug administration and time. It should, therefore, be possible to develop kinetic models for such drug interactions. Although awareness of this fact exists (5, 14–16), there have been relatively few systemic attempts to establish these models.

The intent of the present studies was to illustrate, using tolbutamide as an example, how pharmacokinetic analysis leads to further insights regarding the causes, possible mechanisms, and assistance in the design of experiments aimed at elucidating various facets of drug interactions and how predictive pharmacokinetic models of drug interactions can be developed, which have potential utility in deciding appropriate dosage regimens when combined drug therapy is required.

Together with the anticoagulants, the interactions with oral hypoglycemic agents constitute some of the most adverse clinical cases of drug interactions. Interactions with the sulfonylurea oral hypoglycemic agent, tolbutamide, are the most commonly reported. Hypoglycemic crises have been reported when patients, stabilized on tolbutamide, have added sulfaphenazole, dicoumarol, phenylbutazone, or phenyramidol to their drug regimen (17, 18). In each case cited, clear chemical data exist showing a slowing of tolbutamide elimination, and it appears that these interactions involve inhibition of tolbutamide oxidation to hydroxytolbutamide (Fig. 1). Tolbutamide is thought to be converted to hydroxytolbutamide by NADPH-linked microsomal enzymes (19). This oxidation appears to be almost quantitative in man. Hydroxytolbutamide is further metabolized to carboxytolbutamide, presumably via tolbutamide aldehyde, by enzymes in the cytoplasmic soluble fraction. Almost all the tolbutamide administered can be found as hydroxy and carboxytolbutamide in the urine of man, with only a little being excreted unchanged (20). The soluble enzymes probably responsible for the oxidation of hydroxytolbutamide and tolbutamide aldehyde include alcohol dehydrogenase, which is NAD-linked, and aldehyde dehydrogenase, also NAD-linked and/or xanthine-oxidase dependent. Administered separately, hydroxytolbutamide possesses hypoglycemic activity in man, whereas carboxytolbutamide does not (21). The half-life of tolbutamide is normally between 4 and 8 hr, and the oxidation of tolbutamide is the rate-limiting step in elimination of this drug and its metabolites from the body.

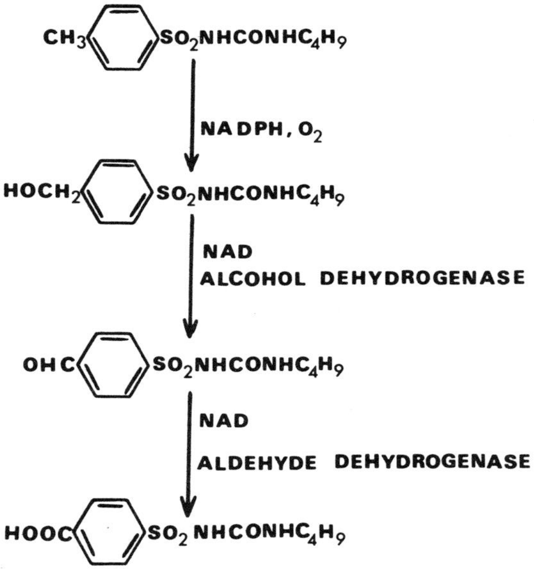

FIG. 1. Proposed scheme describing tolbutamide metabolism.

Subsequent oxidation steps are very rapid, and, when administered separately, hydroxy and carboxy metabolites have half-lives of 40 min and 20 min, respectively (21). Accordingly, the hydroxytolbutamide levels are always too low to significantly contribute to the hypoglycemic effects following tolbutamide administration. Also, a few hours after tolbutamide administration, the rate of urinary excretion of the sum of the two metabolites equals the rate of tolbutamide oxidation and offers a very sensitive measure of changes in the rate of tolbutamide oxidation.

The best studied interaction is that between the sulfonamide, sulfaphenazole, and tolbutamide. Sulfaphenazole is reported to impair tolbutamide elimination and increase the half-life of tolbutamide from the normal 4 to 8 hr to values ranging from 24 to 74 hr (21, 22). The clinical crises probably arise when the dosage regimen is unaltered and tolbutamide accumulates to an undesirable extent upon chronic administration in the presence of sulfaphenazole. Figures 2 and 3 illustrate the situation when sulfaphena-

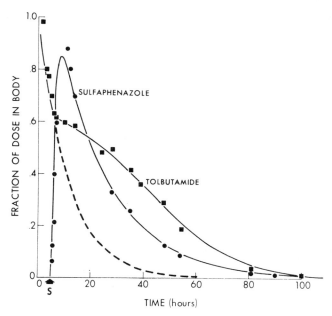

FIG. 2. Tolbutamide-sulfaphenazole interaction kinetics in man. The experimental data (tolbutamide, sulfaphenazole) and the analogue computer generated curves (solid lines) describe the interaction between sulfaphenazole and tolbutamide. The subject received an i.v. bolus of 1 g tolbutamide and a 1 g oral suspension of sulfaphenazole (Sulfabid ®) 5.5 hr later. For convenience the amount of the two drugs in the body is expressed as a fraction of the administered dose. The half-life of tolbutamide in the absence of sulfaphenazole is approximately 7 hr. The dotted lines depict the anticipated rapid decline of tolbutamide when administered alone. The degree of inhibition of tolbutamide oxidation continuously changes with the amount of sulfaphenazole in the body. Block is maximal at peak sulfonamide plasma levels. The half-life of sulfaphenazole in this subject is 12 hr (23). Reproduced with permission of the copyright owner.

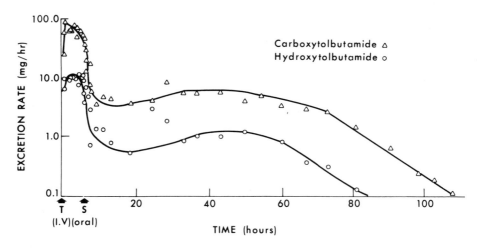

FIG. 3. Tolbutamide-sulfaphenazole interaction kinetics in man. The excretion-rate data of hydroxytolbutamide and carboxytolbutamide for the same subject whose plasma data is portrayed in Fig. 2. At peak plasma sulfaphenazole levels the inhibition of tolbutamide oxidation is almost complete, and with essentially no formation of hydroxytolbutamide, the excretion rate of both this metabolite and carboxytolbutamide rapidly fall, reflecting the very short, 20 to 40 min, half-lives of these species. Beyond 10 hr after the tolbutamide bolus the rate of excretion of these tolbutamide metabolites equals the rate of tolbutamide oxidation. As the sulfaphenazole body levels decline, the degree of inhibition of tolbutamide oxidation diminishes and the excretion rate of the metabolites increases. However, even though the inhibition continually diminishes, so also does the amount of tolbutamide in the body, and after 50 hr the excretion rate of metabolites continually declines, albeit slowly (23). Reproduced with permission of the copyright owner.

zole is given orally to a subject approximately 5 hr after receiving an i.v. 1 g bolus of tolbutamide (23). The delay in sulfonamide administration allowed the establishment of the control value for the half-life of tolbutamide. Sulfaphenazole markedly prolonged tolbutamide-plasma levels with an anticipated sudden drop in the excretion rate of the metabolites. At maximum sulfonamide-plasma levels the block in tolbutamide oxidation was almost complete, and the half-lives determined from the corresponding sharply descending portion of the hydroxy and carboxytolbutamide urinary-excretion rate plot approximated the half-lives of these metabolites when administered alone (21). As the ratio of hydroxy to carboxytolbutamide in the urine remained unchanged in the presence of sulfaphenazole, it appears that this sulfonamide does not influence the oxidation or renal clearance of hydroxytolbutamide in the dose range studied. Neither does sulfaphenazole appear to possess hypoglycemic activity itself, nor does it potentiate the hypoglycemic activity of an i.v. 1 g tolbutamide bolus (17). Also, whereas sulfaphenazole influences tolbutamide oxidation, separate studies show that tolbutamide does not alter the kinetics of sulfaphenazole elimination, which is principally by N^1-glucuronidation and N^4-acetylation (24).

Body burdens of tolbutamide in man normally range between 0.5 and 2 g. This is within the dose range (0.5 to 6 g), where tolbutamide elimination is dose independent and the elimination half-life (and hence rate constant, k_T) remains constant (25). These data imply that the concentration of tolbutamide at the metabolic site, in therapeutic settings, is well below the Michaelis-Menten constant of the oxidative enzyme system. Assuming that sulfaphenazole only acts as an inhibitor of the conversion of tolbutamide to hydroxytolbutamide, and remembering that, in man, this step virtually accounts for tolbutamide elimination, a simple expression can be developed to describe the elimination kinetics of tolbutamide in the presence of the inhibitor (23),

$$\text{Rate of tolbutamide elimination} = \frac{k_T T}{1 + (I/K_I)} \qquad (1)$$

where T and I are the amounts of tolbutamide and sulfaphenazole in the body, and the inhibitor constant, K_I may be defined as the amount of inhibitor that diminishes the effective elimination rate constant by one-half (or prolongs the half-life twofold). According to the above equation, by measuring all the chemical species involved, and determining k_T in the absence of sulfaphenazole, K_I may be estimated. However, relating inhibition kinetics to the amount of drug and inhibitor in the body is only a first approximation, and a more precise quantitative description of the inhibitory process requires relating the phenomenon to the concentration of drug and inhibitor at the metabolic site. Nonetheless, Eq. 1 is sufficiently accurate to allow a good fit of the observed data using an estimated value for K_I of 200 mg sulfaphenazole (Fig. 2). This value of K_I is small compared to the 1 to 2 g daily dose usually recommended for this sulfonamide.

Knowing the K_I for sulfaphenazole and the other relevant pharmacokinetic data, the clinical situation can be modeled. Usually, 0.5 g tolbutamide and 1.0 g sulfaphenazole are given orally twice daily. Initially when only tolbutamide is given, expected plateau levels are reached within four half-lives (26) or 30 hr (Fig. 4). When sulfaphenazole is given, it accumulates likewise and by blocking tolbutamide oxidation causes a rise in the plateau level of the sulfonylurea to approximately seven times its normal value. Also, regardless of whether only sulfaphenazole or both drugs are stopped, it will be 2 to 3 days before tolbutamide returns to its previous level. This analysis explains much of the tolbutamide data seen clinically when both drugs are given concomitantly for extended periods (17, 22).

The average amount of tolbutamide at the new plateau and the time to reach this value is governed by the new half-life of tolbutamide in the presence of a steady level of the inhibitor [$T\frac{1}{2}$ (tolbutamide, inhibited)]. Estimates of these parameters are gained from two equations (27):

$$\bar{A} = \frac{1.44 \times \text{dose} \times \text{half-life}}{\text{dosing interval}}, \qquad (2)$$

$$T^{1/}_{2} \text{ (tolbutamide, inhibited)} = T^{1/}_{2} \text{ (tolbutamide, normal)}$$
$$\times \left(1 + \frac{\text{average amount of inhibitor at plateau}}{K_I} \right), \qquad (3)$$

where $\bar{A}$ is the average amount of drug in the body at the plateau when given on a fixed-dose fixed-interval regimen. If sulfaphenazole ($T^{1/}_{2} = 10$ hr (23, 24) $K_I = 200$ mg) is given 1.0 g twice daily, according to the first equation, the average amount of inhibitor at the plateau is 1.5 g and is reached within 2 days ($4 \times T^{1/}_{2}$). Substituting this average amount of the inhibitor into the second equation indicates that the new half-life for tolbutamide is seven to eight times longer than normal (i.e., from 35 to 40 hr instead of 5 hr). Now it will take approximately 6 days (4×1.5 days) to reach the new plateau when the average amount of tolbutamide is seven to eight times the average plateau level in the absence of the inhibitor (Fig. 4). It is apparent also that,

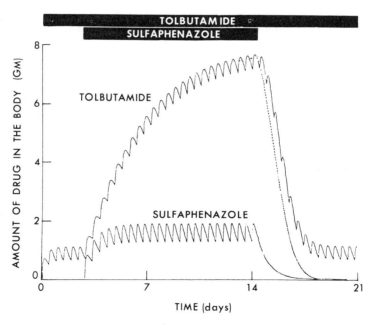

FIG. 4. Tolbutamide-sulfaphenazole interaction kinetics in man. Analogue computer simulations of the clinical situation when tolbutamide (1 g, twice daily) is given in the absence and presence of sulfaphenazole (1 g twice daily). The solid black bars denote the duration of each drug regimen. Having a short half-life (4 to 8 hr) plateau levels of tolbutamide are reached within 2 days. The sulfaphenazole also rapidly reaches plateau concentration (half-life 10 to 12 hr). In the presence of sulfaphenazole, the amount of tolbutamide in the body continues to rise until output once again equals input. Upon cessation of sulfaphenazole, the decline of tolbutamide, whether continued (solid line) or stopped at the same time as sulfaphenazole (dotted line) takes several days before falling into the accepted therapeutic range (23). Reproduced by permission of copyright owner.

to maintain the normal amount of tolbutamide in the body, the dosage regimen of this sulfonylurea would have to be reduced eightfold. In any individual, the degree of interaction will depend upon the dosage regimen and pharmacokinetics of each drug and the K_I in that individual. At present the variation of K_I within the population is unknown.

Tolbutamide elimination in man is a special case in that almost all is removed via one pathway. Inhibiting this pathway has a pronounced effect on tolbutamide levels. The more general situation is where drug is eliminated by several pathways. Considering the more general case, a model of drug inhibition interactions can be developed in an analogous manner to that developed for describing the tolbutamide-sulfaphenazole interaction in man. The equations are similar to those derived for schedules of drugs in patients with varying degree of renal impairment. The information required is the fraction of the dose in the body eliminated by the particular pathway of interest in the absence of inhibitor (f_m) and the ratio of the amount of inhibitor (I) to the inhibitor constant (K_I). When a fixed regimen is administered, the ratio (R) of the half-life of the drug in the presence ($T\frac{1}{2}$ inhibitor) and absence ($T\frac{1}{2}$ normal), of the inhibitor, which is also the ratio of the average steady-state amount of drug before ($\overline{Ab}$ normal) and after inhibition ($\overline{Ab}$ inhibited) is given by (23)

$$R = \frac{T\frac{1}{2} \text{ (inhibited)}}{T\frac{1}{2} \text{ (normal)}} = \frac{\overline{Ab} \text{ (inhibited)}}{\overline{Ab} \text{ (normal)}} = \frac{1}{[f_m/(1 + I/K_I)] + (1 - f_m)} \quad (4)$$

It follows from the above equation that for drugs with $f_m \leqslant 0.5$ the maximum value for R, when inhibition of the pathway is virtually complete $(I \gg K_I)$, is two. And, unless the therapeutic index of a drug is small, an alteration in the dosage regimen of a drug, when coadministered with the inhibitor, is probably unwarranted. Also, if the dosage regimen of a drug is maintained whose f_m is > 0.5, an adverse reaction may be seen before the new plateau is reached or, if seen at the plateau, it will take some time ($4 \times T\frac{1}{2}$ inhibited) after initiation of the inhibitor regimen.* Alternatively, to prevent drug accumulation, the dosage schedule of the drug will have to be reduced to $1/R$ of the normal regimen. The situation will be more complex when the concentration of drug at the metabolic site exceeds its K_m value, and when both drugs are competitors of one or more of the other's pathways.

Tolbutamide, an acid, is significantly bound to plasma and presumably tissue proteins. Its hypoglycemic activity probably is a function of the unbound concentration in the plasma and tissue waters. Sulfaphenazole, dicoumarol, and phenylbutazone are also acids, highly bound to plasma

---

* When the inhibitor $T\frac{1}{2}$ is longer than the $T\frac{1}{2}$ of the drug at the plateau level of the inhibitor ($T\frac{1}{2}$, inhibited) and both are given on a fixed-dose fixed-interval regimen, then the accumulation kinetics of the drug becomes controlled by the inhibitor $T\frac{1}{2}$.

and tissue proteins, and are capable of displacing tolbutamide and one another from albumin in *in vitro* experiments (19). Because of these associations, protein-binding displacement has been intimated as a contributory cause of the enhanced hypoglycemic experience when these drugs are used in combination with tolbutamide. Certainly, the extent of binding in plasma often has to be considered. Christensen et al. (17) noted that, at approximately the same plasma-tolbutamide concentration the hypoglycemic effect was more pronounced when methyl-sulfaphenazole, an inhibitor of tolbutamide elimination, was added to a reduced daily regimen of the sulfonylurea. This observation may be explained by the higher unbound concentration in the presence of the methyl-sulfaphenazole. However, it is unlikely that the contribution of displacement alone to tolbutamide therapy is major, compared to inhibition of oxidation, as many other sulfonamides, which substantially displace tolbutamide from albumin neither prolong its half-life nor potentiate its effect (22, 28). Nonetheless, it is worthwhile to consider certain aspects of displacement.

Appreciable drug displacement occurs when a major portion of the same binding sites are occupied by the displacing agent. In plasma, tolbutamide is primarily bound to albumin (29). Consequently, to displace tolbutamide from plasma albumin requires that the plasma concentration of the displacer at least approaches or exceeds 0.6 mM, the concentration of plasma albumin. For a substance of molecular weight of 300, this corresponds to 180 mg/l. This plasma concentration is seen with sulfonamides and salicylates, which are commonly given in gram doses and which possess small volumes of distribution. It is also approached with phenylbutazone. Although the normal dose of this anti-inflammatory agent is 100 mg, owing to its long half-life, phenylbutazone accumulates to well over 1 g in the body when given three times daily. Plasma concentrations exceeding 0.6 mM can also be achieved following the rapid intravenous bolus (< 10 sec) of quite modest doses. These events are likely fleeting, however, as displacer mixes with the vascular system and distributes out into the tissues. The rapid injection of even larger doses (> 14 mg/kg) of displacer, which reside primarily in plasma, will produce significant rises in the unbound-drug concentration but only transiently as displaced drug moves out into the large tissue water space down the newly created concentration gradient (30). However, such a transient rise in the unbound concentration of tolbutamide in plasma may be sufficient to cause additional insulin release and depression of the blood glucose.

An appreciable increase in the fraction of unbound, and presumably pharmacologically active, drug in the body will occur only if drug is normally substantially bound to and is displaced from both plasma and tissue-binding sites. Displacement from plasma sites alone is inconsequential. Thus, the fraction of a drug in the body bound to plasma proteins is $3\beta/Vd$, where 3 is the plasma volume in liters, Vd the volume of distribution of the drug, also expressed in liters, and β is the fraction of drug in plasma bound to plasma proteins. For tolbutamide, $\beta \approx 0.95$ and Vd $= 10$ l (19) in man, which means that approximately 30% in the body resides on the plasma proteins. Nonetheless, even in the extremely unlikely event of it being completely displaced off its plasma-binding sites ($\beta \rightarrow$ O), with a dramatic drop in the total plasma concentration, this 30% added to the remaining 70% would only increase the unbound concentration in the body by 42%. This increase is small compared to the normal changes in the unbound concentration as tolbutamide is eliminated. Any substantial increase in unbound concentration above that anticipated from plasma displacement automatically implies that tissue binding is significant and that tissue displacement must have occurred.

Experiments in sheep point to the possibility of significant tissue displacement of tolbutamide. At 60 μg/ml, 84% of drug in plasma is bound to plasma proteins ($\beta = 0.84$) and the volume of distribution is 11 1/50 kg animal. At the end of a 3-hr infusion of sulfadimethoxine, at the rate of 2 g/hr, the unbound plasma concentration had risen twofold, whereas β had increased to 0.5 (Fig. 5). Calculations, analogous to those described pre-

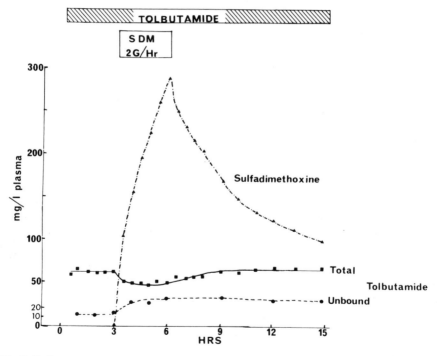

FIG. 5. Tolbutamide-sulfadimethoxine interaction in sheep. Tolbutamide is infused at a constant rate (95 mg/hr) throughout the experiment. Initially, both total- and unbound-plasma concentrations remain constant but as sulfadimethoxine displaces tolbutamide from binding sites, total levels fall and unbound concentrations rise. Failure of the unbound tolbutamide concentration to return to presulfonamide level suggests that sulfadimethoxine may also inhibit tolbutamide elimination.

viously, clearly indicate that plasma displacement alone accounts for only a small fraction of the increase in the unbound concentration.

So far, much of the comments refer to situations where drug is given only once in the absence and presence of displacer. The more common clinical picture is where both are given on a multiple-dose regimen. The experiment in the sheep where tolbutamide is infused continuously, while sulfadimethoxine is infused over several hours, attempts to mimic the clinical situation. In this regard, it is interesting to note the failure of the unbound concentration to return to the presulfonamide levels (Fig. 5). In the sheep, the hepatic extraction ratio is only 0.01, a value estimated from a clearance for tolbutamide of 30 ml/kg/hr and a knowledge that only 15% of the drug is excreted unchanged *(personal observation)*. For drugs, such as tolbutamide, which have a low hepatic extraction ratio, clearance *(CL)* should be dependent on the unbound plasma concentration *(C_f)* such that

$$CL = \alpha\, CL_{\max},\tag{5}$$

where α is the fraction of drug unbound in plasma. Clearance increases with displacement and is maximum *($CL_{\max}$)* when all drug in plasma is unbound ($\alpha = 1$). This equation is analogous to the one describing the influence of protein binding on the renal clearance of a drug that is solely cleared by glomerular filtration and is not reabsorbed, $CL_{\max}$ now being the glomerular filtration rate (31). Upon a constant rate of infusion ($R°$), the steady-state plasma concentration *(C_{pss})* is defined by

$$R° = CL \cdot C_{pss}.\tag{6}$$

By appropriately substituting Eq. 5 into Eq. 6 and realizing that $C_p = C_f/\alpha$, the steady-state equation can be rewritten as

$$R° = CL_{\max} \cdot C_{fss}.\tag{7}$$

Thus, at the steady state the unbound concentration should be constant and independent of the degree of protein binding. Or, stated differently, if a compound only acts to displace a drug, it may cause variations in the unbound-drug concentration between but not at steady state. The fact that, in the constant tolbutamide infusion experiment, the unbound concentration in the presence of sulfadimethoxine did not tend to return to the pre-existing steady-state value (Fig. 5), is therefore taken to suggest that this sulfonamide does more than displace tolbutamide. The elevated unbound concentration implies that $CL_{\max}$ is diminished presumably through inhibition of tolbutamide metabolism.

The effect of sulfadimethoxine on tolbutamide elimination in man is unclear. Sulfadimethoxine is said to either result in no change (28) or shorten (19) tolbutamide elimination half-life. However, because it is determined by clearance and volume of distribution, which are both altered by displacement, half-life is a poor index of events occurring at the metabolite site. More detailed analysis is needed before definitive statements can be made, including measurement of the unbound-drug concentration.

The studies of the interaction of tolbutamide with other drugs stress the importance of measuring both bound and unbound drug and metabolites. Pharmacokinetic analysis aids in the interpretation of such data and allows the establishment of models to describe the temporal changes of the pertinent chemical species. Ultimately, it is hoped that this quantitative kinetic approach can be integrated with and be used to predict the pharmacological sequalae following a given drug interaction.

ACKNOWLEDGMENTS

Much of the work reported in this chapter was supported by U.S. Public Health Service Grants AM 12763–06 and NIGMS 16496, from the National Institutes of Health, National Institutes of General Medical Sciences, and Training Grant 5 TO1 GM 00728.

REFERENCES

1. MacGregor, A. G. (1965): *Proc. Royal Soc. Med. 58*, 943.
2. Melmon, K., Morelli, H. F., Oates, J. A., Conney, A. H., Tozer, T. N., Harpole, B. P., and Clark, T. H. (1967): *Patient Care 1.*
3. Hartshorn, E. A. (1968): *Drug Intelligence 2*, 174.
4. Azarnoff, D. L., and Hurwitz, A. (1970): *Pharmacol. Physicians 4*, 1–5.
5. Yesair, D. W., Bullock, F. J., and Coffey, J. J. (1972): *Drug. Metab. Rev. 1*, 35.
6. Hansten, P. D. (1973): *Drug Interactions*, 2nd. Ed., Lea and Febiger, Philadelphia.
7. Martin, E. W. (1971): *Hazards of Medication*, Lippincott, Philadelphia.
8. Evaluations of Drug Interactions (1973): American Pharmaceutical Association, Washington, D.C.
9. Prescott, L. F. (1969): *Lancet, N. Amer. Ed. 2*, 1239.
10. Morrelli, H. F. (1970): In: *Clinical Pharmacology*, ed. K. H. Melmon and H. F. Morrelli, Chap. 17, MacMillan Press, Washington.
11. Wagner, J. G. (1968): *Ann. Rev. Pharmacol. 8*, 67.
12. Levy, G. (1966): *Clin. Pharmacol. Therap. 7*, 362.
13. Levy, G., and Gibaldi, M. (1972): *Ann. Rev. Pharmacol. 12*, 85.
14. Levy, G., and Yamada, H. (1971): *J. Pharm. Sci. 60*, 215.
15. Sellers, E. M., and Koch-Weser, J. (1971): *Ann. N.Y. Acad. Sci. 179*, 213.
16. Riegelman, S., Rowland, M., and Epstein, W. L. (1970): *J. Amer. Med. Assoc. 213*, 426.
17. Christensen, L. K. (1969): III International Diabetic Symposium. Pharmacokinetics and Mode of Action of Oral Hypoglycemic Agents, Capri, 1969. *Acta Diabetologica Lat. 6 (Suppl. 1), 143.*
18. Hussar, D. A. (1970): *J. Amer. Pharm. Assoc. 10*, 619.
19. Tagg, J., Yasada, D. M., Tanabe, M., and Mitoma, C. (1967): *Biochem. Pharmacol. 16*, 143.
20. Thomas, R. C., and Ikeda, C. J. (1966): *J. Med. Chem. 9*, 507.
21. Schulz, E., and Schmidt, F. H. (1970): *Pharmacol. Clin. 2*, 150.
22. Christensen, L. K., Hansen, J. M., and Kristensen, M. (1963): *Lancet 2*, 1298.
23. Rowland, M., and Matin, S. B. *(in press): J. Pharmacok. Biopharm.*
24. Riess, W., Schmidt, K., and Keberle, H. (1965): *Klin. Wochen. 43*, 740.
25. Duncan, L. J. P., and Baird, J. D. (1957): *Scott. Med. J. 2*, 171.
26. Rowland, M. (1970): *Clinical Pharmacology*, Chap. 2, ed. K. H. Melmon and H. F. Morrelli, MacMillan Press, Washington.

27. Wagner, J. G., Northam, J. I., Alway, C. D., and Carpenter, O. S. (1965): *Nature 207*, 1301.
28. Dubach, U. C., Bückert, A., and Raaflaub, J. (1966): *Schweiz. Med. Wschr. 96*, 1483.
29. Wishinsky, H., Glaser, E., and Perkal, S. (1962): *Diabetes 11*, 18.
30. McQueen, E. G., and Wardell, W. M. (1971): *Brit. J. Pharmac. 43*, 312.
31. Wagner, J. G. (1971): Biopharmaceutics and relevant pharmacokinetics, p. 247, Drug Intelligence, Illinois.

Drug Interactions, edited by P. L. Morselli,
S. Garattini, and S. N. Cohen. Raven Press,
New York © 1974

Interactions with Antiepileptic Drugs Involving Multiple Mechanisms

Henn Kutt

Departments of Neurology and Pharmacology, Cornell University Medical College, New York, New York 10021

INTRODUCTION

Numerous interactions between antiepileptic drugs themselves or between antiepileptic drugs and other therapeutic or chemical agents have been reported in recent years and reviewed elsewhere (1–3). Most of these interactions are manifested by changes of the plasma level of the primary drug after addition of another drug. Although various pharmacokinetic parameters may be involved in causing these changes, an alteration of the rate of drug metabolism is the most frequently implicated mechanism.

It is important to emphasize that the extent of plasma level changes with a given interacting drug combination may vary considerably among the patients taking even the same doses of these agents. Whether or not the plasma level change is clinically significant depends in part on the starting plasma level of the primary drug. When the latter is high, a relatively small increase may result in intoxication. When the starting level is low, a relatively large increase may merely improve the seizure control, but have no adverse effects. Furthermore, with the exception of a few drug combinations, marked plasma level changes occur only in a minority, apparently particularly susceptible individuals. Thus several of the potentially interacting drug combinations may be administered, if clinically indicated, with caution and with relative safety when the primary drug plasma levels are being monitored. Sometimes dosages that are smaller or larger than the average antiepileptic doses need to be used during polypharmacy.

The majority of interactions with antiepileptic drugs reported so far involve diphenylhydantoin for several reasons. (a) Diphenylhydantoin is particularly vulnerable to factors that alter the rate of its biotransformation, as it is eliminated almost entirely in the metabolized form(s). (b) Diphenylhydantoin is one of the most widely used antiepileptic drugs. (c) Adequate methods for determination of diphenylhydantoin concentration have been available for a long time.

INTERACTIONS BETWEEN DIPHENYLHYDANTOIN
AND SOME OTHER COMMONLY USED DRUGS

Table 1 contains data from various studies about drugs that have been observed to increase diphenylhydantoin plasma levels. Disulfiram has caused marked elevation of diphenylhydantoin plasma levels in the majority of patients taking these agents together (4, 5). Sulthiame also caused marked or moderate elevations of diphenylhydantoin plasma levels in the majority of patients (6, 7). Isoniazid caused clinically significant elevations of diphenylhydantoin plasma levels in approximately 10% of patients taking these drugs in combination (8, 20). Bishydroxycoumarin (9), methylphenidate (12, 21, 22, 23), phenothiazines (17), and benzodiazepines (13, 17) have caused marked diphenylhydantoin plasma level elevations only in a few patients out of many taking these drugs together. It is apparent that with the majority of interacting drugs listed in Table 1, clinically significant effects have occurred only in a minority of patients who have taken them.

The mechanisms that determine the extent of diphenylhydantoin accumulation, in individual patients, caused by the interacting drugs are not all clear, and more work is needed to clarify the specific reasons for variations in individual susceptibility.

The available clinical and experimental data about two interactions will now be evaluated and discussed in detail. These include the diphenylhydantoin-isoniazid interaction and the diphenylhydantoin-phenobarbital interaction.

INTERACTION BETWEEN DIPHENYLHYDANTOIN AND ISONIAZID

Clinical Observations

Elevations of previously stabilized diphenylhydantoin plasma levels have been observed in patients after isoniazid has been added to their medication. Marked elevations and clinically evident diphenylhydantoin intoxication occur in about 10% of patients taking this drug combination. Minor elevations occur more frequently (20 to 30% of patients), whereas in at least 50% or more of the patients, no change of diphenylhydantoin plasma level occurs after addition of isoniazid in the commonly used clinical doses of 300 mg isoniazid daily (8, 20, 24). The diphenylhydantoin plasma levels in the apparently susceptible patients usually reached toxic concentrations within 2 to 4 weeks after the onset of isoniazid administration. Concurrent use of aminosalicylic acid seemed to accentuate the isoniazid effect in some patients (24). The clinical problem in the toxic patients was usually solved by a reduction of diphenylhydantoin dosage from the commonly given amount of 300 to 400 mg daily to 100 to 200 mg daily. This resulted in a decline of the diphenylhydantoin plasma level

TABLE 1. *Drugs that have been noted to elevate diphenylhydantoin (DPH) plasma levels and prolong its half-life*

References	Drug	No. of patients	DPH levels[a] before admin. of other drug	DPH levels[a] during admin. of other drug	Increase of plasma half-life of DPH	Probability of marked elevations of DPH level
Kiørboe (4); Olesen (5)	Disulfiram	9	4–20	18–51		high
Hansen et al. (6); Olesen and Jensen (7)	Sulthiame	11 4	4–14	8–28		moderate
Kutt et al. (8)	Isoniazid	34	8–20	34–61	×2	moderate
Hansen et al. (9)	Dicoumarol	6 3	4–20	12–40		low
Solomon and Schrogie (10)	Phenyramidol	5 5	4–10	8–14	×4	low
Christensen and Skovsted (11)	Chloramphenicol	2 3	2–3	7–11	×2	low
Garrettson et al. (12)	Methylphenidate	1	9	28		low
Vajda et al. (13)	Chlordiazepoxide or diazepam				×2.5	low
Siersbaek-Nielsen et al. (14)	Sulfamethizole	4 1	4–20 unknown	11–41 intox.	×2	low
Kutt and Louis (15)	Methylphenidate	6				low
Hansen et al. (9)	Phenylbutazole					low
Frantzen et al. (16)	Sulfaphenazole					low
Kutt and McDowell (17)	Ethosuximide					low
	Chlorpromazine					low
	Prochlorperazine					low
	Chlordiazepoxide					low
Karlin and Kutt (18)	Halothane					low
Kutt (19)	Propoxyphene					low

[a] Expressed as µg/ml.

and stabilization at a new nontoxic but effective range. The signs and symptoms of diphenylhydantoin intoxication disappeared.

Experimental Studies

In order to study the relationships between isoniazid dosage and its effect upon diphenylhydantoin plasma levels, animal experiments were carried out in our laboratory. Groups of rats were given constant doses of diphenyl-hydantoin (50 mg/kg) and varying doses of isoniazid (6 to 50 mg/kg). The animals receiving higher doses of isoniazid achieved higher diphenyl-hydantoin plasma levels (25). Cats were given diphenylhydantoin daily and stable diphenylhydantoin plasma levels were achieved. Then isoniazid was given, and elevations of diphenylhydantoin plasma levels occurred, which were proportional to the dosage and plasma levels of isoniazid (26).

In vitro studies using fortified rat hepatic microsomal systems (for details, see legend of Fig. 1) demonstrated that the addition of isoniazid to the incubation mixtures strongly inhibited diphenylhydantoin metabolism (8, 25). The double reciprocal plot seen in Fig. 1 suggests that this inhibition is of a noncompetitive type. Aminosalicylic acid also inhibited the diphenyl-

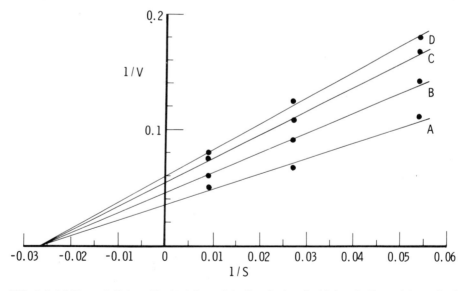

FIG. 1. Inhibition of diphenylhydantoin metabolism by isoniazid. Incubation mixture: 2 ml of 9,000 × g supernatant fraction of rat liver and 3 ml of 0.2 M phosphate buffer, pH 7.4; cofactors: NADP 8.2×10^{-4} M, NAD 9.3×10^{-4} M and ATP 3.9×10^{-3} M. V expressed as nmoles of diphenylhydantoin metabolized per 15 min per 10 mg of protein per ml. S expressed as nmoles of diphenylhydantoin per ml. Curve A: control. Curves B, C, and D: isoniazid added in concentrations of 3.6×10^{-5} M, 1.1×10^{-4} M, and 5.4×10^{-4} M, respectively.

hydantoin metabolism to a small extent. Addition of this agent to incubation mixtures which contained isoniazid as the inhibitor markedly potentiated the isoniazid effects, perhaps by prolonging the stay of isoniazid in the active form. Thus the laboratory experiments demonstrated that isoniazid is an inhibitor of diphenylhydantoin metabolism, and this action could explain the elevation of diphenylhydantoin plasma levels in the patients in whom this occurred.

In order to understand the variations in individual susceptibility in regard to the extent of the diphenylhydantoin-isoniazid interaction, further clinical studies were carried out (8, 26). These revealed that the extent of diphenylhydantoin plasma level elevations by isoniazid was greatest in the very slow isoniazid inactivators, whose isoniazid plasma levels were over 8 μg/ml 3 hr after a test dose of 10 mg of isoniazid per kg. Modest elevation of diphenylhydantoin plasma levels were seen in patients whose isoniazid plasma levels ranged from 6 to 8 μg/ml. In the fast isoniazid inactivators, whose isoniazid plasma level remained below 6 μg/ml 3 hr after the test dose, no elevations of diphenylhydantoin plasma levels were observed. Thus, also in man, the extent of diphenylhydantoin plasma level elevation by isoniazid seemed to be related to isoniazid concentration. Determination of the phenotype in regard to the isoniazid inactivation was found to be helpful for predicting which patients may develop clinically significant isoniazid-diphenylhydantoin interactions, i.e., identifying the susceptible individuals.

INTERACTION BETWEEN DIPHENYLHYDANTOIN AND PHENOBARBITAL

Clinical Observations

Various observations indicate that diphenylhydantoin plasma levels in epileptic patients who are taking diphenylhydantoin alone may become altered after phenobarbital has been added to their medication. Table 2 summarizes data from several clinical studies in which diphenylhydantoin plasma levels have been monitored before and after addition of phenobarbital. In some patients, a decline of diphenylhydantoin plasma level was seen, in others, no change occurred, whereas in still others, a rise of diphenylhydantoin level took place. It has been commented that the higher the starting plasma level of diphenylhydantoin, or the higher the phenobarbital dose (3, 35), the more likely a decline of diphenylhydantoin plasma level will occur. Shortening of the apparent plasma half-life of diphenylhydantoin by phenobarbital has been observed in some patients (36).

The decline of diphenylhydantoin plasma level or the shortening of its apparent plasma half-life is generally believed to result from the stimulation of diphenylhydantoin metabolism by phenobarbital, although possible

TABLE 2. *The effect of phenobarbital (PB) on the plasma level of diphenylhydantoin (DPH)*

Reference	No. of patients	DPH levels before administration of PB (μg/ml)		DPH levels during administration of PB (μg/ml)		DPH level change
		range	average	range	average	
Cucinell et al. (27)	5	7–22	11	4–15	7	down
Buchanan et al. (28)	4	3–12	6.6	1–7	2.6	down
	1	—	7	—	7	none
Kutt et al. (29)	9	5–23	13	4–17	10	down
	11	3–19	9	3–19	9	none
	6	4–18	9	6–22	11	rise
Diamond and Buchanan (30)	4	1.5–6.1	4.4	0.7–4.7	2.9	down
	3	0.9–3.5	3.3	0.9–3.5	3.3	none
	3	0.6–7.5	4.1	1.1–8.1	5.0	rise
Garrettson and Dayton (31)	2	3.3–21	12	0.4–12	6.0	down
	1	—	2.8	—	2.8	none
	1	—	2.8	—	3.9	rise
Morselli et al. (32)	5	4–40	16	1–17	6	down
	2	5–8	6.5	5–8	6.5	none
Hirschmann (33)	1	—	17	—	28	rise
Booker et al. (34)	8	unknown	15.1	unknown	19.5	rise

effects upon other pharmacokinetic parameters, such as absorption, are not known.

Experimental Studies

Pretreatment with phenobarbital has been found to shorten the diphenyl-hydantoin plasma half-life in dogs (35, 37). We have studied the effect of phenobarbital pretreatment on diphenylhydantoin metabolism in rats (38). Sprague-Dawley white male rats weighing 200 g were treated with pheno-barbital dissolved in saline. The dosage was 75 mg per kg daily, for 3 to 7 days, given intraperitoneally. Control animals received saline injections. The animals were sacrificed 24 hr following the last injection. Isolated hepatic microsomes and 9,000 × g supernatant fractions were prepared and incubated with diphenylhydantoin as substrate in the presence of appropriate cofactors (details given in legend of Fig. 2) (38). The pre-

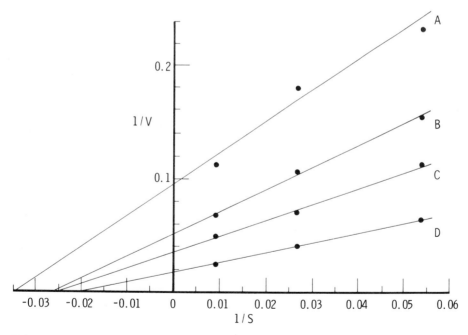

FIG. 2. Stimulation of diphenylhydantoin metabolism by rat hepatic microsomal prepara-tions following pretreatments with phenobarbital (75 mg/kg daily) for 7 days. Incubation mixture: 0.5 ml of Hepes buffer pH 7.4, 0.25 ml of soluble fraction; 0.5 ml of enzyme; 1.72 μmole of NADP; 12.5 μmole of glucose-6-phosphate; 12.5 μmole of MgSO$_4$; and water to make a final volume of 2.5 ml. V expressed as nmoles of diphenylhydantoin metabolized per 2 mg of microsomal protein per ml per 10 min. S expressed as nmoles of diphenyl-hydantoin per ml. Curve A: control microsomes. Curve B: control 9,000 × g supernatant fraction. Curve C: phenobarbital treatment microsomes. Curve D: phenobarbital treat-ment 9,000 × g supernatant fraction.

treatment for 7 days nearly doubled the V_{max} for diphenylhydantoin metabolism by both the isolated microsomes and the $9,000 \times g$ supernatant as compared to the preparations from control animals (see Fig. 2). Pretreatment for 3 days increased the V_{max} by approximately 50%. The apparent K_m was increased by phenobarbital pretreatments. Thus it is clear that pretreatment with phenobarbital increases the diphenylhydantoin metabolizing enzyme activity per mg of microsomal protein in rats, although this increase may not be as marked as seen with some other substrates. Stimulation of diphenylhydantoin metabolism by phenobarbital in rat hepatic microsomal preparations has been also observed by other investigators (39).

On the other hand, phenobarbital inhibited diphenylhydantoin metabolism when it was added to incubation mixtures containing fortified rat hepatic $9,000 \times g$ supernatant fraction from untreated control animals (40). Figure 3 suggests that this inhibition was of competitive type. Competitive inhibition of diphenylhydantoin metabolism by phenobarbital *in vitro* was noted also by Gabler and Hubbard (41).

Further evidence that phenobarbital can interfere with formation of the diphenylhydantoin enzyme complex was obtained in our studies of substrate-induced difference spectra (42). Addition of diphenylhydantoin to isolated rat hepatic microsomes suspended in Hepe's buffer, pH 7.4, pro-

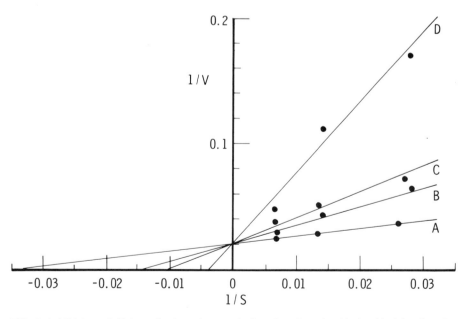

FIG. 3. Inhibition of diphenylhydantoin metabolism by phenobarbital added *in vitro*. Incubation mixture as in Fig. 1. Curve A: control; curves B, C, and D: phenobarbital added in concentrations 5.9×10^{-4} M, 1.1×10^{-3} M and 2.3×10^{-3} M, respectively.

duced a type I spectral response. The K_s was approximately 30 μM and the δA_{max} ranged from O.D. 0.02 to 0.04 with 3 mg of microsomal protein per ml. Addition of phenobarbital, also a type I substrate, as a modifier to the microsomal suspension before adding diphenylhydantoin reduced the δA_{max} of the diphenylhydantoin-induced difference spectra, as seen in Fig. 4; and Fig. 5 suggests that this interference was competitive in nature. The δA_{max} of the diphenylhydantoin-induced difference spectra was also reduced with the microsomes obtained from rats pretreated with phenobarbital, as compared to microsomes obtained from rats injected with saline. This was attributed to phenobarbital found in small quantities in the microsomes, following the pretreatments (43).

Thus it appears that phenobarbital can have a dual effect upon diphenylhydantoin metabolism. On one hand, it can induce the production of the diphenylhydantoin-metabolizing enzyme, but on the other hand, it can inhibit the action of this enzyme. The net result in the clinical situations probably depends upon the balance between these two effects. It may be assumed that when no change of diphenylhydantoin plasma level occurs after addition of phenobarbital to the patient's medication, these factors are

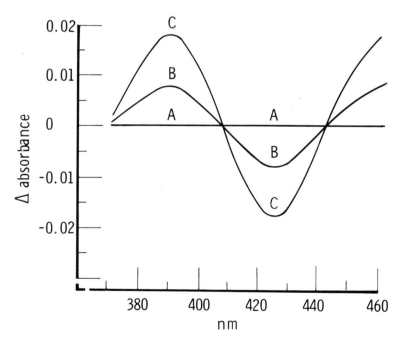

FIG. 4. Diphenylhydantoin-induced difference spectra with nonreduced rat hepatic microsomes from untreated animals. Curve A: baseline. Curves B and C: diphenylhydantoin added to sample cuvette; final concentration 123 μM. In the experiment that rendered curve B, phenobarbital (1.22 $\times$ 10^{-4} M) was added to microsomes as modifier before addition of diphenylhydantoin.

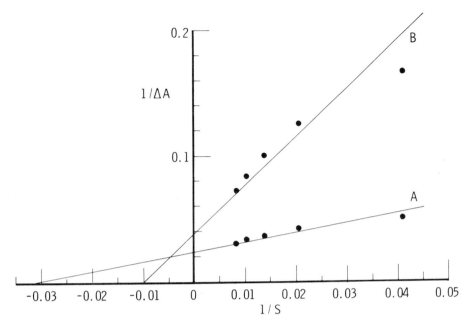

FIG. 5. Reduction of δA_{max} of diphenylhydantoin-induced difference spectra by phenobarbital as modifier. Study mixture: isolated rat hepatic microsomes 3 mg of microsomal protein per ml in 0.1 M Hepes buffer pH 7.4. δA expressed as O.D. × 1,000 between 390 and 425 nm. S expressed as nmoles of diphenylhydantoin per ml. Curve A: control. Curve B: phenobarbital added to microsomes (1.22×10^{-4} M).

in balance, when a decline is seen, the induction is evident, and when a rise of diphenylhydantoin plasma level takes place, the inhibition prevails.

The factors that regulate these balances are not all clear, but the patient's previous drug intake history may play a role in that he may already be maximally induced. Also the drug dosages may be important, as well as the genetic make-up of the patient, with regard to the extent of the enzyme inducibility by phenobarbital. The latter point is relevant because work from Vesell's laboratory (44) has shown that the extent of inducibility of the metabolism of aminopyrine by phenobarbital can be genetically determined in man.

SUMMARY

Some interactions with antiepileptic drugs manifest in plasma level changes. Thus elevation of diphenylhydantoin level may be caused by disulfiram, sulthiame, bishydroxycoumarin, benzodiazepines, and isoniazid among others. The extent of these elevations varies considerably among individual patients.

The diphenylhydantoin-isoniazid interaction was studied in detail. In rat hepatic microsomal preparations isoniazid in concentrations of 3.6×10^{-5} M inhibited diphenylhydantoin metabolism by 20% and in concentrations of 5.4×10^{-4} M by 64%. The type of inhibition was noncompetitive. The extent of diphenylhydantoin plasma level elevations by isoniazid in patients was greatest in the very slow isoniazid inactivators, whose isoniazid plasma levels were over 8 μg/ml 3 hr following a test dose of 10 mg/kg of isoniazid.

Studies of phenobarbital-diphenylhydantoin interactions revealed that phenobarbital added to rat hepatic microsomal preparations in concentrations of 6×10^{-4} M inhibited diphenylhydantoin metabolism by 12% and in concentrations of 1.2×10^{-3} M by 36%. Conversely, pretreatment of rats with phenobarbital (75 mg/kg) for 7 days increased the diphenylhydantoin metabolism per mg of microsomal protein by 100%. This dual action may explain why in some patients a decline, in others an elevation, and still in others no change of diphenylhydantoin plasma levels occurs after onset of administration of phenobarbital.

Thus interactions with antiepileptic drugs may be caused by induction or inhibition of their biotransformation. Genetic make-up of the patient may determine in which individuals clinically significant interactions take place.

REFERENCES

1. Kutt, H. (1972): In: *Antiepileptic Drugs*, p. 169, Raven Press, New York.
2. Buchanan, R. A., and Sholiton, L. I. (1972): In: *Antiepileptic Drugs*, p. 180, Raven Press, New York.
3. Cucinell, S. A. (1972): In: *Antiepileptic Drugs*, p. 319, Raven Press, New York.
4. Kiørboe, E. (1966): *Epilepsia 48*, 246.
5. Olesen, O. V. (1966): *Acta Pharmacol. Toxicol. 24*, 317.
6. Hansen, J. M., Kristensen, M., and Skovsted, L. (1968): *Epilepsia 9*, 17.
7. Olesen, V., and Jensen, N. (1969): *Dan. Med. Bull. 16*, 154.
8. Kutt, H., Brennan, R., Dehejia, H., and Verebely, K. (1970): *Amer. Rev. Resp. Dis. 101*, 377.
9. Hansen, J. M., Kristensen, M., Skovsted, L., and Christensen, L. K. (1966): *Lancet 2*, 265.
10. Solomon, H. M., and Schrogie, J. J. (1967): *Clin. Pharmacol. Ther. 8*, 554.
11. Christensen, L. K., and Skovsted, L. (1969): *Lancet 2*, 1397.
12. Garrettson, L. K., Perel, J. M., and Dayton, P. G. (1969): *J. Amer. Med. Assoc. 207*, 2053.
13. Vajda, F. J. E., Prineas, R. J., and Lovell, R. R. H. (1971): *Brit. Med. J. 1*, 346.
14. Siersbaek-Nielsen, K., Mølholm Hansen, J., Skovsted, L., Lumholtz, B., and Kampmann, J. (1973): *Clin. Pharmacol. Ther. 14*, 148.
15. Kutt, H., and Louis, S. (1972): *Drugs 4*, 227.
16. Frantzen, E., Hansen, J. M., Hansen, O. E., and Kristensen, M. (1967): *Acta Neurol. Scand. 43*, 440.
17. Kutt, H., and McDowell, F. (1968): *J. Amer. Med. Assoc. 203*, 969.
18. Karlin, J. M., and Kutt, H. (1970): *J. Pediatr. 76*, 941.
19. Kutt, H. (1971): *Ann. N.Y. Acad. Sci. 179*, 704.
20. Murray, F. J. (1962): *Amer. Rev. Resp. Dis. 86*, 729.
21. Mirkin, B. L., and Wright, F. (1971): *Neurology 21*, 1123.
22. Kupferberg, H. J., Jeffrey, W., and Hunninghake, D. B. (1972): *Clin. Pharmacol. Ther. 13*, 201.

23. Solow, E. B., and Green, J. B. (1972): *Neurology 22*, 540.
24. Kutt, H., Winters, W., and McDowell, F. (1966): *Neurology 16*, 594.
25. Kutt, H., Verebely, K., and McDowell, F. (1968): *Neurology 18*, 706.
26. Brennan, R. W., Dehejia, H., Kutt, H., Verebely, K., and McDowell, F. (1970): *Neurology 20*, 687.
27. Cucinell, S. A., Conney, A. H., Sansur, M. S., and Burns, J. J. (1965): *Clin. Pharmacol. Ther. 6*, 420.
28. Buchanan, R. A., Heffelfinger, J. C., and Weiss, C. F. (1969): *Pediatrics 43*, 114.
29. Kutt, H., Haynes, J., Verebely, K., and McDowell, F. (1969): *Neurology 19*, 611.
30. Diamond, W. D., and Buchanan, R. A. (1970): *J. Clin. Pharmacol. 10*, 306.
31. Garrettson, L. K., and Dayton, P. G. (1970): *Clin. Pharmacol. Ther. 11*, 674.
32. Morselli, P. L., Rizzo, M., and Garattini, S. (1971): *Ann. N.Y. Acad. Sci. 179*, 88.
33. Hirschmann, J. (1969): *Med. Welt. 5*, 705.
34. Booker, H. E., Tormay, A., and Toussaint, J. (1971): *Neurology 21*, 383.
35. Burns, J. J., Cucinell, S. A., Koster, R., and Conney, A. H. (1965): *Ann. N.Y. Acad. Sci. 123*, 273.
36. Kristensen, M., Hansen, J. M., and Skovsted, L. (1969): *Acta Med. Scand. 185*, 347.
37. Frey, H. H., Kampmann, E., and Nielsen, C. K. (1968): *Acta Pharmacol. Toxicol. (Kobenhavn) 26*, 284.
38. Kutt, H., and Fouts, J. R. (1971): *J. Pharmacol. Exp. Ther. 176*, 11.
39. Gerber, N., Weller, W. L., Lynn, R., Rangno, R. E., Sweetman, B. J., and Bush, M. T. (1971): *J. Pharmacol. Exp. Ther. 178*, 567.
40. Kutt, H., and Verebely, K. (1970): *Biochem. Pharmacol. 19*, 675.
41. Gabler, W. L., and Hubbard, G. L. (1972): *Biochem. Pharmacol. 21*, 3071.
42. Kutt, H., Waters, L., and Fouts, J. R. (1970): *Chem. Biol. Interact. 2*, 195.
43. Kutt, H., Waters, L., and Fouts, J. R. (1971): *J. Pharmacol. Exp. Ther. 179*, 101.
44. Vesell, E. S., and Page, J. G. (1969): *J. Clin. Invest. 48*, 2202.

Drug Interactions, edited by P. L. Morselli,
S. Garattini, and S. N. Cohen. Raven Press,
New York © 1974

Increased Rates of Drug Oxidation in Man

A. Breckenridge, M.L'E. Orme, H. Wesseling, M. Bending, and R. J. Lewis

Department of Clinical Pharmacology, Royal Postgraduate Medical School, Du Cane Road, London W.12, England and Veterans' Administration Hospital, 4150 Clement Street, San Francisco, California 94121

INTRODUCTION

Factors that alter rates of drug oxidation in man have been intensively studied over the past decade. In this chapter we consider three aspects of increased rates of drug oxidation. First, the subject of interindividual variation in enzyme induction is discussed, and it is suggested that induction is a dose-dependent phenomenon. Second, as an attempt to overcome the problems of interactions between inducing agents and the oral anticoagulant warfarin, studies on the effect of administration of phenobarbital on the rate of elimination of the enantiomers of warfarin are reported. Thirdly, to suggest that not all increased rates of drug oxidation in man are due to enzyme induction, studies of a novel effect of hydrocortisone on rates of drug oxidation are presented.

ENZYME INDUCTION, A DOSE-DEPENDENT PHENOMENON

Many investigations have classified drugs as inducers or noninducers of liver microsomal enzyme activity based on studies at one dose level. We have carried out studies in which several dose levels of inducing agents have been given to man and the rat and a dose-response relationship investigated.

Six patients on long-term treatment with the oral anticoagulant warfarin were given a fixed dose (100 mg) of secobarbital nightly for 33 days and the effect on anticoagulant response and plasma-warfarin concentration studied. The pattern of these studies has been described elsewhere in detail (1). Anticoagulant control was measured by the thrombotest method of Owren (2) and plasma-warfarin concentrations by a method specific for unchanged warfarin (3). In these six patients, barbiturate administration resulted in a fall in plasma-warfarin concentration that ranged from 5 to 64.5% of control values (Fig. 1). Three months later, the dose of secobarbital was increased to 200 mg nightly, in separate studies in two patients who showed the smallest fall in plasma-warfarin concentration (5 and 15.3%) when given 100 mg

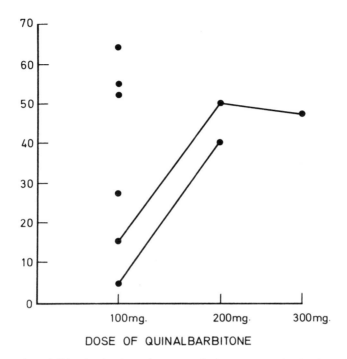

FIG. 1. Percentage fall in steady-state plasma-warfarin concentration in six patients given various doses of secobarbital (quinalbarbitone) nightly for 33 days.

secobarbital nightly. This caused a greater change in plasma-warfarin concentration, which fell by 40.5 and 51%, respectively. Administration of secobarbital, 300 mg nightly, caused no greater decrease in plasma-warfarin concentration than that produced by 200 mg secobarbital in one patient studied after a further period of 3 months (Fig. 1).

To account for the variable fall in plasma-warfarin concentration produced by secobarbital administration, plasma-barbiturate concentrations were measured 12 hr after dosing and the mean values for the last 2 weeks after administration correlated with the percentage fall in plasma-warfarin concentration (Fig. 2). It can be seen that there is a poor correlation between these two parameters. Likewise it was found that the initial rate of warfarin metabolism (calculated by dividing the steady-state plasma-warfarin concentration by the daily dose) correlated poorly with the fall in plasma-warfarin concentration in the nine studies.

To study dose-response curves to other inducing agents, a series of studies in rats was conducted. Dose-response curves were obtained for six barbiturates given at six dose levels for 4 days to groups of six rats. The drugs studied and the doses used were as shown in Table 1. On the 5th day, *in vitro* enzyme activity was assessed by measuring the maximal velocity

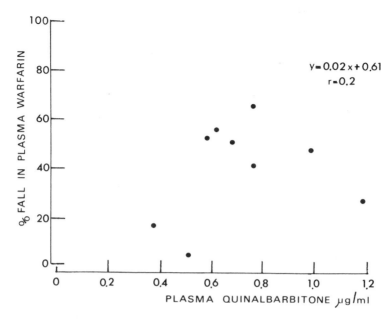

FIG. 2. Correlation of change in plasma warfarin concentration with plasma secobarbital (quinalbarbitone) concentration [by permission of the publishers of *Clin. Pharm. Therap.* (1)].

(V_{max}) of N-demethylation of ethylmorphine in the isolated liver microsomal fraction as described elsewhere (4). A mean value was calculated for each sub-group and expressed as a percentage of the control value. Figure 3 shows these percentage changes. For all six barbiturates, dose-dependent induction could be shown. Phenobarbital and dichlorophenobarbital appeared to be more potent inducing agents than secobarbital and amylobarbital, which in turn are more potent than barbital and thiopental. These lines in Fig. 3 are obviously nonparallel and thus no formal statistical analysis of variance could be done. The plasma half-life of these six barbiturates was measured in groups of eight rats given the drugs by intraperitoneal injection in a dose of 30 mg/kg; further, the liver/plasma ratio was measured 60 min

TABLE 1. *Doses of barbiturates administered to rats (μM/kg day)*

Amobarbital	30.0–533.6
Barbital	13.6–434.3
Dichlorophenobarbital	1.2–217.2
Phenobarbital	3.9–157.2
Secobarbital	31.5–503.8
Thiopental	10.3–166.1

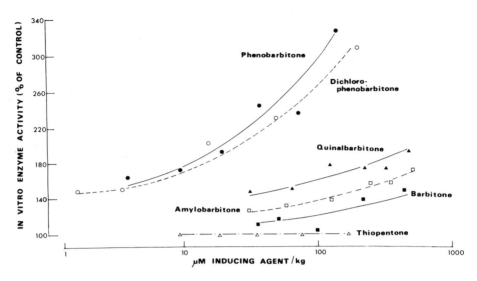

FIG. 3. Change in *in vitro* microsomal enzyme activity in rats pretreated with varying doses of six barbiturates.

after drug administration. As shown in Table 2, there was a relatively poor correlation between the plasma half-life of the drug and its ability to induce liver microsomal enzyme activity. There appeared to be a slightly better correlation between liver/plasma ratio and inducing potency. To study the relationship between the inducing potency and the lipid solubility of the barbiturates, their partition between heptane and water was measured. A 0.2 mM solution of each drug in buffer pH 7.4 was agitated in heptane for 5 min. After extraction into 0.45 M NaOH, the barbiturate concentrations in the organic and aqueous phases were measured. From Table 2, it can be seen that there is little correlation between inducing potency and relative lipid solubility.

These studies clearly illustrate that it is more informative to study in-

TABLE 2. *Plasma half-life, liver/plasma ratio and lipid solubility of six barbiturates*

Drug	$T\frac{1}{2}$ (hr)	Liver/ plasma	Lipid solubility
Phenobarbital	4.9	3.1	.035
Dichlorophenobarbital	32.1	4.6	.039
Secobarbital	0.7	2.0	.31
Amobarbital	0.6	1.6	.25
Barbital	13.1	0.8	.19
Thiopental	1.9	1.7	7.3

ducing agents by constructing dose-response curves than by using data derived from studies at a single dose level. The animal studies, while clearly showing that phenobarbital and dichlorophenobarbital are more potent than the other barbiturates, suggest that there is only a limited correlation between any of the physical parameters studied and inducing potency. In man, the dose response curves to secobarbital again illustrate the importance of taking into consideration the dose of the agent used. In one patient the top of the dose-response curve appeared to have been reached when 200 mg secobarbital was given; a twofold increase in dose from 100 mg produced a change from an insignificant effect to a maximal effect.

EFFECT OF ADMINISTRATION OF INDUCING AGENTS ON THE ENANTIOMERS OF WARFARIN

Warfarin contains an asymetric carbon atom and thus exists as two enantiomers: (S) (−)warfarin and (R) (+)warfarin. Commercial warfarin is a racemic mixture whose pharmacology has been intensively studied: the rate and route of metabolism and the anticoagulant potency differs both in the rat (5) and man (6). The principle metabolic products of (R)warfarin are (R,S)warfarin alcohols, formed by reduction and 6-hydroxy warfarin formed by oxidation; the principle product of (S)warfarin is 7-hydroxy warfarin, formed by oxidation (6). Since (S)warfarin is several times more potent than (R)warfarin, it seemed possible that clinically significant drug interactions might be mediated by alteration in the metabolism of (S)warfarin only.

Thus three male volunteers were given first (R) then (S)warfarin in a dose of 0.5 mg/kg by mouth 10 days apart. (R) and (S)warfarin were a gift from Ward Blenkinsop Pharmaceuticals Ltd. These subjects had taken no other drugs for at least 1 month. The day prior to dosing, each subject was given 20 mg vitamin K_1 by mouth. After dosing, blood samples were taken over 100 hr and the plasma half-life of unchanged warfarin determined using a least-squares method. Subjects were then given phenobarbital 120 mg nightly (two subjects) or antipyrine 300 mg twice daily (one subject) for 44 days. After 30 days, the plasma half-life of one enantiomer was measured, and after 40 days, the plasma half-life of the other.

The apparent volume of distribution (VD) was calculated using the area under the plasma concentration time curve as described elsewhere (7). The plasma clearance of warfarin was also calculated (8).

From Table 3, it can be seen that in each of the three patients studied, the plasma half-life of (R)warfarin was longer than that of (S)warfarin. There was no difference in the VD, and thus the clearance of (R)warfarin was less than (S)warfarin in all three subjects. Administration of phenobarbital (patients 1 and 2) and antipyrine (patient 3) caused a shortening of the

TABLE 3. *Plasma half-life and plasma clearance of the enantiomers of warfarin before and during administration of inducing agents*

Patient		Control		Induced	
		$T \frac{1}{2}$ (hr)	Clearance (ml/hr/kg)	$T \frac{1}{2}$ (hr)	Clearance (ml/hr/kg)
1	R	30.1	3.2	21.2	4.8
	S	20.4	5.5	12.4	7.2
2	R	43.0	2.7	21.5	3.6
	S	18.0	5.2	11.1	8.4
3	R	39.6	2.1	27.7	3.6
	S	21.0	3.5	12.3	7.8

half-lives of both (R) and (S)warfarin and no significant change in the apparent volume of distribution. Thus the clearance of both enantiomers was increased by administration of inducing agents. This gives no support to the use of either enantiomer in clinical practice to avoid the problems encountered in drug interactions between warfarin and inducing agents.

EFFECT OF HYDROCORTISONE ON RATES OF DRUG OXIDATION IN MAN

Recent studies in our laboratory have shown a hitherto undescribed immediate effect of hydrocortisone on the plasma half-life of antipyrine (9).

Antipyrine (900 mg) was taken orally by three fasting normal adults. Over the next 6 hr, blood samples were obtained at hourly intervals. Hydrocortisone hemisuccinate was then given as a single injection 3 mg in 2 ml saline and thereafter infused at a rate of 3 mg/hr for 6 hr. During this time, plasma samples were taken every 30 min. The experiment was repeated 2 weeks later in these subjects, except that the hydrocortisone loading dose was given and the infusion started 2 min prior to antipyrine administration. The infusion of hydrocortisone caused an immediate reduction in the plasma half-life of antipyrine in each of the three subjects. An example is shown in Fig. 4A where the plasma half-life of antipyrine altered from 15.7 to 8.0 hr. When hydrocortisone infusion was started before the administration of antipyrine, the half-life of antipyrine which was 8.1 hr during the infusion, immediately lengthened to 15.1 hr on stopping the hydrocortisone (Fig. 4B). The figure also shows the plasma concentrations of hydrocortisone measured before and during the infusion. At no time did the plasma concentration exceed the highest values found in normal subjects at 9 A.M. (10). A similar alteration was found in the other subjects studied. The apparent volume of distribution of antipyrine was calculated from experiments in which hydrocortisone was given after and before antipyrine. The values did

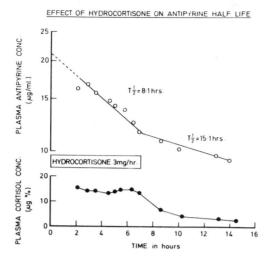

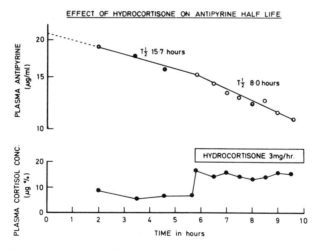

FIG. 4. The effect of an infusion of hydrocortisone 3 mg/hr on the rate of decline of antipyrine concentration and on the plasma hydrocortisone (cortisol) concentration following an oral dose of antipyrine. (top) Hydrocortisone infusion started after antipyrine dosing. (bottom) Hydrocortisone infusion started before antipyrine dosing [by permission of the publishers of the *British Journal of Pharmacology* (9)].

not change significantly. Neither did the administration of hydrocortisone increase the excretion of unchanged antipyrine in urine.

We have demonstrated a similar effect of hydrocortisone on antipyrine elimination in the dog (when antipyrine was given by intravenous infusion), but *in vitro* studies with dog liver have not shown any difference between biopsy samples taken before and during steroid infusion.

The mechanism of this effect of hydrocortisone remains to be elucidated. It is not due to a change in antipyrine absorption, since the effect was seen when hydrocortisone was given before or after antipyrine, and also when antipyrine was given by intravenous infusion to the dog. Since there was no change in the apparent volume of distribution of antipyrine, we must conclude that the rate of metabolic clearance of antipyrine was increased. Our inability to show this effect *in vitro* suggests that either intact cells or the intact organism is necessary to demonstrate this effect of hydrocortisone.

This observation has many implications in studies of drug oxidation in man, and may have important therapeutic applications. From the immediacy of the effect, it is suggested that enzyme induction may not be the underlying mechanism.

ACKNOWLEDGMENTS

We wish to thank Dr. D. S. Davies and Mr. L. Davies for help in these studies. This work was in part supported by the Medical Research Council.

REFERENCES

1. Breckenridge, A., Orme, M. L'E., Davies, L., Thorgeirsson, S. S., and Davies, D. S. (1973): *Clin. Pharmacol. Ther. 14,* 514.
2. Owren, P. A. (1959): *Lancet 2,* 754.
3. Lewis, R. P., Ilnicki, L. P., and Carlstrom, M. (1970): *Biochem. Med. 4,* 376.
4. Breckenridge, A., Orme, M. L'E., Thorgeirsson, S., Davies, D. S., and Brooks, R. V. (1971): *Clin. Sci. 40,* 351.
5. Breckenridge, A., and Orme, M. L'E. (1972): *Life Sci. 2,* 337.
6. Lewis, R. J., Trager, W. F., Chan, K. K., Breckenridge, A., Orme, M., Rowland, M., and Schany, W. (1974): *J. Clin. Invest. (in press).*
7. Wagner, J. G., Northam, J. I., Alway, C. D., and Carpenter, O. S. (1965): *Nature 207,* 1301.
8. Alexanderson, B. (1972): *Europ. J. Clin. Pharmacol. 4,* 82.
9. Breckenridge, A., Burke, C. W., Davies, D. S., and Orme, M. L'E. (1973): *Brit. J. Pharm. 47,* 434.
10. Burke, C. W. (1969): *Brit. Med. J. 2,* 798.

Drug Interactions, edited by P. L. Morselli, S. Garattini, and S. N. Cohen. Raven Press, New York © 1974

Hemodynamic Drug Interactions: The Effects of Altering Hepatic Blood Flow on Drug Disposition

Alan S. Nies, David G. Shand, and Robert A. Branch

School of Medicine, Vanderbilt University, Nashville, Tennessee 37232

INTRODUCTION

One drug may affect the absorption, distribution, or elimination of another drug by numerous mechanisms. In view of the central role of the circulation in transporting a drug from the site of administration, to the sites of action, and to the organs of elimination, it is not surprising that alteration of blood flow is one way to affect the kinetics of drugs and indeed be a point where two drugs can interact. Thus the hemodynamic effects of one drug can alter the disposition of another. Specifically, it is now clear that hepatic blood flow is an important determinant of the elimination of certain drugs, such that the disposition of these drugs can be affected by drug-induced changes in blood flow to the liver. These hemodynamic drug interactions have, as yet, been investigated only in experimental animals; however, there is little doubt that they also occur in man.

INFLUENCE OF HEPATIC BLOOD FLOW ON DRUG ELIMINATION

The importance of hepatic blood flow to drug elimination is related to the ability of the liver to extract drug from the blood, that is, the higher the hepatic extraction of the drug, the greater the influence of hepatic blood flow on drug clearance. If the extraction of a drug is quantitative on a single passage through the liver, then hepatic blood flow determines the hepatic clearance of that drug. For drugs with hepatic extraction ratios of less than 1.0, the influence of hepatic blood flow on drug elimination is less but may still be important.

Because the hepatic extraction ratio is dependent on flow, no simple one-to-one correlation exists between drug clearance and blood flow. The precise relationship between drug clearance, hepatic blood flow, and the drug-eliminating mechanisms of the liver is understood best by referring to the perfusion-limited pharmacokinetic model of Rowland et al. (1).

Assuming that (a) the drug is eliminated by a first-order process, (b) the drug in the hepatic venous blood and the liver is in equilibrium, and (c) the volume of distribution is constant, then the following relationship is valid.

Hepatic drug clearance = Hepatic blood flow (Q) × Hepatic extraction ratio,

$$= Q\left[\frac{\text{Intrinsic hepatic clearance}}{Q + \text{intrinsic hepatic clearance}}\right] \tag{1}$$

The intrinsic hepatic clearance (Cm) is a function of the rate constant for drug elimination, the hepatic volume, and the partition of the drug into the liver from the blood. Cm is a measure of the optimal activity of the hepatic elimination process (metabolism and biliary secretion) and indeed is equal to the maximum drug clearance achievable when hepatic blood flow is not rate limiting. Cm is thus a distinctive property of a particular drug and will remain unchanged unless there are changes in hepatic enzyme activity, biliary secretory capacity, volume of liver or drug binding, or partition into the liver.

The relationship in Eq. 1 indicates that Cm and flow are the two independent variables, whereas actual drug clearance and hepatic extraction ratio are dependent on both flow and Cm. Using this model, one can calculate Cm from any two of the measurable parameters (flow, extraction, and drug clearance) and, from this, compute the expected changes in actual drug clearance associated with changes in liver blood flow or Cm.

As hepatic blood flow increases, actual drug clearance increases to a plateau value. The height of the plateau clearance and the flow at which it is obtained is dependent upon the Cm. However, physiologic restrictions on hepatic blood flow *in vivo* dictate which portion of the curve in Fig. 1 is

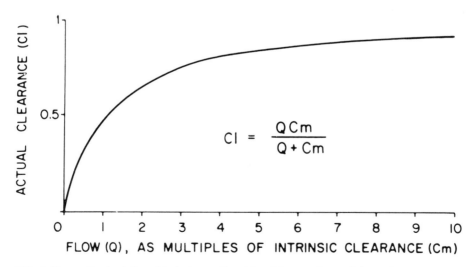

FIG. 1. Theoretical relationship between liver blood flow and actual drug clearance. Both flow and actual clearance have been calculated and computed as multiples of intrinsic metabolic clearance using Eq. 1 in the text. Reprinted from *Drug Metab. and Dispos.* with permission (2).

operative for any given drug. When Cm is very large relative to flow, Eq. 1 simplifies to clearance = flow and the plateau is not attained *in vivo*. When flow is much greater than Cm, clearance is equal to Cm and is independent of flow. For intermediate conditions, when Cm and flow are of the same order of magnitude, clearance is partially flow dependent. Figure 2 shows the expected effects of altering hepatic blood flow from 0.5 to 2 times normal for a series of drugs with different extraction ratios (and thus different Cm values) at normal flow. For drugs with high hepatic extraction ratios (and hence high intrinsic hepatic clearances) actual drug clearance is flow dependent over the range of alteration of hepatic blood flow achievable *in vivo*. The lower the extraction ratio, the less effect flow has on drug clearance, and for drugs with very low extraction ratios, actual drug clearance is nearly independent of flow. Thus, significant hemodynamic drug interactions will occur only with high clearance drugs that have a normally high hepatic extraction ratio.

So far we have discussed only the theoretical aspects of altering hepatic blood flow. Experimental evidence is available, however, to substantiate this theoretical analysis. *In vitro* blood flow through the isolated perfused rat liver can be precisely controlled and drug clearance calculated. Using such a system and propranolol as a test drug, we have found the effects of flow on drug clearance to be those predicted by the theoretical model (2). In this system the two isomers of propranolol are handled identically.

In vivo the clearance of propranolol also substantiates the validity of the model (3). In the monkey, the kinetics and hemodynamic effects of DL-

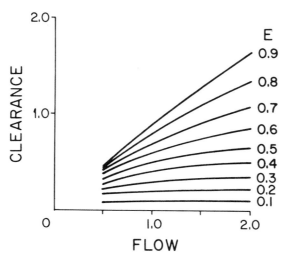

FIG. 2. Theoretical effects of altering hepatic blood flow from one-half to twice normal on the clearance of drugs with various extraction ratios *(E)* at normal flow. Normal flow represented as 1.0. Reprinted from *Drug Metab. and Disp.* with permission (2).

propranolol were compared to those of D-propranolol. Hemodynamic effects were seen with the beta adrenergic-blocking drug, DL-propranolol, which decreased blood flow to all organs except the brain, whereas D-propranolol was without effect (4). Hepatic blood flow was thus 35% lower during administration of DL-propranolol than D-propranolol. In addition, the clearance of DL-propranolol, which has a hepatic extraction of 0.50 in the monkey, was 25% lower than the clearance of D-propranolol. Since *in vitro* experiments indicated that the two isomers of propranolol were equally well extracted by the liver, the discrepancy in drug clearance between D- and DL-propranolol *in vivo* is explained best by the decreased delivery of DL-propranolol to the liver as a consequence of beta-adrenergic blockade. Indeed the calculated Cm values for the two isomers in the monkey are identical and the magnitude of the difference in clearance of racemic versus D-propranolol is that predicted by the model from Eq. 1. With the theoretical analysis confirmed by these *in vitro* and *in vivo* experiments as a basis, one can examine more complex examples of altering hepatic blood flow, including the hemodynamic drug interactions.

HEMODYNAMIC DRUG INTERACTIONS RESULTING FROM DECREASED LIVER BLOOD FLOW

Just as DL-propranolol decreases hepatic blood flow and affects its own clearance, so does it also decrease the clearance of drugs administered simultaneously. The magnitude of this effect depends upon the Cm as reflected by the initial hepatic extraction of the drug. Two drugs that illustrate the principles involved are lidocaine, which has a high hepatic extraction of 0.7 to 0.9 in the dog, and should thus have flow dependent clearance and oxyphenbutazone, which has a low extraction of <0.15 in the dog, and should have an elimination less dependent on flow.

When propranolol is given to a dog who is also receiving lidocaine the clearance of lidocaine is diminished by an amount equal to the decrease in hepatic blood flow and extraction ratio remains relatively constant (Fig. 3). This results in a 50% prolongation in the half-life of lidocaine (5).

With oxyphenbutazone, on the other hand, propranolol decreases clearance relatively less than the reduction in hepatic blood flow and hepatic extraction of oxyphenbutazone rises when blood flow is reduced. Thus the half-life of oxyphenbutazone is prolonged less than 30% (6).

These results with lidocaine and oxyphenbutazone represent two points on a spectrum of drugs likely to be susceptible to hemodynamic drug interactions. For drugs with hepatic extraction ratios and hence Cm less than that of oxyphenbutazone (such as antipyrine and diphenylhydantoin), hepatic blood flow is not an important factor in elimination and such drugs are not subject to hemodynamic drug interactions. However, if the extrac-

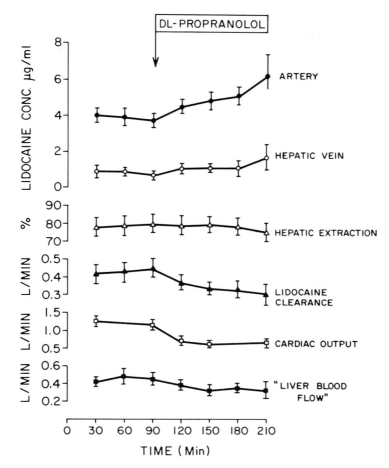

FIG. 3. The effects of DL-propranolol on the disposition of lidocaine during steady-state conditions in the dog. The decrease in lidocaine clearance induced by propranolol can be explained by a decreased hepatic blood flow. Each point represents the mean ± SE ($n = 6$). Reprinted from *J. Pharmacol. Exp. Ther.* with permission (5).

tion ratio is higher than that for oxyphenbutazone, hemodynamic drug interactions may be expected to occur.

DRUG INTERACTIONS RESULTING FROM INCREASED LIVER BLOOD FLOW

Some vasoactive drugs such as glucagon (7) and isoproterenol (8) will increase hepatic blood flow and will thus increase the hepatic clearance of high-extraction drugs. Thus the clearance of lidocaine and propranolol have been shown to be increased by drug-induced increases in hepatic blood flow (Fig. 4). The magnitude of the increase in clearance achievable by this means is that predicted by the model in Eq. 1.

A most interesting example of enhanced drug clearance due to increased hepatic blood flow is appreciated by analyzing the effects of phenobarbital treatment. The ability of phenobarbital to increase the rate of elimination of many drugs and endogenous compounds is usually attributed to an enhanced activity of the drug metabolizing enzymes. However phenobarbital also increases liver blood flow, which, we have seen, may play the major role in determining the elimination of high clearance drugs. In fact, for drugs, endogenous compounds, or other substances with a high Cm and extraction ratio approaching 1.0, no degree of induction of the drug metabolizing enzymes can affect drug clearance, which is entirely flow dependent. In contrast, for drugs with a low Cm, the effects of changes in flow will be relatively insignificant.

To test this hypothesis, we investigated the effects of phenobarbital in the monkey on the clearance of two drugs: antipyrine, which has a low Cm, and propranolol, which has a high Cm. Phenobarbital treatment resulted in a 34% increase in hepatic weight and a proportional increase in hepatic blood flow. The clearances of both propranolol and antipyrine were increased. The

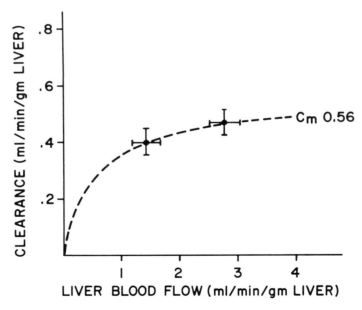

FIG. 4. The effects of glucagon on hepatic blood flow and propranolol clearance in the monkey. The dashed line is predicted from Eq. 1 in the text, bars are standard errors. Note the close fit to the theoretical line. Reprinted from *J. Pharmacol. Exp. Ther.* with permission (7).

mechanism of this increased clearance was analyzed by the pharmaco-kinetic model (Fig. 5). Antipyrine, with an initially low Cm, had an increase in Cm of 300% after phenobarbital treatment. Because of the relatively low Cm, however, the increase in hepatic blood flow was a minor factor in the effect of phenobarbital on antipyrine clearance. In fact from Fig. 5 it can be appreciated that 91% of the increase in antipyrine clearance was due to the increased enzyme activity and only 9% could be attributed to the in-creased flow. This is in contrast to the effects of phenobarbital on pro-pranolol clearance in the same animals. The Cm for propranolol, which is relatively high, was increased by phenobarbital by only 75%. Because of the high Cm, the effects of increased flow played the major role in enhancing drug clearance. Indeed only 43% of the increase in actual drug clearance was due to enhanced enzyme activity, whereas 57% of the change could be attributed to increased hepatic blood flow. These considerations apply to hepatic drug clearance and can be applied to total body clearance when there is little extrahepatic metabolism as appears true for antipyrine (9) and propranolol (3).

These results with phenobarbital allow certain important predictions and generalizations to be made regarding enzyme induction. The clearance con-cept is very useful in understanding the results of treatment with an enzyme inducer. Drug clearance, unlike half-life, provides a measure of efficiency of the elimination process and is often related to physiological parameters that include organ blood flow and drug extraction by an organ. Half-life, on the other hand, must be related to the volume of distribution to determine

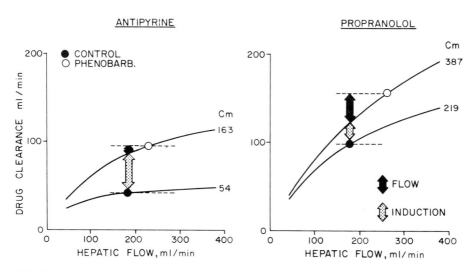

FIG. 5. Relative contributions of increased hepatic blood flow and enzyme induction to the enhanced clearance of antipyrine and D-propranolol caused by phenobarbital treat-ment in the monkey. The lines are those predicted by Eq. 1. See text for explanation.

TABLE 1. *Theoretical effects of twofold increases in hepatic blood flow or intrinsic hepatic clearance* (Cm) *on the actual hepatic clearance of drugs with different initial hepatic extraction ratios*

	Initial hepatic extraction ratio		
	0.2	0.5	0.8
Relationship of *Cm* and flow *(Q)*	$Cm = \dfrac{Q}{4}$	$Cm = Q$	$Cm = 4Q$
Percent increase in clearance when *Cm* doubled	67	33	11
Percent increase in clearance when *Q* doubled	11	33	67

the efficiency of elimination. Furthermore, drug clearance determines the concentration of drug in the blood, which is often related to drug effect. The effects of charges in enzyme activity (i.e., Cm) will depend upon the relative values of hepatic blood flow and the initial Cm. The theoretical effects of a twofold increase in Cm or hepatic blood flow on the hepatic clearance of three drugs with a low (0.2), intermediate (0.5), or high (0.8) hepatic extraction ratio are shown in Table 1. It is evident that the effects of any given degree of enzyme induction on actual drug clearance will be smaller the higher the initial Cm of the drug in contrast to the effects of flow changes, which will be greater the higher the initial Cm. These predictions seem also to apply to endogenously produced substances that are eliminated by the liver. Thus the clearance of aldosterone (10) and cortisol (11) have been shown to be flow dependent.

The ability of phenobarbital to increase both enzyme activity and hepatic blood flow accounts for the enhanced disposition of many exogenous and endogenous substances cleared by the liver. However, the dominant mechanism for the enhanced clearance depends upon the initial ability of the liver to extract the drug (i.e., the intrinsic hepatic clearance). Thus the effects of phenobarbital cannot always be attributed to enzyme induction particularly with high-clearance substances. For example, the enhanced clearance of indocyanine green, which has a high extraction ratio (12), may be as much a result of enhanced flow as induction of a transport protein, ligandin (13). Interestingly 3-methylcholanthrene and 3-4-benzpyrene also induce ligandin (14) but do not alter hepatic blood flow (15) and should not enhance indocyanine green clearance to a degree comparable to phenobarbital. To summarize, it is clear that for proper interpretation of drug interactions with phenobarbital one must know the initial hepatic clearance or extraction of the interacting drug. In this way the contributions of enhanced enzyme activity and increased hepatic blood flow to drug clearance can be predicted.

CONCLUSIONS AND CLINICAL CORRELATIONS

There is evidence that hepatic blood flow in man also is an important determinant of the clearance of high extraction drugs and endogenous substances (10, 16, 17). It is therefore obvious that the experiments cited in this review have probable direct application to clinical situations. In fact the experiments comparing D and DL-propranolol have been performed in man and have shown that the half-life of D-propranolol is shorter than that of L- or DL-propranolol (18). These results are exactly those predicted by the animal experiments.

Any drug that alters hepatic blood flow can change the clearance of other drugs. Since ill patients receive many drugs including vasoactive agents, the physician should be aware of the potential of hemodynamic drug interactions. At the present time the hepatic extraction or clearance of many drugs is unknown, but at least lidocaine and propranolol, two drugs with toxic potential, have flow dependent clearance, and it is likely that further investigation of commonly used drugs will reveal more examples.

An interesting possibility would be the use of a drug that increases hepatic blood flow to enhance the clearance of other drugs that have been taken in overdose. Very lipid-soluble drugs are largely distributed to the tissues and blood concentrations are quite low, so that hemodialysis does little to alter drug elimination. However, the hepatic clearance of these drugs may be high and increasing hepatic blood flow by an agent such as glucagon could augment drug clearance. In fact glucagon has been used for its cardiac effects in treating propranolol and imipramine toxicity (19, 20), but the beneficial effects may extend beyond the cardiac effects to actually enhancing the elimination of the toxic drug.

In summary, the effects of altering hepatic blood flow can be manifest in a variety of ways. A drug can affect its own clearance or the clearance of other drugs by pharmacologically altering hepatic blood flow and the magnitude of the effect on drug clearance depends upon the initial hepatic extraction of the drug. Thus decreased or increased clearance can result from hemodynamic drug interactions. In addition complex interactions such as those with phenobarbital can be understood and predicted only by considering the effects on hepatic blood flow as well as enzyme induction. These considerations apply to all species studied and represent a generally predictable phenomenon.

REFERENCES

1. Rowland, M., Benet, L. Z., and Graham, G. G. (1973): *J. Pharmacokin. Biopharm. 1*, 123.
2. Branch, R. A., Nies, A. S., and Shand, D. G. (1973): *Drug Metab. Disp. 1*, 687.
3. Nies, A. S., Evans, G. H., and Shand, D. G. (1973): *J. Pharmacol. Exp. Ther. 184*, 716.
4. Nies, A. S., Evans, G. H., and Shand, D. G. (1973): *Amer. Heart J. 85*, 97.
5. Branch, R. A., Shand, D. G., Wilkinson, G. R., and Nies, A. S. (1973): *J. Pharmacol. Exp. Ther. 184*, 515.
6. Branch, R. A., Shand, D. G., and Nies, A. S. (1973): *J. Pharmacol. Exp. Ther. 187*, 133.
7. Branch, R. A., Shand, D. G., and Nies, A. S. (1973): *J. Pharmacol. Exp. Ther. 187*, 581.
8. Benowitz, N., Rowland, M., Forsyth, R., and Melmon, K. L. (1973): *Clin. Res. 21*, 467.
9. Woodbury, D. M. (1970): In: *The Pharmacological Principles of Therapeutics* (ed. L. S. Goodman, and A. Gilman), p. 334, Macmillan, New York.

10. Camargo, C. A., Dowdy, A. J., Hancock, E. W., and Luetscher, J. A. (1965): *J. Clin. Invest. 44*, 356.
11. Englert, E. Jr., Nelson, R. M., Brown, H., Nielson, T. W., and Chou, S. N. (1960): *Surgery 47*, 982.
12. Caesar, J., Shaldon, S., Chiandussi, L., Guevara, L., and Sherlock, S. (1961): *Clin. Sci. 21*, 43.
13. Klaassen, C. D., and Plaa, G. L. (1968): *J. Pharmacol. Exp. Ther. 161*, 361.
14. Reyes, H., Levi, A. J., Gatmaitan, Z., and Arias, I. M. (1971): *J. Clin. Invest. 50*, 2242.
15. Ohnhaus, E. E., Thorgeirsson, S. S., Davies, O. S., and Brechenridge, A. (1971): *Biochem. Pharmacol. 20*, 2561.
16. Thomson, P. D., Melmon, K. L., Richardson, J. A., Cohn, K., Steinbrunn, W., Cudihee, R., and Rowland, M. (1973): *Ann. Int. Med. 78*, 499.
17. Stenson, R. E., Constantino, R. T., and Harrison, D. C. (1971): *Circulation 43*, 205.
18. George, C. F., Fenyvesi, T., Conally, M. E., and Dollery, C. T. (1972): *Eur. J. Clin. Pharmacol. 4*, 74.
19. Parmley, W. W., and Sonnenblick, E. H. (1971): *Amer. J. Cardiol. 27*, 298.
20. Ruddy, J. M., Seymour, J. L., and Anderson, N. G. (1972): *Med. J. Aust. 1*, 630.

Drug Interactions, edited by P. L. Morselli,
S. Garattini, and S. N. Cohen. Raven Press,
New York © 1974

Intentional Beneficial and Accidental or Undesirable Drug Interactions in Anesthesia

W. Hugin

University Institute of Anesthesiology, Cantonal Hospital, 4000 Basel, Switzerland

The best weapon against unfavorable drug interactions is the use of the smallest number of drugs that will provide the appropriate response. In contrast, hospitalized patients often receive multiple powerful medications to which the anesthetist will add. A modern anesthetic will often comprise six or more different agents. This polypharmacy not only increases the risk of hazardous interactions but may also complicate the problem of determining which drugs are responsible for unexpected and undesirable effects. It is difficult enough to perceive adequately the warning signs of toxicity of one or two agents. When many drugs are used, this ordinarily difficult job becomes impossible (1). Thus, in this regard, the fewer drugs used the better.

In contrast, there is a sound rationale for combining two or more medicaments based on physiological or biochemical considerations. One of the earliest and still regularly used interactions in anesthesiology has been the premedication with atropine. It is still sound practice to antagonize the cholinergic effects caused by some irritating vapors such as ether, as well as the vagal inhibition of the heart due to endotracheal manipulations or due to succinylcholine. There is evidence also that the negative inotropic effects of anesthetics such as halothane or thiopental can be compensated for, at least partially, by increasing the pulse rate with atropine given i.v. immediately before the anesthetic (2).

Another classical interaction with predictable results comes from the mixture of a local analgesic with a vasopressor, at least in such agents that would cause local vasodilatation.

These two interactions have definitely made anesthesia safer and are therapeutically desirable. In addition, anesthesia offers a nice example for the fact that in certain circumstances pharmacological purism may be at a disadvantage when compared with the use of drug combinations causing controllable interactions:

Up to the time of World War II, muscular relaxation during general anesthesia was mostly achieved by breathing a high concentration of a strongly acting vapor such as ether. The price paid for the advantage of muscular flaccidity was high, and consisted of a number of undesirable side effects of the anesthetic, from which the patient suffered often more than from the combined effects of his disease and operation.

The introduction of specific muscle relaxants in the 1940s represented real progress, making possible things which were not thought of before. The overall effects of deep general anesthesia were broken down into different components, each of which was effected by a separate specific agent. *d*-Tubocurarine was one of them. It occupies the same receptors as acetylcholine at the myoneural junction, but the complex with the receptor is biologically inert. In the presence of *d*-tubocurarine, acetylcholine is unable to trigger the depolarization mechanism. This complex of a receptor with agonist and antagonist is reversible. In addition, the anesthetist makes use of this property to overcome the effects of *d*-tubocurarine at the end of an operation by blocking cholinesterase and thus accumulating acetylcholine.

Because of the law of mass action, acetylcholine will take more of the receptor sites and striated-muscle activity will be restored. This interaction is necessary for the prompt reversal of curarization and expeditiousness in a busy operating suite. But this situation is unfortunately connected with strong muscarinic effects, calling for use of an anticholinergic. Atropine in rather large doses is routinely given before pharmacological reversion of the muscle relaxation. The important progress brought about by curare was not possible by the addition of just one drug but by introducing intentional interactions among three drugs. Anyhow, the excellent results are proof that this combination of drugs, each one exerting strong and specific effects, is beneficial. Control of muscular activity involves control of breathing, and this in combination with minimal side effects of light general anesthesia is an important factor in the maintenance of circulatory stability. It is not an overstatement to claim that the rapid expansion of modern surgery is very much connected with the purposeful application of drug interactions in which the relaxants come into play.

More links have been added to this chain of interactions, some of which may involve unwanted effects.

Coincident with the increasing use of benzodiazepin derivates, both as premedications and as inducing agents in anesthesia, a higher incidence of prolonged postoperative respiratory depression was noticed in patients to whom curare-like drugs had been administered (3). Investigations showed that *diazepam* had a profound effect upon the action of the muscle relaxants. The neuromuscular block increased severalfold in degree and duration, whereas the block by succinylcholine was reduced markedly. Diazepam probably acts by reducing acetylcholine release at the presynaptic membrane.

Certain antibiotics such as streptomycin, neomycin, and others exert weak nondepolarizing neuromuscular blocking action. Infrequently, these medicaments cause skeletal muscle paralysis by their direct action and significantly enhance and prolong the neuromuscular block produced by curare-like drugs.[1]

Finally, it has been shown that the two types of relaxants, the competitive and the depolarizing, are antagonists (4). The essential difference between the two types is the ability to occupy the receptor site. Relaxants that react with the receptor without occupying it act as depolarizers. Once they become bound to the receptor they act as curare-like drugs. All this is dependent on temperature, acid-base equilibrium, and ionic changes and influences in a complex way the ease with which depolarization and repolarization can be affected. The neuromuscular block by curare-like drugs is an impressive example of changes of affinity between drug and receptor under different pH conditions. Whereas acidosis potentiates this effect it is opposed by alkalosis (5).

Furthermore, it was observed that ventricular arrhythmias frequently followed the administration of succinylcholine to fully digitalized patients and that once these arrhythmias occurred they could be abolished by *d*-tubocurarine (6). In the incompletely digitalized patient without electrocardiographic evidence of digitalis, succinylcholine can produce changes that are characteristic of digitalization, such as prolonged P-R interval, depressed S-T segment, and T-wave changes. It seems that the two types of relaxants favor in a contrary way the entry and efflux of cations through the myocardial membrane.

Whereas some drugs used in anesthesia exert their effect by a specific chemical relation to receptors, the inhalational anesthetics in contrast act at relatively high concentrations, obviously on unspecific sites and their effects can be reversed by high pressure. It is therefore rather unlikely that they cause important interactions on receptor sites. On the other hand, there are interactions at the site of uptake.

On inhalation of an anesthetic gas or vapor, the concentrations of the agent in the alveoli and blood gradually approach the inspired concentration. One of the determining factors of equilibration is the alveolar ventilation. This is of particular importance in the more soluble anesthetics, such as diethylether or methoxyflurane. Carbon dioxide increases the speed of induction by augmenting the ventilation (7) somewhat also by increasing cerebral blood flow (8). This interaction shortens considerably the induction time and use is made in overcoming the difficulties of the second stage.

In combining nitrous oxide–oxygen with a strongly acting vapor, another interaction comes into play: the so-called second gas or concentration effects. Nitrous oxide being absorbed causes an increased tracheal inflow of anesthetic gas and vapor (9). Also the uptake of a large volume of nitrous

---

[1] The best way to cope with this situation is to withhold these antibiotics until some 4 to 6 hr have elapsed after the operation.

oxide in the beginning of anesthesia leaves a higher concentration of the second agent in the alveoli.

Space limitations prohibit the enumeration of many other drug interactions in clinical anesthesia,[2] some of which are definitely beneficial, others are of questionable value. Artificial hibernation, ataract-algesia, neurolept-analgesia, the mineralized and "dissociative states" are but a few expressions for drug combinations that exert a kind of additive depressing effects on the central nervous system. As a matter of fact most of these combinations are still due the proof of their superiority in the sense of providing a higher degree of safety for the patient.

The persistent drinker and particularly the patient who is a narcotic addict may exhibit symptoms through lack of medication and develop a dangerous withdrawal syndrome during anesthesia. In this way, a vanishing interaction may become just as detrimental as an oncoming one. As long as the patient is in a waking state, the syndrome is not difficult to diagnose: weakness, tremor, anxiety, and sweating are leading symptoms, which may combine with cardiovascular instability. In the state of anesthesia however, serious cardiovascular collapse or even convulsions may be the first indication of difficulty, with a fair chance of misinterpretation. A normal dose of a narcotic analgesic given i.v. for trial, will then rapidly reverse the withdrawal syndrome.

A wide variety of preoperatively used drugs interact with anesthetics. These interactions may be detrimental to the maintenance of homeostasis during surgery. The most frequently given classes of medicaments are psychotropics, diuretics, and anticholinesterases.

Anticholinesterases are frequently used in the treatment of glaucoma, leaving a much reduced activity of both, pseudo- and true cholinesterases (10).

The short duration of action of succinylcholine is due to rapid hydrolysis by pseudocholinesterase. If this enzyme's activity is markedly reduced, the otherwise short-acting relaxant will cause prolonged apnea.

Thiazide diuretics cause increased losses of sodium and potassium (11). Potassium depletion can result in two adverse effects during anesthesia: prolongation of curarization (12) and arrhythmias in patients receiving digitalis. Proper digitalization is not easily achieved in advanced heart disease. The range between therapeutic effect and toxicity is narrow, one of the reasons being that the response depends on a critical balance among electrolytes: sodium, potassium, and calcium. This balance in the myocardium is easily upset by thiazide diuretics used in the treatment of congestive heart failure.

Among psychotropic drugs are some with prominent alpha-adrenergic blockade, e.g. chlorpromazine, causing marked hypotension during anes-

---

[2] Connected with enzyme induction, protein binding, or interplay at receptor sites.

thesia. In addition, phenothiazines have additive effects when combined with hypnotics, narcotics, or anesthetics (13).

It is not difficult to cope with these interactions if we know about them in advance (14). Unfortunately many patients taking medicaments do not know which drug they take and finding out from the general practitioner is sometimes difficult and time consuming. One of the important reasons for a preoperative visit by the anesthetist is to interrogate the patient about present and past drug intake (15). But often we leave the patient knowing as little as that he uses some white tablets or some little red pills. This is a renewed plea for the introduction of a system that allows the identification of drugs by the size, shape, and color of tablets and pills.

There are no unpredictable interactions between the traditional sedatives and drugs likely to be given during anesthesia. Long term use of these, however, will lead to a certain degree of tolerance to many anesthetics. The interaction between alcohol and barbiturates has been the cause of tragedies not only in the hospital, but also outside. This is why we have become very careful with the increasing numbers of general anesthesias given on an out-patient basis. We hand a form to all ambulant patients, who will be put asleep, on which they sign having understood that they are not allowed to drink alcohol or drive a vehicle or do dangerous work until the next day.

A particularly important group of drugs comprises the monoamine oxidase (MAO) inhibitors, which influence a wide variety of other enzymes. Substances affected include barbiturates, narcotics, acetanilid, cocaine, and others. Interactions between MAO inhibitors and indirectly acting sympathomimetics have resulted in *hypertensive crisis*. Deaths from intracranial hemorrhage and acute heart failure have been reported. Interaction with barbiturates has resulted in prolonged sleep time and coma with pethidine in hyperpyrexia and severe hypertension. Even if not all patients receiving MAO inhibitors have adverse reactions during anesthesia it is theoretically desirable to withdraw the drug for some 2 to 3 weeks before elective surgery. But this must not be done at the risk of recurrence of undesirable symptoms, such as suicidal depression or violence. An alternative is for the anesthetist to avoid drugs likely to overact in the presence of MAO inhibition. In such a situation as well as in emergencies, it is best to omit barbiturates and narcotics as well as inhalation agents, which increase the circulating level of catecholamines, such as ether or cyclopropane. Phentolamine, which has been used successfully to combat accidentally induced hypertension in patients on MAO inhibitors (16), must be at hand.

Similarly, in antihypertensive therapy the dangers of continuing therapy must be weighed against the dangers of withdrawing drugs to which the body has become physiologically accustomed. These include cardiac failure, cerebrovascular accidents, and renal failure. Whereas the hypertensive patient may run a greater than average risk from anesthesia and surgery, any benefit to be obtained from withdrawal of medication, which may take up to 2 weeks to be effective, may be more than outweighed by the disadvantage of loss of control of the hypertension. Both treated and inadequately treated hypertensive patients tend to develop hypotension during anesthesia, while normotensive and adequately treated hypertensives cause little concern. Whereas treated hypertensive patients have a normal systemic peripheral resistance and blood volume, the untreated hypertensives, who have an increased peripheral resistance and possibly a reduced blood volume, will be much more affected by drugs and anesthetics that reduce peripheral resistance. Therefore untreated hypertension constitutes a serious risk and withdrawal of antihypertensive drugs is unnecessary and potentially dangerous in patients who are about to undergo surgery. Looked at it in this way, psychotropic and antihypertensive drugs lead to tolerable interactions with anesthesia, provided one knows exactly which drugs the patient is taking and provided the anesthetist is well prepared to adapt his technique.

Genetic defects leading to complications during anesthesia embrace a host of clinical conditions, from rare diseases like familial dysautonomia to the more common such as diabetes mellitus. Most of these disorders are diagnosed before the patient is listed for operation, and he will receive proper treatment and the anesthetist will be prepared. Undiagnosed conditions that alter the patient's pharmacological responsiveness to drugs pose a greater threat. This group may include acute intermittent porphyria (17), glucose-6-phosphate dehydrogenase deficiency, and perhaps even fulminant hyperthermia.

One of the genetically controlled enzymes of greater practical importance is pseudocholinesterase, which may be present in reduced quantities or in an atypical variety with very low or lacking activity (18). Some of the nongenetic factors that can lower plasma cholinesterase activity are severe liver disease, burns, irradiation, and procaine. In a state of atypical or lowered plasmacholinesterase activity, succinylcholine may produce full muscular paralysis of several hours duration and a very slow recovery (19).

Regarding the widespread polypharmacy in seriously ill patients undergoing operation and anesthesia, drug interactions are no exception (20). Fortunately most of them are benign or there are physiological compensating mechanisms. In my field of activity the most frequent disturbances are a deepening and prolongation of unconsciousness, lowering of blood pressure, and lowering of body temperature. In clinical practice, anesthetists are quite familiar with these changes and even the worst of central nervous system depression (with apnea and loss of reflexes) can be managed without permanent sequellae provided the oncoming complication is recognized in good time.

More serious are hypertensive or hyperthermic reactions and cardiac arrhythmias, which call for immediate treatment. But again, we are equipped with efficient means for a rapid reversal. The problem is more one of immediate recognition and correct interpretation.

Except for the most urgent emergencies and some other extraordinary cases, we should find time to inform ourselves about a potentially serious drug condition and consequently adapt our technique or care using compensatory means that are readily available. In modern literature some nicely prepared "danger lists for anesthetists" (21) are much appreciated assistance in the prevention of undesirable drug interactions.

REFERENCES

1. Beecher, K. H. (1950): *Ann. Surg. 131*, 4.
2. Hugin, W. (1961): *Der Anaesthesist 10*, 2.
3. Feldman, S. A. (1970): *Brit. Med. J. 2*, 335.
4. Walts, L. F., and Dillon, J. B. (July, 1969): Anesthesiology.
5. Baraka, A. (1964): *Brit. J. Anaesth. 36*, 272.
6. Dowdy, E. G., and Fabian, L. W. (1963): *Anesth. Analg. Curr. Res. 42*, 501.
7. Eger, E. I. II. (1964): *Brit. J. Anaesth. 36*, 155.
8. Goldberg, M. A., Barlow, C. F., and Roth, L. J. (1961): *J. Pharmacol. Exp. Therap. 131*, 308.
9. Epstein, R. M., Rackow, H., and Salanitre, E. (1964): *Anesthesiology 25*, 364.
10. Eilderton, T. E., Farmati, O., Zsigmond, E. K. (1968): *Canad. Anaesth. Soc. J. 15*, 291.
11. Mudge, G. H. (1965): In: *Pharmacological Basis of Therapeutics*, ed. 3, Goodman and Gilman, New York.
12. Taylor, G. J. (1963): *Anesthesiology 18*, 9.
13. Jenkins, L. C., and Graves, H. B. (1965): *Canad. Anaesth. Soc. J. 12*, 121.
14. Katz, R. L., Weintraub, H. D., and Papper, E. M. (1964): *Anesthesiology 25*, 142.
15. Anton, A. H., and Gravenstein, J. S. (1968): *Intern. Anesth. Clin. 6*, 312.
16. Bethune, H. C., Burrell, R. H., and Culpan, R. H. (1963): *Lancet 2*, 1923.
17. Ward, R. J. (1965): *Anesthesiology 26*, 212.
18. Doenicke, A., Gürtner, T., Kreutzberg, G., Remes, I., Spiess, W., and Steinbereithner, K. (1963): *Acta Anaesth. Scand. 7*, 59.
19. Hart, S. M., and Mitchell, J. V. (1962): *Brit. J. Anaesth. 34*, 207.
20. Godwin, E. (1968): *Hospital Medicine 2*, 412.
21. Grogono, A. W., and Jones, E. P. (1968): *Anesthesiology 23*, 2.

Drug Interactions, edited by P. L. Morselli,
S. Garattini, and S. N. Cohen. Raven Press,
New York © 1974

Decreased Plasma Half-Lives of Antipyrine and Phenylbutazone in Workers Occupationally Exposed to Lindane and DDT

Birgitta Kolmodin-Hedman

Department of Clinical Pharmacology at Karolinska Institutet and the Department of Occupational Health, National Board of Occupational Health and Safety, 100 26 Stockholm, Sweden

INTRODUCTION

Previously it has been shown in animal experiments that exposure to chlorinated hydrocarbon pesticides induces the microsomal hydroxylating enzymes in the liver. In 1963, Hart and co-workers (1, 2) reported shortening of hexobarbital sleeping times in rats exposed to chlordane, which was sprayed in the animal stall. Chronic feeding of rats with DDT produced similar and long-lasting effects. Street and Blau (3) have shown that dieldrin is also capable of inducing. The no-effect level of DDT on aldrin epoxidation in rats was found by Gillett (4) to be 2.5 ppm. Kinoshita et al. (5) found that 1 ppm of DDT induced drug oxidation *in vitro*. High single doses i.p. of α-benzene hexachloride enhanced the metabolism of acetanilide and paranitrophenol (6). Schwabe and Wendling (7) found that 5 mg of γ-HCH (lindane) decreased pentobarbital sleeping times.

This report describes studies in humans exposed to a mixture of pesticides mainly lindane and DDT. For details the reader is referred to the original papers. One feasible way to assess the activity of liver microsomal enzymes in man is to estimate the plasma-elimination rate of drugs that are (a) metabolized in the liver, (b) not excreted unchanged to any great extent in the urine, (c) not appreciably bound to plasma proteins.

ANTIPYRINE

Since antipyrine fulfills these criteria it was used in our initial work.

Subjects

Exposed to Lindane

Twenty-six Swedish male workers sprayed a solution of 4% lindane, 1% pyrethrum, 0.125% piperonylbutoxide, and 2.5% malathion in kerosene.

Previously they had been exposed occupationally also to DDT during a period of 5 years. They did not have any fixed place of work. Gloves and respirators were not used regularly. They worked from daily to once weekly and the employment period varied from 1 to 15 years. Thus dermal and respiratory exposure occurred. Plasma levels of pesticides could not be analyzed at that time adequately. The state of health of the men was checked by history, physical examination, and routine laboratory tests.

Exposed to DDT

Personnel from six pine and fir nurseries were examined. Twenty-three subjects were examined during exposure. Fifteen persons were re-examined 8 months after exposure. They planted and replanted fir and conifer plants that were dipped in a 1% solution of DDT during spring and summer months. A few of the subjects prepared this solution, thus handling dry DDT powder. The plasma levels of *p,p'*-DDE and *p,p'*-DDT on the same test days were determined.

Controls

The control subjects consisted of office personnel, 15 men and 18 women. No one admitted any drug consumption during the 2 months preceding the study. The controls came from the same geographical area. In the DDT-exposed material, the subjects served as their own controls 8 months after exposure.

Methods

Antipyrine was given as a single oral dose of 10 or 15 mg/kg and blood samples were drawn 3, 6, 9, and 12 hr after taking the drug. Antipyrine was estimated spectrophotometrically according to Brodie and associates (8).

Results

The results are given in Table 1. In the men exposed to lindane and DDT the mean was 7.7 hr, SD 2.6 hr. In the controls no sex difference was found in the half-lives. The distribution of the half-lives had a mean of 13.1 hr, SD 7.5, median 11.5, and a range 5.2–35.0 hr. The groups differed significantly in a Wilcoxon test $0.01 < p < 0.001$ (9).

The half-lives in the persons exposed intermittently to DDT are given in Table 2. The mean was 9.8 hr and SD 2.8 during exposure and the same, i.e., 10.9 ± 3.8 hr 8 months after exposure. The DDE and DDT levels were 15 ± 8 ng/ml and 10 ± 9 ng/ml, respectively during exposure on the same day as the antipyrine study. Eight months after exposure, the mean DDE

TABLE 1. *Plasma half-lives of antipyrine in workers exposed to lindane and DDT in hours*

	Exposed	Controls
Mean	7.7	13.7
SD	2.6	7.5
Range	2.7–11.7	5.2–35.0
n	26	33

and DDT values were 16 ± 7 and 10 ± 3 ng/ml, respectively. These do not differ significantly from the former and are only slightly higher than those in unexposed subjects (10). These circumstances probably explain why the half-life values did not differ between the two study periods and why they are not significantly shorter than in unexposed individuals.

PHENYLBUTAZONE

Phenylbutazone is oxidized to oxyphenbutazone. It is highly bound to plasma proteins (11). The plasma half-life is an indicator of its rate of metabolism and is shortened by phenobarbital treatment (12). The plasma half-lives of phenylbutazone were significantly shorter in men occupationally exposed to DDT than in controls. The levels of DDT and DDE in serum were 506 ± 88 and 573 ± 60 ppb, respectively (13).

Phenylbutazone half-lives after a single oral dose were studied in the men exposed to lindane and DDT.

Subjects and Methods

Some of the previously examined men were excluded because of an earlier diagnosis of gastritis and/or peptic ulcer. Thus the remaining 14 men exposed to lindane participated. Lindane exposure in this investigation was checked by measuring the plasma levels on the first test day. Office personnel of the same sex and age participated as controls.

TABLE 2. *Plasma half-lives of antipyrine in workers intermittently exposed to DDT*

	During exposure (hr)	Plasma levels of *p,p'*-DDE (ng/ml)	Plasma levels of *p,p'*-DDT (ng/ml)	8 months after exposure (hr)	Plasma levels of *p,p'*-DDE (ng/ml)	Plasma levels of *p,p'*-DDT (ng/ml)
Mean	10.9	15	10	9.8	21	7
SD	3.8	8	9	2.8	12	6
n	15	23		15	21	

Phenylbutazone was given in a dose of 5 mg/kg body weight and blood samples were drawn 24, 48, 96, and 120 hr after administration. Phenylbutazone was estimated spectrophotometrically according to Burns et al. (11).

Results

The results are shown in Table 3. The half-lives differed significantly from controls $p < 0.05$. The mean was 51.5, SD $\pm$ 14.8 and 63.9, SD $\pm$ 11.7 respectively. The plasma levels of lindane and p,p'-DDE and p,p'-DDT were determined. The exposed men differed significantly $p < 0.001$ from the nonexposed concerning lindane. The mean was 18.4, SD $\pm$ 26.8, and median 5, whereas controls had levels below the sensitivity of the method. In one subject a value of 0.2 ng/ml was found. The DDE levels did not differ significantly between the exposed group and the controls and were 33 $\pm$ 27 and 19 $\pm$ 11 ng/ml, respectively. DDT levels were mostly under the detection limit. No relationship was found between plasma half-lives and plasma levels of lindane, $r = 0.39$ (14).

OXAZEPAM

Hunter et al. (15) used the urinary excretion of D-glucaric acid, an end product of the glucuronidation pathway, as an indicator of induction and showed an increase in men occupationally exposed to endrine. Sisenwine et al. (16) showed that the main metabolite of oxazepam in man is the glucuronide. Little is known about the induction in man of glucuronidation with the exception of bilirubin and phenobarbital (17).

Subjects and Methods

Thirteen men exposed to lindane were examined and 13 controls (office personnel) of the same age and sex. Oxazepam was given orally in a single

TABLE 3. *Plasma half-lives of phenylbutazone in workers exposed to lindane*

	Exposed			Controls		
	PT$^{1}/_{2}$ (hr)	Lindane in plasma (ng/ml)	DDE in plasma (ng/ml)	PT$^{1}/_{2}$ (hr)	Lindane in plasma (ng/ml)	DDE in plasma (ng/ml)
Mean	51.5	18.4	33	63.9	0.02	19
SD	14.8	26.8	27	11.7	0.06	11
n	14	14	14	12	12	11
		Median 5				

dose of 0.2 mg/kg body weight. Blood was drawn at 8, 24, 48, 56, and 72 hr after administration. Oxazepam was determined with a GLC-method according to Vessman et al. (18).

Results

The plasma levels of lindane were analyzed on the first test day. The mean was 6.9 ± 3.0 ng/ml in the exposed men and zero in the controls. The results of the oxazepam half-lives are given in Table 4. In the group exposed to lindane the mean was 9.5 ± 1.7 and in the controls 10.5 ± 3.5 and these values did not differ significantly.

ESTIMATION OF PESTICIDES

Estimation of chlorinated pesticides in blood as a measure of exposure is used by several authors (19–22). Blood levels of lindane seem to reflect the degree of acute exposure (20). Plasma levels of DDE reflect a chronic exposure to DDT (19, 21). In this study, a new GLC-method for estimating low levels of chlorinated pesticides has been developed (23). The verification of DDE peaks was performed with mass fragmentography. Figure 1 shows a gas chromatogram in a person exposed to lindane. Figure 2 shows the mass fragmentographic picture in a person with high DDE value and Fig. 3 shows the good correlation between the DDE values obtained with the two techniques ($r = 0.99$).

DISCUSSION

In men exposed to lindane the half-lives of antipyrine and phenylbutazone were decreased compared to controls. The exposure was measured as plasma levels of lindane. If the mechanism is the same as that in animals, then pharmacokinetic observations indicate an induction of the liver microsomal enzymes.

TABLE 4. Plasma half-lives of oxazepam in workers exposed to lindane

	Exposed			Controls		
	$PT\frac{1}{2}$ (hr)	Lindane in plasma (ng/ml)	DDE in plasma (ng/ml)	$PT\frac{1}{2}$ (hr)	Lindane in plasma (ng/ml)	DDE in plasma (ng/ml)
Mean	9.5	6.9	18	10.5	0	18
SD	1.7	3.0	10	3.5	–	7
n	13	13	13	13	13	13

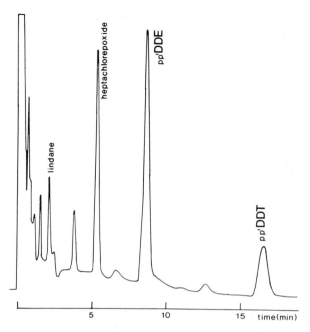

FIG. 1. Decreased plasma half-lives of antipyrine and phenylbutazone in workers occupationally exposed to lindane and DDT.

If the mechanism is the same as that in animals, then the pharmacokinetic observations indicate an induction of the liver microsomal enzymes.

The exposure was measured as plasma levels of lindane with the exception of the first antipyrine study in spray men. In a later step, the antipyrine half-lives in two other groups of spray men exposed to lindane coming from the south of Sweden were investigated and the lindane levels in plasma determined. The mean levels were 7.5 and 9.9 ng/ml respectively (10). In these groups, the antipyrine half-lives were not decreased *(unpublished data)*. In the phenylbutazone study, the mean plasma level of lindane was 18.4 ng/ml and here the half-lives of phenylbutazone differed significantly from controls. A threshold level of lindane in plasma for induction would thus be expected to lie above 10 ng/ml in humans. In the oxazepam study, the mean lindane level was 6.9 ng/ml. An alternative here is that the glucuronidation pathway is less inducible than hydroxylation processes in man. In rats, we have shown that hexobarbital sleeping times are shortened after feeding lindane, regularly with doses of 4 ppm in the food and occasionally down to $1/_2$ ppm (24) corresponding to mean lindane levels in plasma of 42 ng/ml and 8 ng/ml respectively *(to be published)*. Concerning DDT it was shown in the study of conifer nursery workers that mean plasma levels of 15 ng/ml of *p,p'*-DDE and 10 ng/ml of *p,p'*-DDT did not decrease antipyrine half-lives.

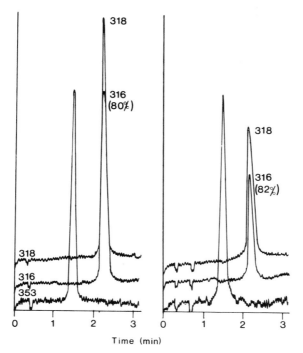

FIG. 2. Decreased plasma half-lives of antipyrine and phenylbutazone in workers occupationally exposed to lindane and DDT.

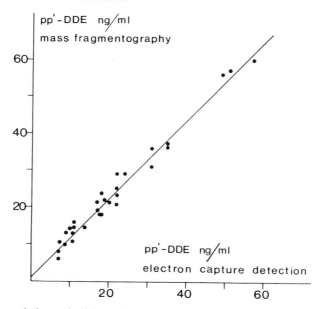

FIG. 3. Decreased plasma half-lives of antipyrine and phenylbutazone in workers occupationally exposed to lindane and DDT.

The "no-effect" levels of DDT in food with respect to liver enlargement in rats was 3.2 ppm (30), whereas 0.5 mg/kg in food increased the hexobarbital oxidation in this species (7).

The antipyrine plasma half-lives did not correlate with the phenylbutazone plasma half-lives in our study. In noninduced twins, the single oral dose half-lives of antipyrine and phenylbutazone were not correlated (26, 27). Davies and Thorgeirsson (28) found that the single oral dose plasma half-lives of antipyrine were correlated with the plasma half-lives of phenylbutazone after repetitive doses. Vesell et al. (29) found in his twin studies that persons starting with a long half-life of antipyrine were more induced with phenobarbital than those with a short one.

Many authors regard the induction of liver microsomal enzymes as an adaptation to the exposure to foreign lipid soluble compounds and not as a sign of liver damage (25, 30). Our men, some of them exposed for 15 years to lindane and for 5 years to DDT, were clinically healthy as judged by history, physical examination, and laboratory tests. They only showed a change of the lipoprotein pattern, namely hyperalphalipoproteinemia (31).

SUMMARY

In 26 men occupationally exposed mainly to lindane and DDT, antipyrine had a significantly shorter plasma half-life than in 33 control subjects.

Phenylbutazone plasma half-lives were shorter in 14 men exposed mainly to lindane compared to age and sex-matched controls. Oxazepam plasma half-lives in 12 men exposed mainly to lindane did not differ significantly from those in controls. The lindane exposure of the men was checked by measuring the plasma levels of lindane with an improved gas chromatographic method. The plasma levels of the occupationally exposed men ranged between 0 and 90 ppb and were significantly higher than in control subjects.

REFERENCES

1. Hart, L. G., and Fouts, J. R. (1963): *Proc. Soc. Exp. Biol. Med. 114*, 388.
2. Hart, L. G., Shultice, R. W., and Fouts, J. R. (1963): *Toxicol. Appl. Pharmacol. 5*, 371.
3. Street, J. C., and Blau, A. D. (1966): *Toxicol. Appl. Pharmacol. 8*, 497.
4. Gillett, J. W. (1968): *J. Agr. Food Chemistry 16*, 295.
5. Kinoshita, F. K., Frawley, J. P., and Dubois, K. P. (1966): *Toxicol. Appl. Pharmacol. 9*, 505.
6. Koransky, W., Magour, S., Noack, G., and Schulte Hermann, R. (1969): *Naunyn Schmied. Arch. Exp. Path. Pharmak. 263*, 281.
7. Schwabe, U., and Wendling, I. (1967): *Arzn. Forsch. 17*, 614.
8. Brodie, B. B., Axelrod, J., Soberman, R., and Levy, B. B. (1949): *J. Biol. Chem. 179*, 25.
9. Kolmodin, B., Azarnoff, D. L., and Sjöqvist, F. (1969): *Clin. Pharmacol. Therap. 10*, 638.
10. Kolmodin-Hedman, B., Palmér, L., Götell, P., and Skerfving, S. (1973): *Work-environm. Health 10*, 100.
11. Burns, J. J., Rose, R. K., Chenkin, T., Goldman, A., Schulert and Brodie, B. B., *J. Pharmacol. Exp. Therap. 109*, 346.

12. Whittaker, J. A., Price-Evans, D. A. (1970): *Brit. Med. J. 4*, 323.
13. Poland, A., Smith, D., Kuntzman, R., Jacobson, M., and Conney, A. H. (1970): *Clin. Pharmacol. Therap. 11*, 724.
14. Kolmodin-Hedman, B. (1973): *Europ. J. Clin. Pharmacol. 5*, 195.
15. Hunter, J., Maxwell, J. D., Stewart, D. A., Williams, R., Robinson, J., and Richardson, A. (1972): *Nature 237*, 399.
16. Sisenwine, S. F., Tio, C. O., Shroder, S. R., and Ruelius, H. W. (1972): *Arzn. Forsch. 22*, 682.
17. Yaffe, S. J., Levy, G., Matsuzawa, T., and Baliah, T. (1966): *New Engl. J. Med. 275*, 1461.
18. Vessman, J., Freij, G., and Strömberg, S. (1972): *Acta Pharm. Suecia 9*, 447.
19. Dale, W. E., Curley, A., and Cueto, C. (1966): *Life Sci. 5*, 47.
20. Milby, T. H., Samules, A. J., and Ottoboni, F. (1968): *J. Occupat. Med. 10*, 584.
21. Nachman, G. A., Freal, J. J., Barquet, A., and Morgade, C. (1969): *Health Lab. Sci. 6*, 148.
22. Radomski, J. L., Deichmann, B., Rey, A. A., and Merkin, T. (1971): *Toxicol. Appl. Pharmacol. 20*, 175.
23. Palmér, L., and Kolmodin-Hedman, B. (1972): *J. Chromatogr. 74*, 21.
25. Hoffman, D. G., Worth, H. M., Emmerson, J. L., and Anderson, R. C. (1970): *Toxicol. Appl. Pharmacol. 16*, 171.
26. Vesell, E. S., and Page, J. G. (1968): *Science 159*, 1479.
27. Vesell, E. S., and Page, J. G. (1968): *Science 161*, 72.
28. Davies, D. S., and Thorgeirsson, S. S. (1971): *Ann. N.Y. Acad. Sci. 179*, 411.
29. Vesell, E. S., and Page, J. G. (1969): *J. Clin. Invest. 48*, 2202.
30. Remmer, H. (1972): *Europ. J. Clin. Pharmacol. 5*, 116.
31. Carlsson, L. A., and Kolmodin-Hedman, B. (1972): *Acta. Med. Scand. 192*, 29.

Drug Interactions, edited by P. L. Morselli, S. Garattini, and S. N. Cohen. Raven Press, New York © 1974

Drug Interactions in the Human Fetus and in the Newborn Infant

P. L. Morselli,[1] M. Mandelli,[2] G. Tognoni,[1] N. Principi,[2] G. Pardi,[3] and F. Sereni[2]

[1] *Istituto di Ricerche Farmacologiche "Mario Negri," Via Eritrea, 62–20157,* [2] *the Department of Child Health, and* [3] *the Department of Obstetrics and Gynecology, University of Milano, Medical School, Milano, Italy*

INTRODUCTION

Most of the data available on drug metabolism in the human fetus come from *in vitro* studies during early stages of pregnancy (8 to 25 weeks), whereas only a few refer to the perinatal period. These studies indicate that the enzyme systems responsible for drug degradation are less active in fetuses than in adults (Pikkarainen and Räihä, 1967; Di Toro, Lupi, and Ansanelli, 1968; Yaffe, Rane, Sjöqvist, Boréus, and Orrenius, 1970; Ackermann and Rane, 1971; Pelkonen, Jouppila, and Vorne Kärki, 1971; Idänpään-Heikkila, Jouppila, Poulakka, and Vorne, 1971; Rane and Ackermann, 1972; Fouts, 1973; Juchau, Lee, Louviaux, Symms, Krasner, and Yaffe, 1973; Pelkonen, Vorne, Jouppila, and Kärki, 1971).

These *in vitro* data do not provide direct indications on drug metabolic degradation during late fetal life and on neonatal drug metabolism. Furthermore, the information that can be derived from them is not easily applicable to clinical situations.

Recent concerns on toxic effects of drugs, either administered to the newborn or to the mother in late pregnancy (Marx, 1973), stress the need to conduct more investigations into drug disposition in the neonate, particularly when several drugs are given according to the practice of polytherapy.

In this report we present some observations on diazepam metabolism in premature and full-term newborns who received, directly or through the mother, either diazepam alone or combined with phenobarbital. The results obtained are indicative of an induction of diazepam metabolism in the case of combined treatment.

The data presented here confirm our previous observations on benzodiazepine metabolism in human newborns (Morselli, Principi, Tognoni, Reali, Belvedere, Standen, and Sereni, 1973; Sereni, Mandelli, Principi, Tognoni, Pardi, and Morselli, 1973) and are in agreement with the report of Stern, Khanna, Levy, and Yaffe (1970) who observed an increased excretion of salicilamide in newborns following phenobarbital treatment.

METHODOLOGY

A first group of observations was performed on newborn infants and children who, for therapeutic reasons, had to receive either diazepam or phenobarbital and diazepam. A second group of observations refers to newborn infants whose mothers received diazepam during the 24 hr preceding delivery. In three of the cases considered, the mothers received phenobarbital treatment for various lengths of time during gestation.

Urines were collected for the 24 to 48 hr following drug administration, and plasma samples were collected on occasion for clinical laboratory test analyses.

Quantitative chemical analysis of plasma and urine concentrations of diazepam and of its metabolites was carried out according to a GLC procedure previously described (Morselli et al., 1973).

DIAZEPAM PLASMA DISAPPEARANCE RATE IN NEWBORN INFANTS AND CHILDREN

Diazepam plasma levels after an i.m. administration of 0.33 mg/kg were followed in four premature infants (28 to 34 weeks) and in five children (4 to 8 years). As reported before (Morselli et al., 1973), the apparent plasma half-life for diazepam in the children group was of 18 ± 3 hr (mean $\pm$ SE), whereas in the premature group individual values ranged from 38 to 120 hr with a mean of 75 ± 37 hr.

The kinetic data are summarized in Table 1. It can be noted that prematures showed a reduced apparent volume of distribution and a very significantly reduced drug clearance in respect to children. In the same groups, remarkable differences were present also for the plasma levels of N-demethyldiazepam, the demethylated derivative of diazepam.

As reported in Fig. 1., *N*-demethyldiazepam was already present in the plasma of the children group 1 hr after diazepam administration with a peak value at 24 hr; however in the premature group the compound was not

TABLE 1. *Diazepam apparent kinetic parameters in premature newborns and children*

	T $\frac{1}{2}$ (hr)	T. B. Cl. (ml/hr/kg)	Vd (1/kg)	AUC (ng/ml · hr)
Prematures	75.33 ± 37.53	27.49 ± 8.53^a	1.80 ± 0.29	$6,322 \pm 1164^b$
Children	17.38 ± 3.01	102.10 ± 9.72	2.60 ± 0.53	$3,015 \pm 148$

$^a p < 0.01$ in respect to children.
$^b p < 0.05$ in respect to children.
Diazepam was administered i.m. at the dose of 0.3 mg/kg and plasma samples collected in the following 48 hr.
T $\frac{1}{2}$—apparent plasma half-life; T. B. Cl.—total body clearance; Vd—volume of distribution; AUC—area under the curve of plasma levels.

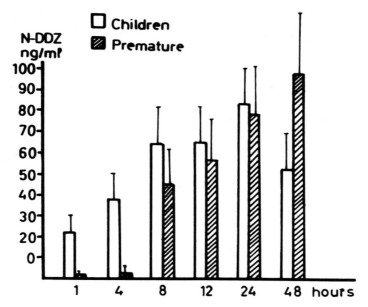

FIG. 1. N-Demethyldiazepam (N-DD2) plasma levels in premature infants and children after administration of 0/3 mg/kg i.m. of diazepam.

measurable up to 4 hr, and its plasma concentrations were still increasing after 48 hr.

The data suggest that in premature infants there is a slower N-demethylation rate when compared to children, and a reduced metabolic degradation of N-demethyldiazepam to oxazepam and, possibly, other metabolites.

In a second series of observations, the apparent disappearance rate of diazepam from plasma was followed in 11 full-term newborns whose mothers received diazepam during the 24 hr preceding the delivery. Plasma levels were determined within the first 48 to 72 hr of life, and the data are reported in Table 2.

In full-term newborns the apparent plasma half-life of diazepam varied from 21 to 40 hr with a mean value of 31 ± 2 hours. It may be noted that the diazepam apparent plasma half-life was not related to the drug concentration at birth.

DIAZEPAM AND DIAZEPAM METABOLITES URINARY EXCRETION IN NEWBORN INFANTS AND CHILDREN

Diazepam and N-demethyldiazepam were excreted as such only in traces in the three age groups (premature infants, full-term infants, and children) after a single diazepam administration of 0.33 mg/kg i.m.

TABLE 2. Apparent plasma half-life (T$\frac{1}{2}$) of diazepam (DZ) in full-term newborns[a]

Case	Gestational age (weeks)	Body weight at birth (kg)	DZ at birth (ng/ml)	Kel (h^{-1})	Apparent plasma T$\frac{1}{2}$ (hrs)
TS-3-PE	40	3.50	272	0.021	33.0
TS-5-PE	40	3.80	165	0.023	30.1
TS-8-PE	40	4.20	129	0.023	30.1
PT-01-OS	40	3.90	86	0.023	30.1
TS-6-PE	37	2.50	66	0.015	45.9
TS-4-PE	38	3.10	58	0.032	21.6
PT-07-OS	38	2.77	55	0.031	22.3
PT-MI-7-OS	40	3.95	37	0.023	30.1
TS-9-PE	40	3.90	35	0.030	23.1
TS-7-PE	40	3.80	34	0.017	40.2
TS-1-PE	38	2.91	29	0.020	34.6
Average (± SE)	39.1 ± 0.3	3.48 ± 0.17		0.023 ± 0.001	31.0 ± 2.2

[a] The drug was administered to the mother in the 24 hr preceding the delivery at the dose of 10 mg i.m.

TABLE 3. Urinary excretion (24 hr) of diazepam metabolites in prematures and full-term infants and in children following administration of diazepam (0.3 mg/kg i.m.) (the data are expressed as percent of the administered dose)

Metabolite		Premature infants (6)[b] (8–21 days)	Full-term infants (5)[b] (4–30 days)	Children (5)[a] (4–7 years)
N DDZ	F	0.05 ± 0.01	0.17 ± 0.04	0.05 ± 0.01
	C	0.57 ± 0.11	0.67 ± 0.22	1.46 ± 0.35
MOX	F	n.d.	n.d.	n.d.
	C	n.d.	0.12 ± 0.09	1.26 ± 0.25
OX	F	n.d.	n.d.	n.d.
	C	n.d.	0.02 ± 0.01	1.77 ± 0.68
Total benzodiazepines		0.62 ± 0.11[a]	0.98 ± 0.29[a]	4.54 ± 1.00
$\frac{(MOX + OX)}{(DZ + N\ DDZ)} =$		—	0.13 ± 0.08[a]	2.25 ± 0.22

[a] $p = 0.001$ in respect to children.
[b] The number of subjects is given in parentheses.
NDDZ = N-demethyldiazepam; MOX = N-methyloxazepam; OX = oxazepam; F = free; C = conjugated; n.d. = nondetectable. The urinary excretion of diazepam was identical in the three groups accounting for 0.5% of the administered dose.

Significant differences were, however, present with respect to the conjugated derivatives (Table 3). No hydroxylated metabolites were detectable in the 24 hr urine of the premature infants group, a limited amount was detectable in the full-term newborn group, while a considerable excretion of hydroxylated derivatives was found in the children group.

Considering the ratio between hydroxylated and nonhydroxylated compounds present in the 24-hr urine of the three groups, remarkable differences were evident, suggesting a reduced hydroxylating activity in both the premature and full-term newborn groups. It may be interesting to recall that in the full-term infant group, hydroxylated metabolites become detectable in the 24-hr urine only after 8 to 10 days of extrauterine age.

The same results were obtained in three full-term newborns whose mothers received diazepam during the 24 hr preceding the delivery (Table 4). In these cases, also, the ratio between hydroxylated (N-methyloxazepam and oxazepam) and nonhydroxylated (diazepam and N-demethyldiazepam) compounds was below 0.4. The main conjugated metabolite found in the 24-hr urine was N-demethyldiazepam, whereas N-methyloxazepam was present only in traces and oxazepam was not detectable.

EFFECTS OF PHENOBARBITAL ADMINISTRATION TO THE MOTHER OR TO THE NEWBORN ON DIAZEPAM METABOLISM IN THE NEWBORN

The diazepam plasma apparent half-life was found to be significantly reduced (in comparison with that previously observed in premature infants and full-term newborns) in three newborns whose mothers had received phenobarbital for various lengths of time during gestation and diazepam in the last 24 hr prior to delivery (Table 5). It should be emphasized that the case MI-21-OS, which presented an apparent plasma half-life of about 12 hr, was a premature newborn.

Many factors could play a role in the observed reduced diazepam plasma half-life after phenobarbital pretreatment, and these data alone cannot be taken as clear evidence of an increased drug metabolism (Morselli, Marc, Garattini, and Zaccala, 1970; Morselli, Rizzo, and Garattini, 1971). However, other data support the suggestion that an increased degradation of diazepam after phenobarbital exposure may occur in the newborn.

Table 6 reports data relative to the urinary excretion of diazepam and of its metabolites in two premature infants who, for convulsive disorders, were under treatment with phenobarbital for 4 and 8 days, and to whom diazepam also had to be administered for a further control of the seizures. A remarkable amount of hydroxylated metabolites was detectable in the 24- and 48-hr urines in both cases, whereas no differences in respect to the previous data were noticed as far as N-demethyldiazepam excretion is con-

TABLE 4. Benzodiazepine urinary excretion in three newborns after diazepam administration to the mothers in the 24 hr preceding delivery

Case	Plasma concen. at birth ng/ml		Plasma DZ T½ (hrs)	Urine (μg/48 hr)						$\dfrac{[MOX + OX]}{[DZ + N\text{-}DDZ]}$
				Free			Conjugated			
	DZ	N-DDZ		DZ	N-DDZ	MOX	N-DDZ	MOX	OX	
TS-3-PE	272	26	33	0.01	0.01	n.d.	8.10	0.51	n.d.	0.060
TS-5-PE	165	65	30	0.01	0.01	n.d.	2.10	0.72	n.d.	0.340
TS-7-PE	34	54	40	0.01	0.01	n.d.	4.95	0.01	n.d.	0.002

DZ = diazepam; N-DDZ = N-demethyldiazepam; MOX = methyloxazepam; OX = oxazepam.

TABLE 5. *Diazepam (DZ) apparent plasma disappearance rate in a premature and in two full-term newborn infants — Effect of phenobarbital administration on the mother*

Case	Birth weight (kg)	Gest. age (weeks)	Plasma DZ $T^{1/_2}$ (hrs)	Barbiturates administered to the mother
MI.21.OS	2.00	33	11.45	Phenobarbital 100 mg/day for the last 8 days of pregnancy.
MI.22.OS	3.75	40	17.77	Phenobarbital 200 mg/day for the last 8 days of pregnancy.
MI. 4.OS	3.95	40	19.94	Phenobarbital 100 mg/day from the beginning of pregnancy.
Mean ± SE	3.23 ± 0.62		16.3 ± 2.5	

All observations were performed during the first 2 days of life.

cerned. Furthermore, it should be underlined that in both cases the ratio between hydroxylated and nonhydroxylated compounds was significantly higher than the one usually observed in children, suggesting a real increase of hydroxylating activity. The fact that the excretion of N-demethyldiazepam conjugated derivative did not increase, and that N-methyloxazepam was also present as a free compound, is, in our opinion, supporting evidence of an increased activity of hydroxylating systems rather than of conjugating mechanisms.

DRUG EXCRETION OF DIAZEPAM METABOLITES IN THE NEWBORN FOLLOWING CHRONIC DIAZEPAM ADMINISTRATION TO THE MOTHER

Reports have appeared in the literature suggesting high hydroxylating activity in the newborn (Horning, Stratton, Wilson, Horning, and Hill, 1971; Horning, Stratton, Nowlin, Wilson, Horning, and Hill, 1973). In most cases the mothers received the drug chronically, and the assumption was based on urinary data only.

In Tables 7 and 8, two examples are reported where, after chronic diazepam administration to the mother, the urinary excretion of diazepam metabolites was followed in the newborn for 48 hr after delivery. In both cases, hydroxylated compounds were present in considerable amounts. However, the fact that in one case (Table 7) the quantity found in the 0- to 24-hr fraction was higher than the 24- to 48-hr fraction and that in the second case (Table 8) N-methyloxazepam was already detectable in the venous cord plasma suggests that the hydroxylated compounds found in the urine of these two newborns were mainly of maternal origin. Preliminary results from this laboratory indicate also that both N-methyloxazepam and ox-

TABLE 6. Urinary excretion of diazepam metabolites after administration of 0.3 mg/kg i.m. of diazepam in two premature infants pre-treated with phenobarbital (data are expressed as percent of administered dose)

Case	Gest. age (weeks)	Age (days)	Birth weight (kg)	Urine fraction	Diazepam and metabolites							$\dfrac{[MOX + OX]}{[DZ + N\text{-}DDZ]}$
					Free			Conjugated				
					DZ	N-DDZ	MOX	N-DDZ	MOX	OX	Total	
MI.2.PU	38	15	2.6	0–24 hr	0.02	0.03	0.02	1.11	2.21	2.00	5.32	3.71
				24–48 hr	0.01	0.09	0.05	0.96	5.53	6.25	12.74	12.3
				Total	0.03	0.12	0.07	2.07	7.74	8.25	18.06	
MI.3.PU	34	4	2.0	0–24 hr	0.04	0.02	0.15	0.06	0.43	0.24	0.73	6.9
				24–48 hr	0.02	0.07	n.d.	0.12	1.13	1.26	2.51	10.7
				Total	0.06	0.09	0.15	0.18	1.56	1.50	3.24	

DZ = diazepam; N-DDZ = N-demethyldiazepam; MOX = methyloxazepam; OX = oxazepam.
Case MI.2.PU received phenobarbital for 8 days at the dose of 15 mg/day (i.m.).
Case MI.3.PU received phenobarbital for 4 days at the dose of 10 mg/day (i.m.).

TABLE 7. Urinary excretion ($\mu g \cdot$ tot) of diazepam metabolites in a newborn whose mother received diazepam chronically for the 10 days preceding the delivery (20 mg/day)

		0–24 hr	24–48 hr
N-DDZ	F	0.08	0.06
	C	0.82	0.54
MOX	F	n.d.	n.d.
	C	1.61	0.65
OX	F	n.d.	n.d.
	C	0.04	0.01
$\dfrac{(MOX + OX)}{(DZ + NDDZ)} =$		1.83	1.10

N-DDZ = N-demethyldiazepam; MOX = methyloxazepam; OX = oxazepam. F = free; C = conjugated.

TABLE 8. Urinary excretion of diazepam and diazepam metabolites in a newborn whose mother received diazepam (20 mg/day) and phenobarbital (500 mg/day) for the 10 days preceding the delivery

		Plasma (ng/ml)				Urine ($\mu g \cdot$ tot)	
		At birth			25 hr Newborn venous		
		Mother venous	Cord venous	Cord arterial		0–24 hr	0–48 hr
DZ	F	80	123	162	37	Traces	Traces
	C	—	—	—	—	—	—
N-DDZ	F	155	140	150	227	0.82	1.24
	C	n.d.	n.d.	n.d.	n.d.	0.54	0.86
MOX	F	12	18	17	32	n.d.	n.d.
	C	24	10	12	47	1.74	5.34
OX	F	n.d.	n.d.	n.d.	n.d.	n.d.	n.d.
	C	n.d.	n.d.	n.d.	n.d.	4.28	8.60
					$\dfrac{[MOX + OX]}{[DZ + N\text{-}DDZ]} =$	4.40	6.89

DZ = diazepam; N-DDZ = N-demethyldiazepam; MOX = methyloxazepam; OX = oxazepam. F = free; C = conjugated.

azepam can easily cross the placenta (Mandelli and Morselli, *unpublished results*).

COMMENTS AND CONCLUSIONS

The data presently available on drug disposition in newborn infants indicate a slower elimination rate of drugs as compared to children or adults (Glatke, 1968; Reinicke, Rogner, Frenzel, Maak, and Klinger, 1970; Sereni, Perletti, Marubini, and Mars, 1968; Sereni, Perletti, Manfredi, and Marini, 1965; Sereni and Principi, 1968; Sereni, Morselli, and Pardi, 1973; Garattini, Marcucci, Morselli and Mussini, 1973).

Whereas for antibiotics the low renal clearance may be the relevant factor, for drugs such as tolbutamide (Nitowski, Matz, and Berzofsky, 1966), barbiturates (Melchior, Svensmark, and Trolle, 1967; Krauer, Draffan, Williams, Clare, Dollery, and Hawkins, 1973), diphenylhydantoin (Mirkin, 1971), nortriptyline (Sjöqvist, Bergfors, Borgå, Lind, and Ygge, 1972), and mepivacaine (Meffin, Long, and Thomas, 1973) the reduced drug-disposition rate in newborns seems to be linked to a reduced activity of liver mixed-function oxidase system, with particular reference to the hydroxylating activity. At variance with these data, recent reports (Horning et al., 1973; Rane and Sjöqvist, 1972) have suggested a relatively high hydroxylating activity in the perinatal period.

The disagreement may be due to the fact that different drugs have been utilized and that measurements of metabolites were essentially performed on the urines. Furthermore, the conclusions were reached without giving consideration to the repeated drug intake by the mothers. The data presented here confirm our previous observations (Sereni et al. 1973; Morselli et al., 1973) and are in good agreement with a recent paper of Meffin et al. (1973) where, on evaluating the urinary excretion of mepivacaine metabolites in newborns after drug administration to the mothers, a low drug hydroxylation was reported, whereas demethylation processes were comparable to the ones observed in adults.

The data presented here clearly demonstrate that diazepam is poorly disposed in the newborns, a fact that may have clinical relevance for the wide use of this drug in obstetrics and pediatrics (Flowers, Rudolph, and Desmond, 1969; Prensky, Raff, Moore, and Schwaab, 1967). Furthermore, side effects in newborns, whose mothers received diazepam prior to the delivery, have recently been described (Owen, Irani, and Blair, 1972; Cree, Meyer, and Hailey, 1973). Whether the low hydroxylation of diazepam is due to a low level of the liver microsomal enzymes or to inhibition by e.g. steroids or growth hormone, remains to be established.

Administration of phenobarbital, either to the mother or to the newborn, leads to an increased rate of diazepam disappearance from plasma and to an increased urinary excretion of hydroxylated derivatives. Also, the ratio between urinary hydroxylated and nonhydroxylated metabolites of diazepam is increased in the newborns receiving phenobarbital directly or through the mothers. The most likely explanation of these findings is that phenobarbital is interacting with diazepam by inducing the hydroxylating activity of liver microsomal enzymes, both in the fetus and in the newborn.

The fact that the fetus, during its intrauterine life, may be exposed to a number of inducing agents, either drugs given to the mother or chemicals introduced by the pollution of our living milieu, poses serious problems of unforeseeable drug interactions during the perinatal period.

ACKNOWLEDGMENTS

This work was supported by a U.S. Public Health Service Grant PO1-GM-18376-02 from the National Institutes of Health and by a CNR-Roma, Contract No. 70.01184.115.4019.

The skillful, technical assistance of Mr. Ettore Mastromatteo is greatly appreciated.

REFERENCES

Ackermann, E., and Rane, A. (1971): The monooxygenase system in the human fetal liver: Subcellular distribution and studies on "in vitro" metabolism of aniline. *Chem. Biol. Interact. 3*, 233–234.

Cree, J. E., Meyer, J., and Hailey, D. M. (1973): Diazepam in labour, its metabolism and effect on the clinical condition and thermogenesis of the newborn. *Brit. Med. J. 4*, 251–255.

Di Toro, R., Lupi, L., and Ansanelli, V. (1968): Glucuronation of the liver in premature babies. *Nature 219*, 265–267.

Flowers, C. E., Rudolph, A. J., and Desmond, M. M. (1969): Diazepam (Valium) as an adjunct in obstetric analgesia. *Obstet. Gynecol. 34*, 68–81.

Fouts, J. R. (1973): Microsomal mixed-function oxidases in the fetal and newborn rabbit. In: *Fetal Pharmacology*, ed. L. O. Boréus, pp. 305–320, Raven Press, New York.

Garattini, S., Marcucci, F., Morselli, P. L., and Mussini, E. (1973): The significance of measuring blood levels of benzodiazepines. In: *Biological Effects of Drugs in Relation to their Plasma Concentrations*, ed. D. S. Davies and B. N. C. Prichard, pp. 211–225, Macmillan, London.

Gladtke, E. (1968): Pharmacokinetic studies on phenylbutazone in children. *Il Farmaco 23*, 897–906.

Horning, M. G., Stratton, C., Wilson, A., Horning, E. C., and Hill, R. M. (1971): Detection of 5-(3,4-dihydroxy-1,5-cyclohexadien-1-yl)-5 phenylhydantoin as a major metabolite of 5,5 diphenylhydantoin (Dilantin) in the newborn human. *Anal. Lett. 4*, 537–545.

Horning, M. G., Stratton, C., Nowlin, J., Wilson, A., Horning, E. C., and Hill, R. M. (1973): Placental transfer of drugs. In: *Fetal Pharmacology*, ed. L. O. Boréus, pp. 355–373, Raven Press, New York.

Idänpään-Heikkila, J. E., Jouppila, P. I., Puolakka, J. O., and Vorne, M. (1971): Placental transfer and fetal metabolism of diazepam in early human pregnancy. *Amer. J. Obstet. Gynecol. 109*, 1011–1016.

Juchau, M. R., Lee, Q. H., Louviaux, G. L., Symms, K. G., Krasner, J., and Yaffe, S. J. (1973): Oxidation and reduction of foreign compounds in tissues of the human placenta and fetus. In: *Fetal Pharmacology*, ed. L. O. Boréus, pp. 321–332, Raven Press, New York.

Krauer, B., Draffan, G. H., Williams, F. M., Clare, R. A., Dollery, C. T., and Hawkins, D. F. (1973): Elimination kinetics of amobarbital in mothers and their newborn infants. *Clin. Pharmacol. Therap. 14*, 442–447.

Marx, J. L. (1973): Drugs during pregnancy: Do they affect the unborn child? *Science 180,* 174–175.

Meffin, P., Long, G. J., and Thomas, J. (1973): Clearance and metabolism of mepivacaine in the human neonate. *Clin. Pharmacol. Therap. 14,* 218–225.

Melchior, J. C., Svensmark, O., and Trolle, D. (1967): Placental transfer of phenobarbitone in epileptic women, and elimination in newborn. *Lancet 2,* 860–861.

Mirkin, B. L. (1971): Diphenylhydantoin: Placental transport, fetal localization, neonatal metabolism, and possible teratogenic effects. *J. Pediat. 78,* 329–337.

Morselli, P. L., Marc, V., Garattini, S., and Zaccala, M. (1970): Metabolism of exogenous cortisol in humans. Influence of phenobarbital treatment on plasma cortisol disappearance rate. *Rev. Eur. Et. Clin. Biol. 15,* 195–198.

Morselli, P. L., Principi, N., Tognoni, G., Reali, E., Belvedere, G., Standen, S. M., and Sereni, F. (1973): Diazepam elimination in premature and full term infants, and children. *J. Perinatal Med. 1,* 133–141.

Morselli, P. L., Rizzo, M., and Garattini, S. (1971): Interaction between phenobarbital and diphenylhydantoin in animals and in epileptic patients. *Ann. N.Y. Acad. Sci. 179,* 88–107.

Nitowski, H. M., Matz, L., and Berzofsky, J. A. (1966): Studies on oxidative drug metabolism in the full-term newborn infant. *Pediat. Pharmacol. Therap. 69,* 1139–1149.

Owen, J. R., Irani, S. F., and Blair, A. W. (1972): Effect of diazepam administered to mothers during labour on temperature regulation of neonate. *Arch. Dis. Childhood 47,* 107–110.

Pelkonen, O., Jouppila, P., Vorne, M., and Kärki, N. T. (1971): Effects of maternal intake of phenobarbital and cigarette smoking on drug metabolism in human foetal liver and placenta. *Acta Pharmacol. Toxicol. 29,* 44.

Pelkonen, O., Vorne, M., Jouppila, P., and Kärki, N. T. (1971): Metabolism of chlorpromazine and p-nitrobenzoic acid in the liver, intestine and kidney of human fetus. *Acta Pharmacol. Toxicol. 29,* 284–294.

Pikkarainen, P. H., and Räihä, N. C. (1967): Development of alcohol dehydrogenase activity in the human liver. *Pediat. Res. 1,* 165–168.

Prensky, A. L., Raff, M. C., Moore, M. J., and Schwaab, R. S. (1967): Intravenous diazepam in the treatment of prolonged seizures activity. *New Engl. J. Med. 276,* 779–784.

Rane, A., and Ackermann, E. (1972): Metabolism of ethylmorphine and aniline in human fetal liver. *Clin. Pharmacol. Therap. 13,* 663–670.

Rane, A., and Sjöqvist, F. (1972): Drug metabolism in the human fetus and newborn infant. *Pediat. Clin. N. Amer. 19,* 37–49.

Reinicke, C., Rogner, G., Frenzel, J., Maak, B., and Klinger, W. (1970): Die wirkung von phenylbutazon und phenobarbital auf die amidopyrin-elimination, die bilirubin-gesamtkonzetration im serum und einige blutgerinnungsfaktoren bei neugeborenen kindern. *Pharmacol. Clin. 2,* 167–172.

Sereni, F., Mandelli, M., Principi, N., Tognoni, G., Pardi, G., and Morselli, P. L. (1974): Induction of drug metabolizing enzyme activities in the human foetus and in the newborn infant. *Enzyme, in press.*

Sereni, F., Morselli, P. L., and Pardi, G. (1973): Postnatal development of drug metabolism in human infants. In: *Perinatal Medicine,* ed. H. Bossart, J. M. Cruz, A. Huber, L. S. Prod'hom, and J. Sistek, pp. 63–77, Huber H. Publ., Bern.

Sereni, F., Perletti, L., and Manfredi, A. (1965): Tissue distribution and urinary excretion of a tetracycline derivative in newborn and older infants. *J. Pediat. 67,* 299–305.

Sereni, F., Perletti, L., Marubini, E., and Mars, G. (1968): Pharmacokinetic studies with a long-acting sulfonamide in subjects of different ages. *Pediat. Res. 2,* 29–37.

Sereni, F., and Principi, N. (1968): Developmental pharmacology. *Ann. Rev. Pharmacol. 8,* 453–466.

Sjöqvist, F., Bergfors, P. G., Borgå, O., Lind, M., and Ygge, H. (1972): Plasma disappearance of nortriptyline in a newborn infant following placental transfer from an intoxicated mother: Evidence for drug metabolism. *J. Pediat. 80,* 496–500.

Stern, L., Khanna, N. N., Levy, G., and Yaffe, S. J. (1970): Effect of phenobarbital on hyperbilirubinemia and glucuronide formation in newborns. *Amer. J. Dis. Children 120,* 26–30.

Yaffe, S. J., Rane, A., Sjöqvist, F. Boréus, L. O., and Orrenius, S. (1970): The presence of monooxygenase system in human fetal liver microsomes. *Life Sci. 9,* 1189–1200.

Drug Interactions, edited by P. L. Morselli,
S. Garattini, and S. N. Cohen. Raven Press,
New York © 1974

Interaction Between Neuroleptics and Tricyclic Antidepressants

Lars F. Gram, Johannes Christiansen, and Kerstin Fredricson Overø*

Psychochemistry Institute and the Department of Clinical Chemistry A, Rigshospitalet, 9, Blegdamsvej, DK-2100 Copenhagen, and* Research Laboratories, H. Lundbeck & Co. A/S, DK-2500 Valby Copenhagen, Denmark

INTRODUCTION

In previous studies we have demonstrated that neuroleptics inhibit the metabolism of tricyclic antidepressants in man (1, 2). It was shown that neuroleptics as perphenazine, chlorpromazine, and haloperidol inhibit the urinary metabolite excretion after a test dose of ^{14}C-imipramine or ^{14}C-nortriptyline. At the same time the plasma level of metabolites decreases and plasma level of unchanged nortriptyline increases.

To study the mechanism of this inhibition of metabolism, changes in the urinary metabolite excretion pattern of ^{14}C-imipramine were studied.

In previous studies, we have studied the excretion and distribution of imipramine metabolites in man (3–5). The presently known pathways of imipramine metabolism in man are shown in Fig. 1.

MATERIAL AND METHODS

Six patients, three men and three women aged 20 to 53, were studied. All patients were newly admitted and had been diagnosed as suffering from schizophrenia.

The patients were given a test dose of ^{14}C-imipramine (3 μC = 50 mg) before and during treatment with perphenazine. After test-dose administration, blood samples were drawn 5 to 8 times during the first 24 hr, and the urine was collected in fractions of 4 to 8 hr intervals. All tests were performed in a general psychiatric ward. The urine sampling was difficult under these circumstances, but by fractionated urine sampling it was possible to discard urine portions known to be incomplete, without discarding the whole test. pH was monitored in all urines (4).

Total radioactivity was measured in plasma. Methods for determination of imipramine and desipramine in plasma were not available at the time of these studies. In urine, metabolites were separated by extraction with

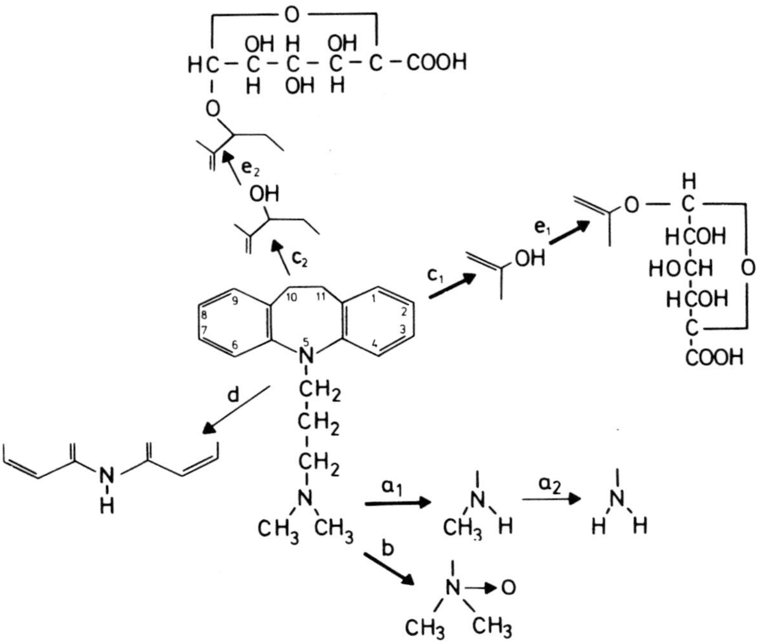

FIG. 1. Biotransformation of imipramine.

ethylene dichloride before and after enzymatic hydrolysis (glucuronidase) of the urine. The metabolites were isolated by two-dimensional thin-layer chromatography and quantified by counting radioactivity in the silica-gel corresponding to the spots on the chromatogram. These methods have been described in detail elsewhere (3–5).

The same interaction was studied after 9 days pretreatment of rats (male Wistar, 200 g) with perphenazine. The changes in urinary metabolite pattern were studied on 24-hr urine.

RESULTS AND DISCUSSION

As seen in previous studies, the perphenazine treatment caused a marked decrease in urinary excretion, and at the same time a decrease in total radioactivity in plasma. In the urine, both the glucuronide fraction and the residual fraction were reduced, whereas the nonconjugated fraction in total was not altered.

Analysis of the metabolites in the nonconjugated fraction showed several changes during treatment with perphenazine (Table 1). The most striking change was a decrease in excretion of 2-hydroxy-desipramine (DMI-OH).

TABLE. 1. *Imipramine metabolites in human urine*[b]

Patient sex, age	K. F. m, 20		E. J. f, 46		I. A. f, 27		N. P. m, 34		M. K. m, 24		K. R. f, 53	
Perphenazine dose (mg/day)	0	60	0	32	0	36	0	48	0	24	0	50[a]
Imipramine	0.0012	0.0076	0.0024	0.0029	0.0013	0.0055	0.0032	0.0044	0.0060	0.0055	0.0001	0.0042
Desipramine	0.0071	0.0184	0.0167	0.0107	0.0015	0.0155	0.0021	0.0077	0.0080	0.0137	0.0001	0.0091
2-Hydroxy-imipramine	0.0014	0.0015	0.0036	0.0007	0.0037	0.0044	0.0054	0.0016	0.0100	0.0091	0.0001	0.0082
2-Hydroxy-desipramine	0.0305	0.0114	0.0483	0.0010	0.0194	0.0027	0.0192	0.0133	0.0370	0.0375	0.0543	0.0552
Imipramine-N-oxide	0.0056	0.0098	0.0087	0.0043	0.0125	0.0280	0.0074	0.0227	0.0026	0.0096	0.0113	0.0135

[a] 50 mg as perphenazine enantate given 14 hr before ^{14}C-imipramine.

[b] Average urinary excretion of imipramine metabolites in man in drug-free period and during perphenazine treatment. Excretion in percent of dose per hour. Results from urine fractions from first 8 hr after test-dose administration were omitted from the calculations.

TABLE 2. *Imipramine metabolites in rat urine*[a]

	Control	Perphenazine pretreated	p
Imipramine	0.168	0.225	N.S.
Desipramine	0.059	0.099	N.S.
2-Hydroxy-imipramine	0.026	0.025	N.S.
2-Hydroxy-desipramine	0	0	·
Imipramine-N-oxide	0.454	1.500	<0.01
Iminodibenzyl	0.139	0.430	<0.01

[a] Urinary excretion of imipramine metabolites in control rats ($n = 6$) and rats pretreated with perphenazine 10 mg/kg/day for 9 days ($n = 6$). Excretion in percent of dose per liter per day.

The excretion of imipramine (IP), desipramine (DMI), and imipramine-N-oxide (IPNO) was increased in most cases. The relative proportion of IP versus IPNO and IP versus DMI indicated that neither N-oxidation nor demethylation was influenced by perphenazine. The excretion of unconjugated 2-hydroxy-imipramine was very low in both control and perphenazine period.

In the rat studies, it was also found that the excretion of glucuronide metabolites and the residual fraction was reduced in perphenazine-treated rats. In the nonconjugated fraction (Table 2), the most striking features were increase in excretion of IPNO and iminodibenzyl (IDB), the dealkylated metabolite. The hydroxy metabolites were present in very small amounts and no definite change could be observed. This is probably due to a very fast glucuronide formation from IP-OH and DMI-OH.

From these data it is therefore possible to draw conclusions concerning the effect of perphenazine on the metabolism of imipramine (Fig. 2). Perphenazine seems to inhibit the hydroxylation resulting in increased amount of IP, DMI, and a corresponding increase in formation of IPNO, and in the rats also of IDB. When studying the ratio IP/DMI in human urine and in rat tissues, it could be concluded that demethylation is not influenced by perphenazine.

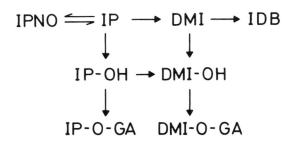

FIG. 2. Pathways in biotransformation of imipramine.

However, the time course of metabolite excretion after oral administration of ^{14}C-imipramine to man deserves special attention in relation to the interaction (Fig. 3). Several striking features of the time course should be observed. The nonconjugated form of IP-OH is excreted in very small amounts. At the same time glucuronide metabolites (IP-O-GA) were excreted in large amounts. The conjugation process therefore seems to be very fast, the ratio IP-OH/IP-O-GA ranging from 1/20 to 1/100.

The N-oxide formation is pronounced in the first hours after test-dose administration and decreases then rapidly during the first day. This most likely reflects changes in the metabolism during the first pass metabolism

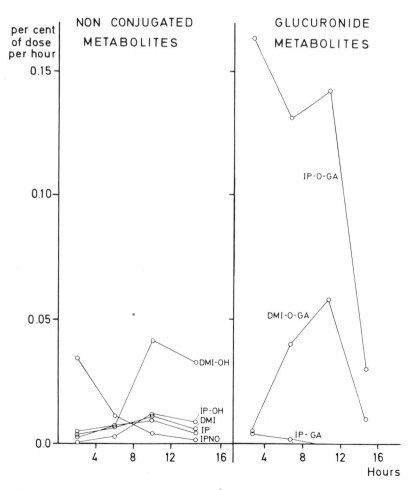

FIG. 3. Time course of metabolite excretion after oral administration of ^{14}C-imipramine (50 mg = 3 μC) to man (subj. M. K., drug-free period).

of imipramine. A saturation of the hydroxylation is likely to occur at this stage and might result in increased N-oxide formation, due to an increased amount of IP. The formation of glucuronide directly from IP (IP-GA) in the first hour after test-dose administration might also be explained in this way. The influence of perphenazine on N-oxide formation appears to be different during this time course. The N-oxidation thus seems to be inhibited in the beginning, i.e., during the first pass metabolism. Later on, the formation of IPNO is increased parallel to increased amounts of IP. In one patient, where the DMI-hydroxylation was almost totally inhibited by perphenazine (Table 1, pat. E. J.), the N-oxidation was also inhibited throughout the whole 24-hr period.

In one patient receiving 24 mg per day and in another receiving perphenazine enantate, 50 mg given the evening before administration of imipramine, the interaction effect was relatively weak.

The effect of perphenazine on metabolism of IP, inhibition of hydroxylation and no or little effect on demethylation and N-oxidation (Fig. 2), reminds very much of the effect of SKF 525A on imipramine metabolism *in vitro* as reported by several groups (6–8).

REFERENCES

1. Gram, L. F., Kofod, B., Christiansen, J., and Rafaelsen, O. J. (1971): In: *Advances in Neuropsychopharmacology*, p. 447, Excerp ta Medica, Amsterdam.
2. Gram, L. F., and Fredricson Overø, K. (1972): *Brit. Med. J. 1*, 463.
3. Christiansen, J., Gram, L. F., Kofod, B., and Rafaelsen, O. J. (1967): *Psychopharmacologia 11*, 255.
4. Gram, L. F., Kofod, B., Christiansen, J., and Rafaelsen, O. J. (1971): *Clin. Pharmacol. Thér. 12*, 239.
5. Christiansen, J., and Gram, L. F. (1973): *J. Pharm. Pharmacol. 25*, 604.
6. Bickel, M. H., and Minder, R. (1970): *Biochem. Pharmac. 19*, 2425.
7. Gigon, P. L., and Bickel, M. H. (1971): *Biochem. Pharmac. 20*, 1921.
8. Nahazawa, K. (1970): *Biochem. Pharmac. 19*, 1363.

Drug Interactions, edited by P. L. Morselli,
S. Garattini, and S. N. Cohen. Raven Press,
New York © 1974

Pharmacokinetic Studies on Interaction
of Rymazolium and Morphine-like Drugs

Susanna Fürst and J. Knoll

Department of Pharmacology, Semmelweis Medical University, Budapest, VIII. Üllöi ut 26,
Hungary

A new morphine derivative, 6-deoxy-6-azido-dihydroisomorphine; Azido-morphine; AM, has been recently described (1–3). Figure 1 shows the chemical structure of the drug in comparison with morphine.

Table 1 summarizes the toxicity data of azidomorphine, administered intravenously, subcutaneously, and perorally, compared with the parent molecule (morphine) and with fentanylcitrate. The action of analgesics on the threshold of nociceptive reaction was evaluated with the hot plate method on rat (4). As can be seen, a new morphine derivative, azidomorphine, is 40 times more toxic than morphine when administered subcutaneously. On the other hand, this compound was found to possess marked analgesic activity in several assays being about 200 times more potent than morphine when tested by hot plate method. The median therapeutic indices were counted on the base of LD_{50}/ED_{50} ratio and were found to be as high as 351, whereas that of morphine was 84 (Table 1).

The time course of the analgesic action of narcotics has been studied also using the hot plate test. Morphine is known to produce its analgesic action in man for 4 to 5 hr. In order to further analyze the relationship between time and action, we have calculated the half-times ($T^{1}/_{2}$) of the effect, especially the half-times belonging to the ED_{50} values of analgesics. The half-time is considered as a period expressed in minutes measured between the peak activity and its decrease to the half, and is calculated graphically, on the basis of time-action curves.

First, we have calculated the half-times belonging to the ED_{50} of azido-morphine (Fig. 2). The time curves of Fig. 2 demonstrate the half-times associated with different doses of the drug. It is clear that the half-times are dose dependent; consequently, the half-time belonging to the ED_{50} can be calculated if the logarithms of the doses are plotted against the half-times of different doses ($T^{1}/_{2}$/min). $T^{1}/_{2}$ was found to be 32 min for azidomorphine (Fig. 2) and 40 min for morphine. In order to prolong the analgesic effect of the two narcotics mentioned above, Rymazolium (1,6-dimethyl-3-carb-ethoxy-4-oxo-6,7,8,9-tetrahydro-homopyrimidazol-methylsulphate) was

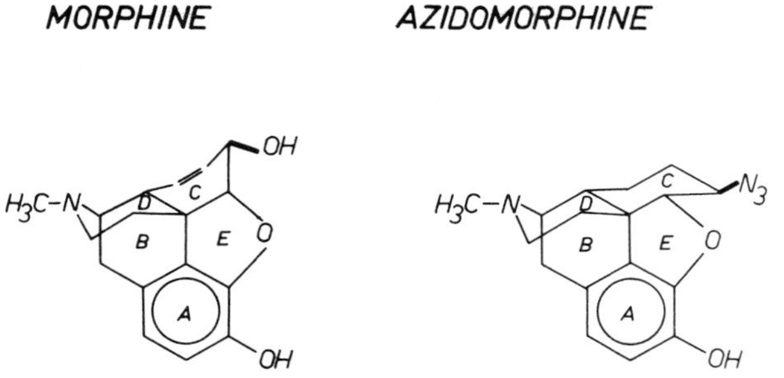

MORPHINE   AZIDOMORPHINE

FIG. 1. Chemical structure of 6-deoxy-6-azido-dihydroisomorphine (azidomorphine) compared with morphine.

used (5–7). This drug was found to be similar to the minor analgesics, differing from those in its ability to potentiate the analgesic effect of narcotics. When Rymazolium is administered together with morphine or azidomorphine in a dose ineffective alone, it potentiates not only the analgesic effect but prolongs the duration of action, too. The half-time of the analgesic effect of azidomorphine (0.025 mg/kg s.c.) is 22 min, that of Rymazolium (50 mg/kg s.c.) 45 min, and that of the combination as long as 105 min (Fig. 3). The same was found for morphine, where the half-time of the effect of the combination (5 mg/kg morphine + 50 mg/kg Rymazolium) was 92 min, whereas that for each component was 45 min.

In conclusion, our results suggest that drugs having the ability to potentiate the effect of narcotic analgesics may increase the duration of effect, too.

In other experiments, the kinetic parameters of azidomorphine on the longitudinal muscle strip of guinea pig ileum and the hot plate method were

TABLE 1. Comparison of analgetic activity (hot plate) and toxicity data of morphine, fentanyl, and 6-deoxy-6-azido-dihydroisomorphine

Compound	$LD_{50}{}^a$ (mg/kg)			$ED_{50}{}^b$ hot plate (s.c.)	$LD_{50}/ED_{50}{}^c$ s.c.
	i.v.	s.c.	p.os.		
6-Deoxy-6-azido-dihydro-isomorphine	8.1	13.0	62.0	37 μg/kg	351
Morphine	360.0	520.0	1200.0	6.2 mg/kg	84
Fentanyl	—	30.0	—	21 μg/kg	1420

^{a} LD_{50} = median lethal dose, calculated graphically.
^{b} ED_{50} = median analgesic activity, calculated graphically.
^{c} LD_{50}/ED_{50} = median therapeutic index.

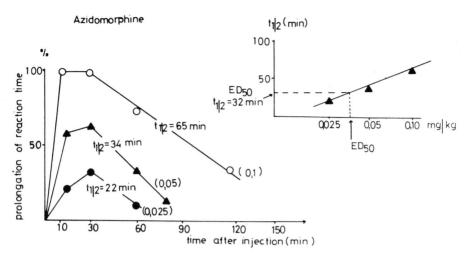

FIG. 2. Time course of analgesic action of azidomorphine measured on the hot plate test (rat). (For $T^{1/2}$ time calculation see text.)

investigated by means of two narcotic antagonists, naloxone and nalorphine.

Gyang and Kosterlitz (8) have shown that all narcotic analgesic drugs have "dual" agonist and antagonist action. They examined the effects of these drugs on the contractions of the longitudinal muscle, stimulated coaxially, and both "narcotic agonist" and "narcotic antagonists" were shown to be partial agonists. Naloxone is the only drug studied so far that

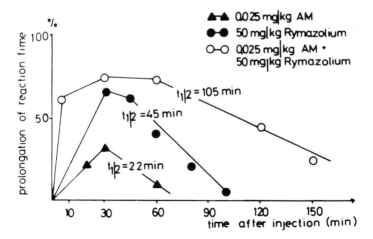

FIG. 3. Time course of analgesic action of azidomorphine, Rymazolium, and their combination. (For $T^{1/2}$ time calculation see text.)

has little or no agonist activity and can therefore be used as a "pure" antagonist (9, 10). Although many attempts have been made to find a narcotic agonist without antagonist activity, this search has not been successful thus far. All the drugs causing tolerance and physical dependence are narcotic agonists. No tolerance was observed after the treatment with narcotic antagonists. Azidomorphine, the new morphine derivative investigated by us (1–3), failed to cause tolerance and physical dependence in rhesus monkeys when administered in therapeutic (analgesic) doses. It seemed of interest, therefore, to study kinetic parameters of this morphine derivative. The presynaptic inhibitory action of narcotics on neuroeffector transmission of longitudinal muscle strip of guinea pig ileum (11) was chosen as a model.

Morphine and morphine-like drugs show a dose-dependent inhibition of the contractions of a longitudinal muscle strip, when low frequency stimulation is applied. The concentration causing 50% inhibition of the twitch (ID_{50}) to characterize agonist activity and the equilibrium constant (K_e) to characterize antagonist activity were estimated as described by Gyang and Kosterlitz (8).

ID_{50} concentration of drug producing 50% inhibition of responses of the longitudinal muscle strip to field stimulation at 0.1 Hz was calculated by a "multiple dose" method. The dose-response curves were plotted as percentage inhibition of the twitch against the log concentration of drug used. Since Gyang and Kosterlitz (8) showed that reproducible dose-response curves in the ileum preparation could be produced for morphine when doses were administered at intervals of 20 min, the preparations were allowed to rest for 20 min between the two consecutive doses of narcotics used.

The mathematical analyses were programmed and performed by a computer.

Azidomorphine has been found to reduce dose dependently the responses of longitudinal muscle of guinea pig ileum to field stimulation at 0.1 Hz. However, it failed to affect the contractions produced by high-frequency stimulation (20 Hz). The inhibitory action of azidomorphine on contractions induced by 0.1-Hz stimulation is due to its inhibitory action on acetylcholine release from nerve terminals of Auerbach plexus. Azidomorphine, 10^{-8} M, reduced the output of acetylcholine by 85.3% when 0.1-Hz stimulation frequency was applied. However, the output in response to 20-Hz stimulation was not affected by azidomorphine. In addition, the presynaptic inhibitory action of azidomorphine on neurochemical transmission of longitudinal-muscle-strip preparation is supported by the fact that the effect of acetylcholine added to the bath was not influenced.

Plotting the inhibitory effect of azidomorphine and morphine against the log concentration of agonists, it was found that naloxone shifted the dose-response curves of azidomorphine to the right. The parallel displacement to the right depended on the concentrations of naloxone.

Since naloxone (NX) and azidomorphine (AM) interact reversibly with a receptor (R) site in the cells

$$AM + R \rightleftharpoons AMR,$$
$$NX + R \rightleftharpoons NXR,$$

and only the AMR combination is pharmacologically effective (12) at equilibrium, the following relationship should hold:

$$DR - 1 = K_e \, (AM)$$

where K_e is the affinity constant of the NX-receptor complex, and DR is the ratio of AM concentrations in the presence and absence of NX required to produce the same effect and (NX) is the concentration of naloxone in solution.

Thus the plot of log $(DR - 1)$ against log of NX concentration should produce a straight line with a gradient of 1 and an intercept on the abscissa corresponding to log K_e (Fig. 4a,b).

Figure 4 illustrates a plot of log $(DR - 1)$ against log (NX) constructed from a series of five experiments. The antagonism between naloxone and azidomorphine and morphine on longitudinal-muscle-strip preparation (Fig. 4a) and on analgesia using the hot plate method (Fig. 4b) was studied.

The slopes of the lines were for AM and for Mo 1.194 ± 0.29 and 0.955 ± 0.31, respectively; none of these values differed significantly from unity indicating a competitive nature of antagonism between naloxone and AM and Mo, respectively. The values of the dissociation constant (K_e) obtained from the intercepts on the abscissa are for azidomorphine-naloxone 9.06 $(8.71 \times 10^{-10}$ M), and for morphine-naloxone 8.48 $(3.31 \times 10^{-9}$ M), respectively. The difference between the two values is significant $p < 0.01$. These data indicate that a higher concentration of naloxone is required to antagonize the agonist effect of morphine than that of azidomorphine. Figure 4b demonstrates the antagonism between naloxone and azidomorphine and morphine as measured by the hot plate method. K_e values for azidomorphine and morphine are 0.023 and 0.118 mg/kg indicating that in this test too a higher amount of naloxone was required to antagonize the agonist effect of morphine than that of azidomorphine ($p < 0.01$).

The use of pA_2 is a convenient method for expressing the activity of an antagonist in terms of the dissociation constant of the antagonist-receptor complex in competitive antagonism. Table 2 shows the kinetic parameters of narcotics studied. Azidomorphine in a concentration of 2.0 nM reduced the contractions of longitudinal muscle strip in response to stimulation at 0.1 Hz by half (ID_{50}).

Apparent differences between azidomorphine and morphine were ob-

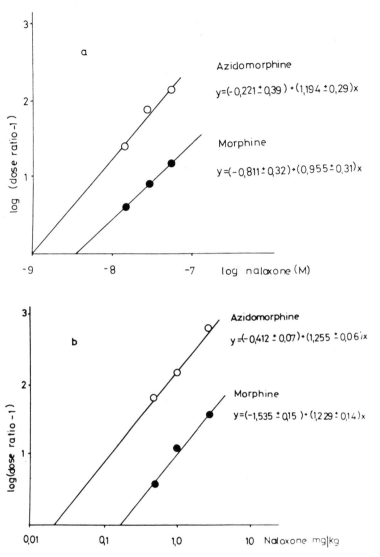

FIG. 4. Competitive nature of the antagonism by naloxone of the depressant effects of morphine and azidomorphine. (a) *Longitudinal muscle* strip of guinea pig ileum. The lines are drawn from the regression equations. Each point represents five independent experiments. The intercept on abscissa *(pA$_a$)* for naloxone-azidomorphine 9.06 and for naloxone-morphine 8.48, i.e., 0.87 nM and 3.31 nM, respectively. (b) *Analgesic action* measured by the hot plate method. Each point represents the average of analgesic effect obtained in a group of 10 rats. The intercept on the abscissa for naloxone-azidomorphine is 0.023 and for naloxone-morphine 0.118 mg/kg. Naloxone and azidomorphine and morphine were administered 30 min prior to the test, since it has been shown that the maximal activity of naloxone and morphine (13) and also azidomorphine was reached at 30 min. All the drugs used were administered subcutaneously.

TABLE 2. *Kinetic parameters of azidomorphine and different morphine derivatives*

Drug	ID_{50} (nM)	K_e (nM)	$P_a/(ID_{50}/K_e)$
Azidomorphine	2.0 ± 0.55 (11)	ID_{50} (5)	1
Morphine	58.0 ± 6.8 (5)	16.5 ± 1.1 (3)	3.5
Normorphine	68.0 (2)	ID_{50} (2)	1
Nalorphine	46.0 ± 6.5 (3)	9.4 ± 0.5 (3)	4.89
Pentazocine	370 (2)	29.2 (2)	12.7
Naloxone	53.2 (2)	2.5 ± 0.1 (5)	21280

No. of experiments in parentheses.

ID_{50} concentration of drug producing 50% inhibition of responses of the longitudinal muscle strip to field stimulation at 0.1 Hz. The ID_{50} values were calculated by "multiple dose" method of Gyang and Kosterlitz (8).

K_e equals the concentration causing a dose ratio of 2; the dose ratio is obtained:

$$DR = \frac{M_3}{M_2 - M_1},$$

the depressant effect of the drug which is read off a dose-response curve obtained shortly before the starting of the experiment. K_e (equilibrium constant) was calculated from

$$K_e = \frac{a}{DR - 1},$$

where a is the molar concentration of the partial agonist, which produces the inhibition indicated by M_1. Morphine was used as agonist. $P_a/ID_{50}/K_e$ = antagonist potency (10).

served in the hot plate experiments. Figure 5 demonstrates that the analgesic action of morphine was antagonized to a greater extent ($DR = 120.9$) than that of azidomorphine ($DR = 21.4$) when nalorphine was used as antagonist in a dose of 15 mg/kg. The dose ratio (DR) is calculated as a ratio of the ED_{50} values obtained in the presence and absence of antagonist. ED_{50} values were calculated from dose-response curves.

Summarizing our results, in agreement with the findings of others (10), the K_e value for morphine was considerably smaller than its ID_{50} concentration. On the other hand, azidomorphine did not inhibit the effect of morphine in its agonist (ID_{50}) concentration, i.e., it has been shown to be highly potent and compared to morphine, "pure" agonist. The statistically significant differences in pA_2 values (antagonist activity) obtained in longitudinal muscle strip and also in the hot plate method using either morphine or azidomorphine as agonist suggest that some differences regarding drug-receptor interactions between these molecules might exist, leading to the functional differences observed. The fact that azidomorphine was antagonized by naloxone much more easily than by morphine and that the

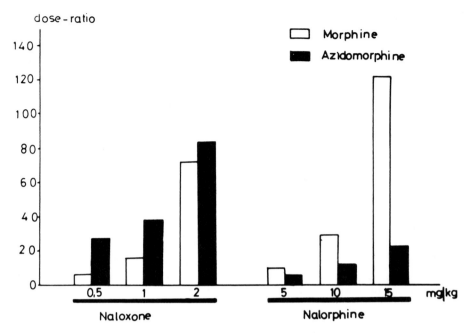

Fig. 5. Antagonistic effect of naloxone and nalorphine on hot plate reaction times obtained in rats treated with morphine and azidomorphine. Antagonism is expressed as dose ratio (for calculation of dose ratio see text). All the drugs used were given subcutaneously 30 min prior to the test. Note the differences in antagonism observed with naloxone and nalorphine when morphine and azidomorphine were applied as agonists.

opposite was observed when nalorphine was used as antagonist support this hypothesis.

REFERENCES

1. Knoll, J., Susanna, Fürst, and Kelemen, K. (1971): *Orvostud. 20*, 266.
2. Knoll, J. (1973): *Pharm. Research Comm. 5*, 175.
3. Knoll, J., Susanna, Fürst, and Kelemen, K. (1973): *J. Pharm. Pharmacol. 25*, 929.
4. Woolfe, G., and McDonald, A. P. (1944): *J. Pharmac. Exp. Ther. 80*, 300.
5. Knoll, J., Mészáros, Z., Szentmiklósi, P., and Susanna, Fürst (1971): *Arzneimittel Forsch. 21*, 717.
6. Knoll, J., Susanna, Fürst, and Mészáros, Z. (1971): *Arzneim. Forsch. 21*, 719.
7. Knoll, J., Susanna, Fürst, and Mészáros, Z. (1971): *Arzneim. Forsch. 21*, 727.
8. Gyang, E. A., and Kosterlitz, H. W. (1966): *Brit. J. Pharmac. Chemother. 27*, 514.
9. Földes, F. F., Lunn, J. N., Moore, J., and Brown, I. M. (1963): *Am. J. Med. Sci. 245*, 23.
10. Kosterlitz, J. W., and Watt, A. J. (1968): *Brit. J. Pharmac. Chemother. 33*, 266.
11. Paton, W. D. M. (1957): *Brit. J. Pharmac. Chemother. 12*, 119.
12. Schild. H. O. (1957): *Pharmac. Rev. 9*, 242.
13. Smits, S. E., and Takemori, A. E. (1970): *Brit. J. Pharmac. Chemother. 39*, 627.

Drug Interactions, edited by P. L. Morselli,
S. Garattini, and S. N. Cohen. Raven Press,
New York © 1974

Interaction Between Carbamazepine and Diphenylhydantoin and/or Phenobarbital in Epileptic Patients

Johannes Christiansen and Mogens Dam

Department of Clinical Chemistry A and Department of Neurology, Rigshospitalet, University Hospital, Denmark

Interaction between phenobarbital and diphenylhydantoin has been known for some years. As carbamazepine now is widely used in the treatment of epilepsy, we wanted to investigate whether phenobarbital and diphenylhydantoin had any influence on the plasma level of carbamazepine in patients with epilepsy.

One hundred twenty-three patients were treated with carbamazepine. The material was separated into four groups. In group 1, 30 patients were treated with carbamazepine alone (the number of determinations of plasma carbamazepine was 43). In group 2, 48 patients were treated with carbamazepine and diphenylhydantoin (the number of determinations of plasma carbamazepine was 62). In group 3, 18 patients were treated with carbamazepine and phenobarbital (the number of plasma determinations was 44), and in group 4, 27 patients were treated with all three drugs (the number of plasma determinations in this group was 77).

An ultramicromethod for determination of carbamazepine and metabolites in 10 μl plasma has been used. The method is based on thin-layer chromatography and subsequent *in situ* fluorescence measurement of the chromatogram. The plasma sample is applied direct to the chromatoplate, without extraction. The standard deviation of the method is about 5% relative and the sensitivity is about 20 ng in a 10-μl sample.

Figure 1 shows a scatter diagram of the four groups. The abscissa dose is given in mg/kg body weight, and the ordinate plasma concentration of carbamazepine is given in mg/l.

Figure 2 shows the regression lines calculated from the corresponding values for dose/plasma concentrations in the four groups. The difference between the regression line of group 1 and the other groups is highly significant ($p < 0.001$) the difference between groups 2 and 4 and 3 and 4 is significant as well.

The average plasma level of carbamazepine in patients taking this drug

285

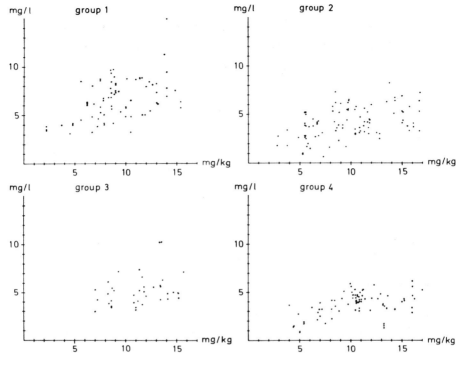

FIG. 1.

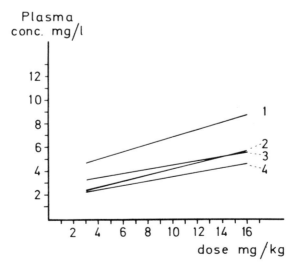

FIG. 2.

Carbamazepine plasma conc. mg/l	clinical			total
	better	unchanged	worsen	
0 - 3	9	5	0	14
3 - 6	35	30	3	68
6 - 9	16	4	0	20
› 9	1	1	0	2

FIG. 3.

alone was about twice the level when they were treated also with diphenyl-hydantoin and phenobarbital, 6.7 mg/1 and 3.7 mg/1.

The administration of diphenylhydantoin and/or phenobarbital to patients in carbamazepine treatment results in a significant decrease in carbamazepine plasma level compared to patients treated with carbamazepine alone. The decrease suggests a change in carbamazepine metabolism in the liver resulting from stimulation of the microsomal enzymes by diphenylhydantoin and phenobarbital. It could, however, also be explained by an effect of diphenylhydantoin and phenobarbital on the binding of carbamazepine to microsomal enzymes. Other possibilities could be changes in absorption, excretion, tissue distribution, or protein binding. Further studies on this subject are in progress.

In order to investigate whether the found drug interaction has any therapeutic consequence, we selected 104 patients with epilepsy and studied the effect of the antiepileptic drugs given. The patients were divided

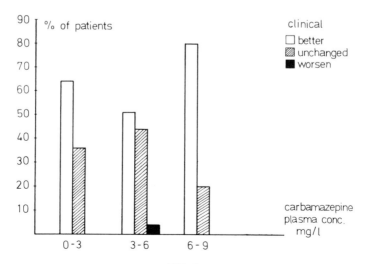

FIG. 4.

in patients with severe epilepsy (seizures once a day to once a week), patients with moderate epilepsy (with seizures once a week to once a month), and patients with mild epilepsy (with seizures less than once a month). If a patient changed from one group to another, he was grouped as better or worse, depending on the new frequency of seizures.

Figure 3 shows the correlation between the clinical effect and the plasma level. Figure 4 shows the same results in percent of the patients. Although the number of patients is small, we conclude that the therapeutic level of carbamazepine is higher than 6 mg/l. Our demonstration of a drug interaction between carbamazepine, phenobarbital and diphenylhydantoin indicates the importance of measuring the plasma carbamazepine in patients with epilepsy. The carbamazepine plasma level should as a rule be higher than 6 mg/l in order to achieve the best clinical result.

Drug Interactions, edited by P. L. Morselli, S. Garattini, and S. N. Cohen. Raven Press, New York © 1974

The Uptake of Diphenylhydantoin by the Human Erythrocyte and Its Application to the Estimation of Plasma Binding

G. R. Wilkinson and D. Kurata

Division of Clinical Pharmacology, Department of Pharmacology, Vanderbilt University, Nashville, Tennessee 37232

INTRODUCTION

There is an increasing awareness that for certain drugs the dosages required to obtain optimal therapeutic effects may differ quite widely between different patients. The "usual" dose or dosage schedule may produce little response in some patients, cause toxicity, often serious, in others, and may be fully satisfactory only in a few. These differences are frequently attributed to interpatient variability in drug absorption, distribution, metabolism, and excretion, which may be caused by genetic and/or environmental factors, the presence of disease states such as renal or hepatic dysfunction, or the concomitant administration of other drugs. If the desired pharmacologic response can be simply and accurately quantitated, as in the case of anticoagulant drugs like warfarin, then optimization of the dose is readily attainable. Unfortunately, however, the majority of drugs do not exhibit such pharmacological properties and "titration" therapy is not possible. In these cases, and particularly where the difference between effective and toxic doses is small, it has been suggested that individualization of therapy should be based upon steady-state blood or plasma concentrations of the drug (1–3).

For such measurements to become useful guides to dosage adjustments, it is necessary to define by suitable clinical studies the therapeutically effective range of plasma concentrations. At present, this has been accomplished for only a few important drugs including the digitalis glycosides (4), certain anticonvulsant (5) and antiarrhythmic drugs (6, 7), propranolol (8), lithium (9) and nortriptyline (10).

The analytical techniques that are presently used to determine drugs in biological fluids measure the total drug concentration in the sample. Yet, it is a fundamental tenet of pharmacology that only the unbound or free circulating drug is available for distribution to the tissues and biophase, and frequently it is observed that plasma binding limits drug elimination by either metabolism or excretion. If the free-drug concentration is approximately a constant fraction of the total concentration, then the total drug level will be indicative of the pharmacologically active drug concentration. However, there is increasing evidence that considerable interpatient variability may exist in drug plasma-binding characteristics. For example, Alexanderson and Borgå (11) have observed a twofold interindividual variation in the binding ratio of plasma proteins for nortriptyline, and whereas the plasma binding of diphenylhydantoin in adults is constant over the therapeutic range at about 93%, in azotemia and uremia the binding may fall to as low as 70 to 75% (12, 13). Consistent with this increase in the free fraction, seizure control in such patients can be attained at total drug levels of about 1 to 3 $\mu g/ml$ (12, 14); much below the commonly accepted therapeutic range of 10 to 20 $\mu g/ml$. In addition, it is well recognized that a drug interaction may potentially involve displacement of a drug from its plasma-binding sites by a second competitive drug (15).

The above considerations suggest that the therapeutic range of drug plasma levels should be defined with respect to the free concentration of the drug in the plasma rather than the total concentration. Further, the most critical drugs for which such an approach would be appropriate are those that are extensively bound to the plasma constituents under "usual" conditions and where a small decrease in binding, at any given total drug concentration, will produce a large change in the fraction of drug that is unbound.

If measurement of the free-drug concentration in the plasma is more significant with respect to the clinical effects than the total plasma concentration, then consideration must be given to methodology for determining it. The classical techniques of equilibrium dialysis and ultrafiltration are frequently used in research for directly determining the free-drug level in plasma. However, utilization of these methods in a routine, service oriented laboratory is problematic. In the first instance, application of the techniques will minimally triple the analytical workload of the laboratory. Additionally, the methods are laborious, tedious, and time-consuming, the latter being quite important when short turn-around times are frequently demanded by the clinician. Finally, it is necessary to balance this additional time and effort against the likelihood that only a small proportion of the samples will exhibit unusual plasma-binding characteristics. Accordingly, a rapid, simple screening technique for identifying those patients in whom unusual drug plasma binding is present would appear highly desirable. Subsequently, the atypical samples could be studied in more detail by other techniques, and such a screen would also function to alert consultant clinical pharmacologists and clinicians that the generally accepted dose/plasma concentration/clinical response relationships may not be appropriate in that particular individual patient. Our initial studies using diphenylhydantoin (DPH) as a model drug and involving the measurement of the blood/plasma drug concentration ratio suggests that this determination may serve such a function.

METHODS AND RESULTS

In vitro studies at room temperature (24°C) were carried out using fresh human heparinized blood. The blood was centrifuged, plasma and buffy layers removed, and the erythrocytes (RBC) washed three times with isotonic buffered saline, pH 7.4. Depending upon the particular experiment the erythrocytes were then resuspended in either plasma, diluted plasma, or isotonic buffer at a hematocrit of 0.5. Radiolabeled DPH was added, the sample allowed to incubate for 30 min and then aliquots were taken for analysis. In addition, plasma binding of DPH was determined by overnight equilibrium dialysis (16) or ultrafiltration (17).

As indicated in the following equation, the blood/plasma concentration ratio is a function of two potential variables, the RBC/plasma concentration ratio and the hematocrit *(H)*.

$$\frac{\text{Blood}}{\text{Plasma}} = (1 - H) + \frac{\text{RBC}}{\text{Plasma}} \cdot H \qquad (1)$$

Using erythrocytes reconstituted in isotonic buffer, constant RBC/buffer and "blood"/buffer concentration ratios were observed with values of about 4.9 and 3.1, respectively (Fig. 1). Since binding in such a system was negligible, the buffer concentrations studied, 0.2 to 22 μg/ml, encompass the

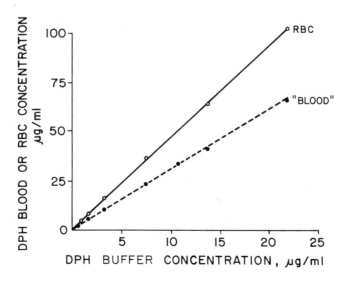

FIG. 1. Effect of DPH buffer concentration upon the "blood" and RBC concentrations in an erythrocyte-buffer system.

TABLE 1. *Effect of various anticonvulsant drugs upon the plasma binding and distribution of DPH[a]*

Drug	Blood / Plasma	Percent unbound[b]
HPPH	0.606	4.78
(5, 14, 40 μg/ml)	0.597, 0.606, 0.611	4.55, 4.79, 4.87
Phenobarbital	0.606	4.78
(22, 55, 111 μg/ml)	0.624, 0.590, 0.595	4.62, 4.55, 4.69
Primidone	0.568	5.76
(5, 25, 50 μg/ml)	0.574, 0.568, 0.586	5.19, 5.25, 5.14
Ethosuximide	0.568	5.76
(20, 100, 200 μg/ml)	0.575, 0.566, 0.580	5.80, 5.42, 5.79

[a] The upper value indicates that obtained in control blood and the three lower figures the values observed at the indicated concentration of the drug under study.
[b] Estimated by ultrafiltration.

probable concentration of unbound DPH that might be observed in patients. The concentration of DPH by the erythrocyte probably reflects membrane or intracellular binding of the drug rather than an active uptake process, since it does not appear to be saturable over the concentration range investigated and competitive inhibition by a close structurally related compound does not occur (Table 1).

According to Eq. 1 if the RBC/buffer concentration ratio is constant, then the hematocrit should influence the blood/plasma concentration in a linear fashion. Using "blood" to which DPH had been added to produce a total concentration of 15 μg/ml, such a relationship was observed for both buffer and plasma reconstituted systems (Fig. 2); however, the slopes of the curves were grossly dissimilar. Since this slope is equal to the RBC/"plasma" concentration ratio minus one, this difference clearly indicates a pronounced effect of plasma upon the uptake of DPH into the erythrocyte.

To demonstrate that binding was responsible for this decreased erythrocyte distribution, the cells were reconstituted in various dilutions of plasma. Such a procedure altered the DPH free fraction, as estimated by ultrafiltration, from about 0.05 to 1.0 at a constant total blood concentration of 15 μg/ml. In response to this perturbation the blood/plasma concentration ratio increased in a linear fashion from a value, at 0% free DPH, of 0.5 to about 3.1 at 100% free DPH (Fig. 3). A similar curve was obtained for the RBC/plasma concentration ratio, its value changing from 0.0 to 4.9 over the same binding range. Additional experiments indicated that the binding of DPH to undiluted plasma was constant over the total plasma concentration range 5 to 55 μg/ml and, therefore, the blood/plasma concentration provides a valid estimate of the extent of plasma binding of DPH over the whole of

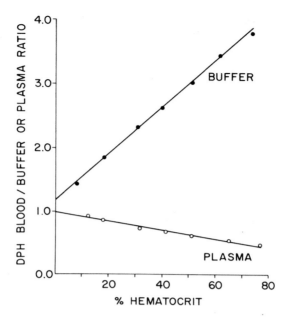

FIG. 2. Effect of hematocrit upon the DPH blood/buffer and blood/plasma concentration ratios.

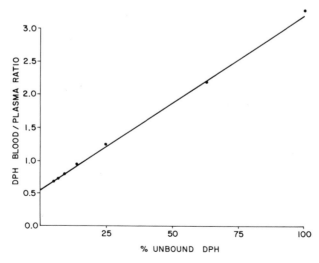

FIG. 3. Relationship between the percentage of unbound DPH in the plasma and the blood/plasma concentration ratio.

TABLE 2. DPH plasma binding and erythrocyte distribution in normal subjects (mean ± standard deviation)

	Blood Plasma	RBC Plasma	Percent unbound[a] u.f.	Percent unbound[a] e.d.	Blood Buffer	RBC Buffer
Male (n = 6)	0.614 ± 0.01	0.227 ± 0.03	5.37 ± 0.19	8.62 ± 0.44	2.917 ± 0.04	4.837 ± 0.08
Female (n = 6)	0.611 ± 0.01	0.217 ± 0.02	5.31 ± 0.18	8.49 ± 0.20	2.901 ± 0.10	4.829 ± 0.20
Total (n = 12)	0.613 ± 0.01	0.222 ± 0.03	5.34 ± 0.18	8.56 ± 0.33	2.909 ± 0.08	4.833 ± 0.16

[a] Measured by ultrafiltration (u.f.) and equilibrium dialysis (e.d.).

the therapeutic concentration range. In blood obtained from 12 normal volunteers, the erythrocyte uptake and the binding of DPH in both plasma and buffer systems were surprisingly constant, and no sex differences were observed (Table 2). The extent of binding exhibited differences according to the method of estimation; a finding previously reported (17). If an RBC/plasma concentration ratio versus free-fraction curve was constructed using values for the latter estimated by equilibrium dialysis, then the straight line had a negative intercept on the ordinate. In contrast, the curve based upon binding measured by ultrafiltration passed through the origin. Such observations would suggest that ultrafiltration is a more valid technique for estimating DPH plasma binding than the presently described equilibrium dialysis and that the latter overestimates the extent of binding by about 3 to 4%.

In common with many other acidic drugs, DPH may be displaced from its plasma-binding sites by other drugs, presumably interacting at these sites. Since the presence of potential displacers in a clinical blood sample would not generally be known, it was considered important to determine whether the blood/plasma concentration ratio technique could detect and accurately quantify the drug interaction. Accordingly, blood containing DPH at a total concentration of 15 μg/ml was incubated for 30 min in the presence of known *in vitro* displacers: salicylic acid, 50 to 550 μg/ml; phenylbutazone, 11 to 111 μg/ml; and sulfamethoxypyridazine, 40 to 220 μg/ml. As reported previously (17), these drugs increased the free fraction of DPH quite significantly, depending upon relative concentrations of DPH and displacing agent, but, more importantly, the changes were associated with changes in the blood/plasma concentration ratio in accordance with the linear relationship established from the plasma dilution experiments (Fig. 4). Significantly, neither the major metabolite of DPH, 5-*p*-hydroxyphenyl-5-phenylhydantoin (HPPH) nor other anticonvulsant drugs, which are commonly administered along with DPH, displaced that drug from its binding sites or affected the blood/plasma concentration ratio when present even in supratherapeutic concentration (Table 1).

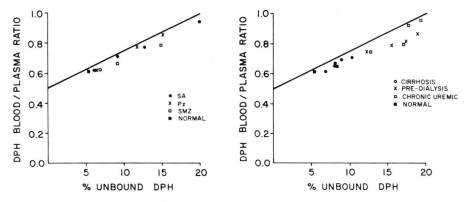

FIG. 4. Alteration in the plasma binding of DPH, and its effect upon the blood/plasma concentration ratio, caused by competitive displacing drugs and various disease states (the solid line represents the mean curve obtained in three normal subjects by diluting the plasma with buffer).

It is now well established that uremia can significantly alter the plasma binding and disposition of DPH (12–14, 18). Additionally, hypoalbuminemia, whether of renal or hepatic causes, leads to an increased propensity to DPH toxicity, and this has been explained upon the basis of a larger than usual free fraction of the drug at any given total plasma concentration (19). Blood from a number of patients with chronic cirrhosis and renal dysfunction exhibited unusually low binding for DPH. However, the disease states did not appear to affect the uptake of the drug into the erythrocytes since the RBC/buffer concentration ratios were not different from these obtained in normal subjects, and the blood/plasma concentration ratio, when corrected to a hematocrit of 0.5, was in good agreement with the values obtained in the plasma dilution experiment (Fig. 4).

Drugs other than DPH also appear to partition into erythrocytes dependent upon the unbound drug concentration. Figure 5 illustrates the findings with two basic compounds, diazepam and propranolol (16, 20). Again there was a linear relationship between the blood/plasma concentration ratio and the extent of binding of the drug, when present in therapeutic concentrations. The difference in the slopes of the curves reflects the difference in the RBC/plasma free concentration ratio for the two drugs, since the slope is equal to the product of that value and the hematocrit. Clearly this partition coefficient of free drug between the plasma and erythrocytes will be the limiting factor for general application of the described technique; the greater its value the more sensitive will be the blood/plasma concentration ratio as an index of plasma binding. The other critical factor, if the technique is used for screening purposes, will be the interpatient variability in the partition coefficient, although results with DPH, diazepam, and propranolol suggest that this may not be too limiting.

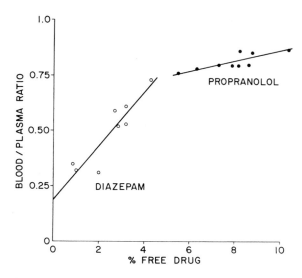

FIG. 5. Relationship between the percentage of unbound drug in the plasma and the blood/plasma concentration ratio for diazepam and propranolol.

SUMMARY AND CONCLUSIONS

The present findings indicate that the blood/plasma concentration ratio closely reflects the plasma binding of DPH. Perturbations of the binding by interindividual genetic or environmental variability, or by the presence of other drugs or pathological disease, such as liver or renal dysfunction, are readily measured by the ratio. Accordingly, the determination of the value may well serve as a simple and rapid technique for assessing the free fraction, and consequently the unbound concentration of DPH in the plasma, thus allowing plasma binding to be accounted for in individualization of therapy of this important anticonvulsant agent.

A suitable screening procedure for the processing of large numbers of samples would probably consist of the following steps:

(a) Collection of blood and measurement of the hematocrit.

(b) Determination in an aliquot of plasma the total DPH concentration by routine analytical methodology.

(c) Addition of a small amount of radiolabeled DPH to an aliquot of blood, incubation, and determination of the blood/plasma concentration ratio of the labeled drug with suitable correction for an abnormal hematocrit.

(d) Estimation of the free fraction of DPH from a calibration curve similar to Fig. 3, and calculation of the free DPH plasma concentration.

The use of trace amounts of radiolabeled DPH has a number of advantages over measuring the DPH concentration by a "cold" method, predominantly the ease, speed, and simplicity of radioisotope counting techniques.

DPH appears to be an ideal drug for testing the validity and value of the described technique since plasma binding is a demonstrable factor in clinical efficacy and toxicity. Such studies are presently being pursued, however, consideration should also be given to other drugs where knowledge of the plasma binding may be an important factor in the individualization of drug therapy.

ACKNOWLEDGMENT

These studies were supported by a grant from The John A. Hartford Foundation, Inc.

REFERENCES

1. Davies, D. S., and Prichard, B. N. C., eds. (1973): *Biological Effects of Drugs in Relation to Their Plasma Concentration,* University Park Press, Baltimore.
2. Vesell, E. S., and Passananti, G. T. (1971): *Clin. Chem. 17,* 851.
3. Koch-Weser, J. (1972): *New Engl. J. Med. 287,* 227.
4. Smith, T. W. (1972): *Circulation 46,* 188.
5. Woodbury, D. M., Penry, J. K., and Schmidt, R. P., eds. (1972): *Antiepileptic Drugs,* Raven Press, New York.
6. Koch-Weser, J., and Klein, S. W. (1971): *J. Amer. Med. Assoc. 215,* 1454.
7. Sokolow, M., and Edgar, A. L. (1950): *Circulation 1,* 576.
8. Coltart, D. J., and Shand, D. G. (1970): *Brit. Med. J. 3,* 731.
9. Baldessarini, R. J., and Stephens, J. H. (1970): *Arch. Gen. Psychiat. 22,* 72.
10. Åsberg, M., Crönholm, B., Sjöqvist, F., and Tuck, D. (1971): *Brit. Med. J. 3,* 331.
11. Alexanderson, B., and Borgå, O. (1972): *Europ. J. Clin. Pharmacol. 4,* 196.
12. Odar-Cedarlöf, I., Lunde, P., and Sjöqvist, F. (1970): *Lancet 2,* 831.
13. Reidenberg, M. M., Odar-Cedarlöf, I., Von Bahr, C., Borgå, O., and Sjöqvist, F. (1971): *New Engl. J. Med. 285,* 264.
14. Blum, M. R., Riegelman, S., and Becker, C. E. (1972): *New Engl. J. Med. 286,* 109.
15. Brodie, B. B. (1965): *Proc. Roy. Soc. Med. 58,* 946.
16. Evans, G. H., Nies, A. S., and Shand, D. G. (1973): *J. Pharmacol. Exp. Ther. 186,* 114.
17. Lunde, P. K. M., Rane, A., Yaffe, S. J., Lund, L., and Sjöqvist, F. (1970): *Clin. Pharmacol. Therap. 11,* 846.
18. Letteri, J. M., Mellk, H., Louis, S., Kutt, H., Durante, P., and Glazko, A. (1971): *New Engl. J. Med. 285,* 648.
19. The Boston Collaborative Drug Surveillance Program (1973): *Clin. Pharmacol. Therap. 14,* 529.
20. Evans, G. H., and Shand, D. G. (1973): *Clin. Pharmacol. Ther. 14,* 494.

Drug Interactions, edited by P. L. Morselli,
S. Garattini, and S. N. Cohen. Raven Press,
New York © 1974

Usefulness of Serum Antiepileptic Drug Levels in the Treatment of Epilepsy

J. Kiffin Penry

Applied Neurologic Research Branch, Collaborative and Field Research, National Institute of Neurological Diseases and Stroke, National Institutes of Health, Bethesda, Maryland 20014

INTRODUCTION

Although the serum concentration of phenobarbital had been determined nearly 30 years earlier, the usefulness of serum antiepileptic drug levels was not fully appreciated until 1960. Buchthal and colleagues (1, 2) advocated the use of serum phenobarbital and diphenylhydantoin levels to diagnose toxicity and to improve clinical control of epileptic seizures. Although their studies on toxicity were accepted and corroborated by other investigators (3), controversy developed over the relationship of serum levels to seizure control. Buchthal and Svensmark (1) presented evidence that patients with a serum diphenylhydantoin level of 10 μg/ml or higher showed a significantly greater reduction of seizure frequency than those with a level of less than 10 μg/ml. On the other hand, Triedman and associates (3) concluded from their studies of serum levels of diphenylhydantoin that there was no relationship between serum concentration and clinical control.

The investigations of Kutt and co-workers in the mid-1960s revealed additional evidence for the therapeutic use of serum antiepileptic drug levels (4). Nystagmus occurred in most patients when the serum concentration of diphenylhydantoin rose above 20 μg/ml (5). Unexpected toxicity appeared with low doses of diphenylhydantoin, resulting from slow biotransformation (long half-life), and clinical control was not achieved because of unexpectedly low serum levels, resulting from rapid biotransformation (short half-life). However, methods for determining serum levels of antiepileptic drugs were not readily available to practitioners providing care for epileptic patients until 1970.

The introduction in 1968 of a gas-liquid chromatographic method (6) for the simultaneous determination of multiple antiepileptic drugs in serum led to the introduction of other gas-liquid chromatographic methods (7, 8). A large number of clinical studies within the past 5 years have clearly demonstrated the value of determining serum antiepileptic drug concentrations for the drugs most commonly used in the treatment of epilepsy (9). Furthermore, clinical investigations currently underway will provide data for most of the less commonly used antiepileptic drugs and several new compounds that have not been marketed.

TOXICITY

The manifestations of neurologic dysfunction are limited in number and may result from many different diseases and drugs. Epilepsy is frequently associated with a lesion of the brain or systemic disorders affecting the nervous system. Consequently, it should not be surprising that patients with antiepileptic drug intoxication, especially children, are investigated for suspected neurologic diseases (10). Symptoms of diphenylhydantoin intoxication may be confused with gastroenteritis, cancer of the gastrointestinal tract, intracranial tumor or abscess, basilar insufficiency, hysteria, and posterior fossa encephalitis (11). Determinations of serum antiepileptic drug concentrations not only prevent unnecessary diagnostic studies, but also yield essential information for prompt and effective treatment.

Serum diphenylhydantoin concentrations above 30 μg/ml usually produce obvious side effects, including slurred speech (12). Nystagmus on lateral gaze usually appears with levels above 20 μg/ml (5). Drowsiness and depressed sensorium appear at much higher levels. A recent study (13) revealed a significant increase in gingival hyperplasia at higher serum concentrations. Failure of earlier studies (14, 15) to demonstrate a relationship between serum diphenylhydantoin concentration and gingival hyperplasia may have resulted from the use of different laboratory methods of measuring serum concentrations.

The dose-related neurotoxic manifestations of primidone and phenobarbital are often indistinguishable from those of diphenylhydantoin, but with the former drugs mild depression of mental function tends to be associated with the other neurotoxic symptoms. Most patients show evidence of toxicity when the serum primidone level is above 15 μg/ml and the serum phenobarbital level is above 40 μg/ml. After chronic administration of primidone, its metabolite, phenobarbital, is always present in the serum at a magnitude of one to four times the amount of primidone (16, 17). Significant amounts of phenylethylmalonamide (PEMA) are also present (18). The toxic ranges for serum levels of primidone and phenobarbital appear to be wider than that for diphenylhydantoin and may result from greater variation in tolerance to the barbiturates.

Dose-related side effects of ethosuximide usually occur when the serum concentration is above 100 μg/ml, but many exceptions have been observed (19). However, when the toxic symptoms of fatigue, lethargy, headache, dizziness, hiccups, and euphoria appear, they are often relieved by minimal lowering of the blood ethosuximide level (20).

Case reports of toxic levels for the other antiepileptic drugs have been presented, but further clinical studies should be conducted to establish the toxic ranges for these drugs.

COMPLIANCE

The most unquestionable and obvious beneficial use of serum antiepileptic drug concentrations is the detection and improvement of compliance with drug ingestion. More than one-third of patients with epilepsy fail to take their medication regularly unless they have been counseled and followed up at regular intervals. About one-third of those patients failing to take their medication regularly ingest so little of the drug that they have either an insignificant serum antiepileptic drug concentration or none at all. Gibberd (21) studied 15 outpatients who were taking a mean daily dose of 225 mg of diphenylhydantoin. The average serum level was 15.7 ± 12.9 μg/ml. For a comparative study, he chose 14 inpatients matched for age who were taking 200 mg of diphenylhydantoin per day. The mean serum level was 28.0 ± 8.1 μg/ml. In a further study of adult outpatients taking diphenylhydantoin, the mean serum concentration was 17.5 ± 14.7 μg/ml before he counseled the patients concerning the ingestion of medication. After appropriate counseling, the mean serum concentration rose to 27.7 ± 7.3 μg/ml. In a group of inpatients and a group of outpatients, both taking ethosuximide, the serum ethosuximide levels were significantly higher in the inpatient group (19, 22).

Although the problem of compliance exists to some degree for all patients who must take chronic medication, it is a special problem for most epileptic patients. More than half of the patients suffering from epilepsy are not directly aware of their seizures and are dependent upon others to tell them what happens when they lose consciousness. Moreover, most of these patients feel well between attacks. Consequently, without special counseling and follow-up, some epileptic patients have a tendency to forget to take the medication or even totally discontinue it when the seizures occur infrequently.

EFFICACY

Reduction of seizure frequency is the primary measure of the efficacy of antiepileptic drugs. Moderation or abbreviation of seizures and behavioral improvement are important but secondary to complete seizure control. Since the early clinical studies of diphenylhydantoin, efficacy has been reported in terms of *complete* or *improved* (significant reduction in seizure frequency) control of seizures.

Therapeutic Dose

From the beginning of modern medical treatment of epilepsy, upon the introduction of phenobarbital (23), the marked variation in therapeutic dose was recognized. Diphenylhydantoin in 200- to 400-mg daily doses was recommended for most patients, but, in a few, seizures were controlled only at higher doses. It became the clinical practice to gradually increase drug doses until the seizures were completely controlled or toxic side effects prevented further increase in dosage. It also became apparent that in some patients seizures were completely refractory to any dose of the drugs. Many clinicians, however, were reluctant to increase the dosage to toxic levels for fear of systemic side effects or blood dyscrasias. Moreover, with the clinician in a mood of reluctance for increasing dosage, vague side effects often provided an excuse to conclude that the drug was either toxic or ineffective. In addition, the vigorous clinician, increasing the dosage to very high levels and provoking a severe reaction, often concluded that the patient was intolerant to the drug. There were many unknown factors between the amount of drug written on the prescription pad and the amount of drug in the brain of the patient.

Therapeutic Range of Serum Concentration

Buchthal and Svensmark (1) were the first to describe a therapeutic range for diphenylhydantoin, as mentioned above. They were able to do this for only two arbitrary blood level ranges (> 10 μg/ml and < 10 μg/ml). Further attempts to define the relationship between serum concentration and seizure control through linear regression analysis failed to show a correlation (3). This should not be too surprising, however, because the values were obtained from the serum concentration of a drug in individual patients rather than from multiple samples at different blood levels in the same patient. Moreover, many of the values plotted came from individuals whose seizures could not be controlled at any blood level of the drug. Ideally, the seizure frequency of individual patients should be measured at varying blood levels. For those with completely controlled seizures at a given blood level, the dose and consequently the blood level should be reduced to see if the seizure frequency increases. Because such clinical experiments are unethical, however, it becomes necessary to rely on less elegant but strictly ethical approaches to the problem.

Gallagher and colleagues (24) have studied blood levels of antiepileptic drugs in a large group of epileptic patients whose medication was adjusted by dosage. A great deal can be learned from their study of the serum:dose relationship for diphenylhydantoin, primidone, and phenobarbital. Although their data do not portray the seizure control obtained, it may be assumed

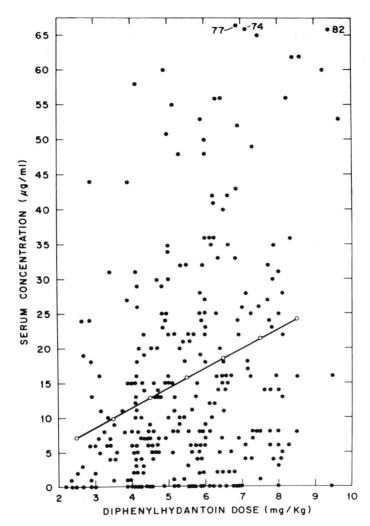

FIG. 1. Linear relationship between serum diphenylhydantoin concentration and dose for a group of outpatients. Most patients are represented by a single point, indicating a wide variation in serum:dose ratio among patients. A dose of 5 mg/kg may vary among patients from 0 to 60 μg/ml resulting from numerous possible causes, beginning with failure of ingestion of the drug to abnormally slow metabolism. (Courtesy of Dr. B. B. Gallagher.)

that maximum control was achieved by adjustment of dosage. Certainly, in the case of diphenylhydantoin (Fig. 1), many individuals were not taking their medication. Also, on very low doses, many patients exhibited very high blood levels. If 5 mg/kg is used as a guide for the initiating dose, it should be apparent from studying Fig. 1 that there is no way to predict the

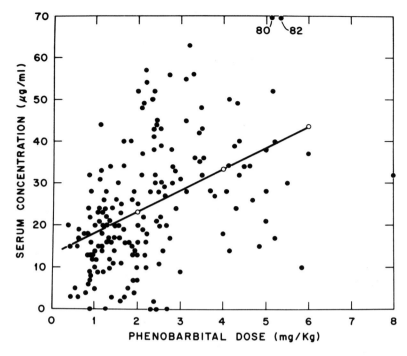

FIG. 2. Linear relationship between serum phenobarbital concentration and dose for a group of outpatients. Note the wide variation among patients, but with fewer zero values than in Fig. 1, probably resulting from better absorption and a much longer half-life than for diphenylhydantoin. (Courtesy of Dr. B. B. Gallagher.)

blood level for an individual. Consequently, it becomes necessary to measure the serum concentration. Note the slope of the regression line in Fig. 1 as compared to Figs. 2 and 3, where there is a high degree of serum:dose correlation. The poor correlation of diphenylhydantoin and the greater number of zero blood levels is related in part to the poor solubility and the very high pKa of the drug.

The findings of Solow and Green (25) in a study of another large group of epileptic patients were similar to those of Gallagher and co-workers (24).

A recent study by Sherwin and colleagues (26) provided further statistical evidence supporting the adjustment of serum concentrations to a therapeutic range for patients with uncontrolled seizures. In 70 patients receiving ethosuximide, with medication prescribed by dose, 38% of those with uncontrolled seizures had serum ethosuximide concentrations below the 95% confidence limits. Appropriate adjustment of the serum ethosuximide concentration resulted in a reduction of seizures in 48% of the patients whose seizures were previously uncontrolled.

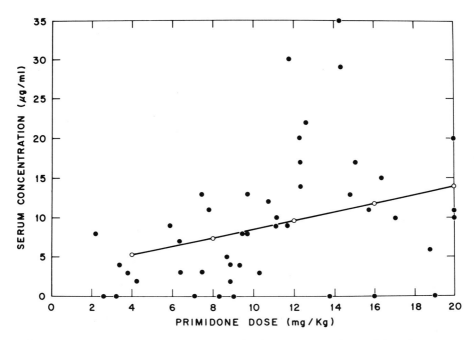

FIG. 3. Linear relationship between serum primidone concentration and dose for a group of outpatients. Note that the correlation between dose and concentration is less than for diphenylhydantoin and phenobarbital, resulting from the biotransformation of primidone to phenylethylmalonamide (PEMA) and phenobarbital, which are also present in the serum. Numerous low values of primidone levels compared with those of phenobarbital probably result from a short half-life. (Courtesy of Dr. B. B. Gallagher.)

In a different population of 352 patients, Green and colleagues (27) adjusted the serum concentrations of diphenylhydantoin, phenobarbital, and primidone and compared their results of seizure control with those previously obtained by adjusting dosage without benefit of serum concentrations. The adjustment of serum concentrations resulted in a statistically significant reduction of seizures.

Although the serum concentration must be adjusted to the individual's need, a therapeutic range is necessary as a starting point, just as a dosage range was originally required. Several studies in the past 5 years have established the therapeutic ranges for diphenylhydantoin (1, 2, 4, 5), phenobarbital (28), primidone (16), and ethosuximide (19). The toxic levels and serum half-lives of the most commonly used antiepileptic drugs are listed in Table 1. Some patients may be completely controlled at levels either lower or higher than the therapeutic range, but therapeutic range is a starting point for individual adjustment of the serum concentration.

TABLE 1. *Pharmacologic properties of four antiepileptic drugs*

| Drug | Therapeutic level | | Toxic level (μg/ml) | Serum half-life (hr) |
	Mean (μg/ml)	Range (μg/ml)		
Phenobarbital	25	20–40	> 40	96 ± 12
Diphenylhydantoin (Dilantin)	12	10–20	> 20	24 ± 12
Primidone (Mysoline)	8[a]	5–11	> 12	18 ± 6
Ethosuximide (Zarontin)	45	40–60	>80	36 ± 6

[a] Phenobarbital concentration in steady state is usually one to four times the level of primidone.

Serum Concentration of Clonazepam

Clonazepam is a potent investigational antiepileptic drug with a dosage range of 0.02 to 0.20 mg/kg for children, and we have studied its efficacy in absence seizures. The skeptics who do not value blood levels contend that serum clonazepam concentration cannot be measured. In Fig. 4, the serum

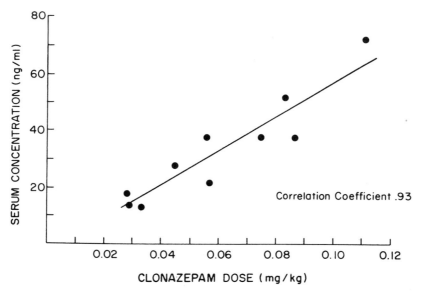

FIG. 4. Linear relationship of serum clonazepam concentration to dose in 10 hospitalized children after 8 weeks of treatment. Even in the minute concentrations of ng, there is a highly significant correlation, even though some variation in serum:dose ratio still exists among patients. Nurse-administered medication eliminated failure of compliance.

clonazepam concentration is measured in nanogram per milliliter, according to the dose in milligram per kilogram for 10 children receiving only clonazepam. The therapeutic serum range has not been established, but it appears from the first 10 patients that it will fall between 20 to 70 ng/ml at steady state. The two children with least improvement had serum concentrations of less than 20 ng/ml, but the one child with a serum level of more than 70 ng/ml, although greatly improved, was incompletely controlled. Serum levels were not adjusted in this study to the point of seizure *control* because it was carried out as part of a double-blind study based on adjustment of dosage.

Clinical Indications for Measuring Serum Concentrations

A reliably determined serum antiepileptic drug concentration is a far better guide to therapy than dose. The medication must be biologically available in the desired amount (29). From the practical point of view, what are the indications for determination of serum concentration? First, when an epileptic patient presents symptoms and signs of intoxication, the serum concentrations of antiepileptic drugs should be determined. It is not possible to distinguish the symptoms and signs of neurologic dysfunction or other intoxicants from the toxic effects of antiepileptic drugs. Second, when the therapeutic dose has been prescribed and complete seizure control is not achieved, the physician should make sure that the drug is biologically available and within the therapeutic range by measuring serum concentration. Moreover, it may be necessary to determine the response of the patient at different concentrations. Third, when a patient is receiving multiple antiepileptic drugs and is experiencing toxicity or uncontrolled seizures, the physician cannot change the dosage of the appropriate drug without knowing the serum concentrations of all drugs present. When the patient has responded completely to a therapeutic dose of an antiepileptic drug, a serum concentration should be determined to make certain that the patient is taking the medication and to record that individual's serum:dose ratio. If seizures then recur in the future, the cause of recurrence can be more accurately determined.

CONCLUSION

Any drug must be biologically available to be effective. The serum antiepileptic drug concentration is a better guide than dose in the treatment of epileptic patients. Serum antiepileptic drug levels at steady state are altered by failure of compliance, poor absorption of the drug, or interaction with other drugs, among other factors. Application of new knowledge about the pharmacology of antiepileptic drugs and the skilled use of antiepileptic drug levels can improve the care of more than one-third of the patients with epilepsy and increase by more than 10% the number of those patients whose seizures are completely controlled.

REFERENCES

1. Buchthal, F., and Svensmark, O. (1959/1960): *Epilepsia 1*, 373–384.
2. Buchthal, F., Svensmark, O., and Schiller, P. J. (1960): *Arch. Neurol. 2*, 624–630.
3. Triedman, H. M., Fishman, R. A., and Yahr, M. D. (1960): *Trans. Amer. Neurol. Assn. 85*, 166–170.
4. Kutt, H., Winters, W., Scherman, R., and McDowell, F. (1964): *Arch. Neurol. 11*, 649–656.
5. Kutt, H., Winters, W., Kokenge, R., and McDowell, F. (1964): *Arch. Neurol. 11*, 642–648.
6. Pippenger, C. E., and Gillen, H. W. (1969): *Clin. Chem. 15*, 582–590.
7. MacGee, J. (1970): *Anal. Chem. 42*, 421–422.
8. Kupferberg, H. J. (1970): *Clin. Chim. Acta 29*, 283–288.
9. Woodbury, D. M., Penry, J. K., and Schmidt, R. P., eds. (1972): *Antiepileptic Drugs*, Raven Press, New York.
10. Patel, H., and Crichton, J. U. (1968): *J. Pediatr. 73*, 676–684.
11. Frantzen, E., Hansen, J. M., Hansen, O. E., and Kristensen, M. (1967): *Acta Neurol. Scand. 43*, 440–446.
12. Husby, J. (1963): *Dan. Med. Bull. 10*, 236–239.
13. Kapur, R. N., Girgis, S., Little, T. M., and Masotti, R. F. (1973): *Dev. Med. Child Neurol. 15*, 483–487.
14. Melchior, J. C. (1965): *Dev. Med. Child Neurol. 7*, 387–391.
15. Livingston, S., and Livingston, H. L. (1969): *Am. J. Dis. Child. 117*, 265–270.
16. Booker, H. E., and Darcey, B. (1971): *Clin. Chem. 17*, 607–609.
17. Fincham, R. W., Schottelius, D. D., and Sahs, A. L. (1974): *Arch. Neurol. 30*, 259–262.
18. Baumel, I. P., Gallagher, B. B., and Mattson, R. H. (1972): *Arch. Neurol. 27*, 34–41.
19. Penry, J. K., Porter, R. J., and Dreifuss, F. E. (1972): In: *Antiepileptic Drugs*, pp. 431–441, Raven Press, New York.
20. Buchanan, R. A. (1972): In: *Antiepileptic Drugs*, pp. 449–454, Raven Press, New York.
21. Gibberd, F. B., Dunne, J. F., Handley, A. J., and Hazleman, B. L. (1970): *Brit. Med. J. 1*, 147–149.
22. Haerer, A. F., Buchanan, R. A., and Wiygul, F. M. (1970): *J. Clin. Pharmacol. 10*, 370–374.
23. Hauptmann, A. (1912): *Munch. Med. Wochenschr. 59*, 1907–1909.
24. Gallagher, B. B., Baumel, I. P., Mattson, R. H., and Woodbury, S. (1973): *Neurology 23*, 145–149.
25. Solow, E. B., and Green, J. B. (1972): *Neurology 22*, 540–550.
26. Sherwin, A. L., Robb, J. P., and Lechter, M. (1973): *Arch. Neurol. 28*, 178–181.
27. Green, J. B., Hartlage, L., Solow, E., and Baum, E. (1973): *Neurology 23*, 405.
28. Buchthal, F., Svensmark, O., and Simonsen, H. (1968): *Arch. Neurol. 19*, 567–572.
29. Brodie, B. B., and Heller, W. M., eds. (1972): *Bioavailability of Drugs*, Proceedings of the Conference on Bioavailability of Drugs at the National Academy of Sciences of the United States, Washington, D.C., November 22–23, 1971, S. Karges, Basel.

Drug Interactions, edited by P. L. Morselli,
S. Garattini, and S. N. Cohen. Raven Press,
New York © 1974

Factors Influencing Anticoagulant Control — An Epidemiological Study

K. O'Malley,* I. H. Stevenson, and C. Ward

Department of Pharmacology and Therapeutics, University of Dundee, Scotland

INTRODUCTION

The oral anticoagulant warfarin belongs to a relatively small group of
drugs in which the effect of the drug is easily assessed. The therapeutic aim
in this case is clearly defined in terms of objective measurement [ideally,
Thrombotest between 5–10% (1)] and a good dose-effect relationship exists.
It is rather surprising that there is little information on how often this ideal
is attained in practice. In this study, we have used an epidemiological approach to examine the dose and anticoagulant effect achieved (percent time
within defined Thrombotest ranges) in a hospitalized population receiving
warfarin. In an attempt to elucidate some of the contributory factors in
situations where optimum anticoagulation was not achieved, we have looked
at the relationship between anticoagulant control and concomitant drug
therapy. In addition, the influence of the patient's age, sex, and pathology
was also examined.

PATIENTS AND METHODS

The hospital-based drug information system has been described by Coull
et al. (2). All medical inpatients (240) in the Dundee General Hospitals
group who had received warfarin during a 2-year period were identified and
their hospital record studied. Data from 177 patients whose case notes contained complete records of warfarin dose, Thrombotest percent, and details of other drugs taken were analyzed. With patients admitted on more
than one occasion, only data from the first admission (or first admission for
which records were complete) were included in the analysis. The mean daily
dose of warfarin was calculated from all warfarin given, excluding loading
and "tailing-off" doses. The Thrombotest percent values obtained during
the same period (three times weekly) were used to calculate a "Mean

---

* Present address: Clinical Pharmacology Program, Emory University School of Medicine,
Woodruff Memorial Building, Atlanta, Georgia 30322

Thrombotest percent." In using the Thrombotest data, values above 30 and below 5 were arbitrarily given the values 31 and 4 respectively. Two ranges of anticoagulation were selected (Thrombotest 5 to 10% and Thrombotest 5 to 15%) and anticoagulant effect assessed by determination of the percentage time for which patients were outside these ranges during the period of warfarin therapy.

In studying the influence of concomitant drug therapy on anticoagulant control, the drugs prescribed in addition to warfarin were classified into three groups on the basis of their potential to interact with oral anticoagulants. Drugs were allocated to one or another of these groups according to documented evidence in man (3) and animal data from the literature.

Group I—known to interact, e.g., barbiturates, phenylbutazone, and chloralhydrate.

Group II—likely to interact, e.g., ethacrynic acid, ascorbic acid, Mandrax (methaqualone/diphenhydramine).

Group III—no suspicion of interaction, e.g., penicillin, nitrazepam, practolol.

Where drugs from more than one group were prescribed, the therapy was classified as Group I whenever a Group I drug was involved and Group II when Group II and Group III drugs were given.

In the analysis of results, the significance of the difference between means was determined using the Student's t test.

RESULTS

In this study, the case records of 177 patients (87 male and 90 female, ranging in age from 30 to 83) were examined. During the 2,180 treatment days surveyed, one bleeding episode occurred. Figure 1 summarizes the extent of anticoagulation achieved. Only 13 patients were continually (excluding "loading" and "tailing-off" periods) in the optimal Thrombotest range of 5 to 10% and 49 patients in the 5 to 15% range. The great majority of patients (120) spent some time with Thrombotest values $>15\%$, i.e., were "under-anticoagulated." "Over-anticoagulation" occurred much less frequently, 44 patients having Thrombotest values $<5\%$ at some time.

Table 1 lists the groups of drugs given in addition to warfarin according to the classification outlined previously. Only three of the 177 patients studied received no other drugs. The anticoagulant control in patients taking Group II drugs (likely to interact) and Group III drugs (no evidence of interaction) was similar. Patients on Group I (known to interact) drugs spent 72.5 or 44.5% of the time out of control depending on the anticoagulation range selected, values significantly higher than those occurring in the other two groups ($p < 0.02$). The number of drugs prescribed in this

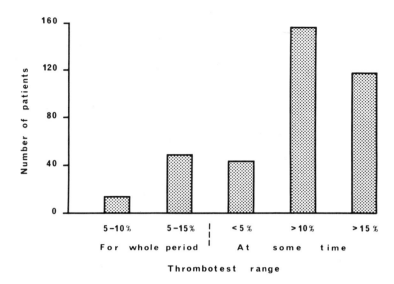

FIG. 1. Anticoagulation achieved in the 177 patients studied—the numbers of patients continually in the 5 to 10% or 5 to 15% Thrombotest ranges or at some time having values <5%, >10%, or >15%.

group was higher than that in patients given only Group III drugs ($p <$ 0.005) but was not significantly different from that in patients given Group II drugs. In the 48 patients in the first group, there was no correlation between the number of different drugs given and anticoagulant control.

A breakdown of the anticoagulant control overall and for different age groups is given in Fig. 2 using the two ranges of anticoagulation, 5 to 10% and 5 to 15% Thrombotest. With both anticoagulation ranges there is an obvious trend in the change of anticoagulant control with age, the mean

TABLE 1. *Concomitant drug therapy and anticoagulant control*

Concomitant drugs	Mean no. of drugs prescribed	No. of patients	Percent time outside anticoagulation range	
			5–10% Thrombotest	5–15% Thrombotest
I	7.3 ± 0.6	48	72.5 ± 3.9	44.5 ± 4.5
II	6.4 ± 0.4	61	57.9 ± 4.3	28.0 ± 3.6
III	4.6 ± 3.4	65	57.4 ± 4.3	27.1 ± 3.4
All patients studied	5.8 ± 2.1	177	60.8 ± 2.5	31.7 ± 2.4

Results are given as means ± SEM.
The allocation of drugs to Groups I, II, and III was as described under "Patients and Methods." The results for percent time spent outside both ranges were significantly higher in the patients on Group I drugs than in those receiving Group II or Group III drugs.

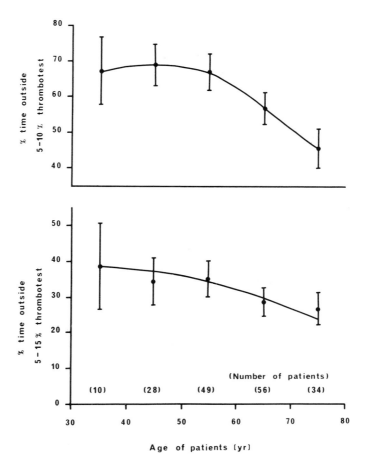

FIG. 2. Anticoagulant control and age—the relationship between age of patients and the percent time spent outside the 5 to 10% and 5 to 15% Thrombotest ranges.

values for the 70+ group being significantly lower in both cases than those for the 4th, 5th, and 6th decades. Anticoagulant control would, therefore, seem to be better in elderly patients.

In Fig. 3, a further breakdown of the age-related anticoagulation data is given. This shows quite strikingly that the proportion of patients in whom Thrombotest values < 5% were obtained increases with age and conversely that values > 10% were encountered most frequently in younger patients. When the data on mean percent time spent at Thrombotest values < 5% or > 10% are considered, the same trend obtained, i.e., that the degree of anticoagulation achieved is greater in old people.

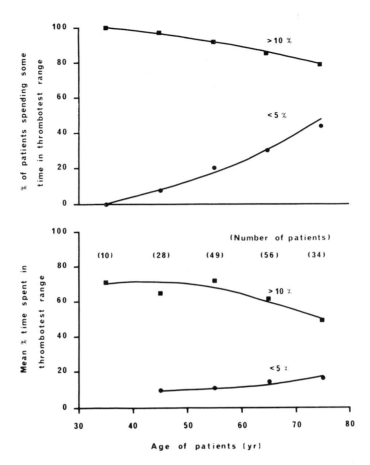

FIG. 3. Anticoagulant control and age — the relationships between age and percent of patients spending some time with Thrombotest values >10% or <5% and between age and mean percent time spent in these ranges.

When the sex of patients in the overall study was considered, no significant difference in anticoagulant control was found. The percentage time which male and female patients spent outside the 5 to 10% range was 62.4 ± 3.6 and 59.3 ± 3.5, respectively, and the corresponding values for the 5 to 15% range was 31.6 ± 3.4 and 31.6 ± 3.3.

In Table 2, results are given for the anticoagulant control in patient groups with different indications for anticoagulant therapy. Only the mean value for the valve prosthesis group in the 5 to 15% range was significantly different from the others. Overall, the results suggest that anticoagulation control does not vary greatly with indication.

TABLE 2. *Anticoagulant control and indication for anticoagulation*

	No. of patients	Percent time outside anticoagulation range	
		5–10% Thrombotest	5–15% Thrombotest
Myocardial infarction	62	60.0 ± 4.2	27.4 ± 3.8
Atrial fibrillation	14	67.9 ± 7.0	35.8 ± 9.8
Valve prosthesis	7	67.8 ± 15.2	58.2 ± 17.4
Deep venous thrombosis and/or pulmonary embolism	75	59.0 ± 4.0	33.8 ± 3.4
Miscellaneous	14	68.8 ± 8.6	26.5 ± 8.6

Results given are means ± SEM.

Anticoagulant Dosage

In considering the effect of concomitant drug therapy on warfarin requirement, doses of warfarin given to patients on the three different types of additional drugs were not compared since the drugs in Group I and II included both antagonists and potentiators of warfarin effect. The warfarin dose and effect were examined in patients given potentiators or antagonists from the Group I drugs (Table 3). There was no significant difference between the doses given, but as might be expected, there was a decreased anticoagulant effect in the group on the antagonist drugs ($p < 0.005$).

Figure 4 shows, relative to age, the mean daily warfarin dose and anticoagulant control achieved (Thrombotest percent) in the 177 subjects studied. The overall trend is for the mean dose to fall after the fifth decade so that in patients over 70 years of age the mean daily dose was 40% lower than in patients 40 to 50 years of age ($p < 0.001$). The trend with the Thrombotest was similar. There was a dramatic fall in Thrombotest percent in the 7th and 8th decades so that in the 8th decade the Thrombotest value was 34% lower than in the 5th decade ($p < 0.001$), i.e., the anticoagulant effect was greater. The combination of lower dose and more marked anticoagulation indicates a marked increase in sensitivity to warfarin in the aged.

TABLE 3. *Effect of interacting drugs (Group I) on warfarin dose and effect*

	Group I potentiators	Group I antagonists
Number of patients	29	19
Warfarin dose (mg)	4.5 ± 0.3	4.9 ± 0.3
Thrombotest percent	11.2 ± 0.8	15.9 ± 1.3

Results are given as means ± SEM.
Allocation of drugs to Group I was as described under "Patients and Methods." The Thrombotest values obtained in the groups were significantly different ($p < 0.005$).

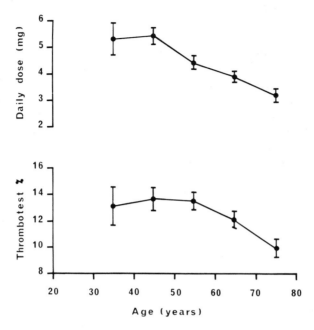

FIG. 4. Mean daily dose of warfarin given and Thrombotest values for patients in the age ranges shown.

There was no difference in the indications for anticoagulant therapy, number of concomitantly administered drugs or patient sex in the young and older group.

No significant differences were found between the warfarin doses given to male and female patients (4.5 ± 0.2 and 4.2 ± 0.2 mg, respectively) or between the Thrombotest percent values obtained (males 13.1 ± 0.3, females 11.7 ± 0.2).

DISCUSSION

In oral anticoagulant therapy, the degree of anticoagulation achieved is readily determined using the Thrombotest and other methods. In this present investigation, the Thrombotest ranges 5 to 10% and 5 to 15% were selected for study. Although not absolutely defined, the optimal Thrombotest range is usually accepted as being 5 to 10% for antithrombotic prophylaxis in, for example, myocardial infarction in patients without any contraindications to intensive therapy. Loeliger et al. (1) have demonstrated this level to be highly beneficial and to be associated with a low incidence of bleeding complications. From their report, at values in excess of 15% there is little or no therapeutic effect in this condition. For prophylaxis against venous thrombosis, particularly in the postoperative period, Owren (4) has reported satisfactory results at levels up to 15% Thrombotest.

In carrying out this study, a hospital-based Drug Information System (2) was used to identify patient populations exposed to warfarin. A retrospective study of these patients case notes has produced a number of surprising and interesting results. Firstly, as indicated in Fig. 1, only 13 of the 177 patients studied were found to be in the optimum Thrombotest range for the entire period (tailing-off and loading dosage period being excluded). Extending the range of Thrombotest values to 5 to 15% brought 49 of the 177 patients within this range of control for the entire period. It should be remembered, however, that for inclusion in the relevant group, all Thrombotest values would have to fall within the required range. From further analysis of this data (Fig. 1) it is clear that the majority of patients was under-anticoagulated at some time – 158 out of the 177 had at some time a Thrombotest value greater than 10%.

The time spent by patients outside of the defined Thrombotest ranges is given in Table 1. The overall patient population was found to have spent 60.8% of the period when they should have been satisfactorily anticoagulated, outside the range 5 to 10% and 31.7% outside the range 5 to 15%. This time varied with concomitant drug therapy (Table 1) and particularly strikingly with age (Fig. 2). The simultaneous administration of Group I drugs (i.e., known to interfere with the action of warfarin) increased the percent time that patients spent outside the optimum Thrombotest range (Table 1). This reinforces previously expressed views (5, 6) regarding the danger of simultaneous drug therapy when patients are anticoagulated with coumarin agents. The extent of concomitant drug therapy in the present study was surprising – only three out of 177 patients receiving no drugs other than warfarin and 48 of them being given drugs for which there is documented evidence of an interaction in man.

When Group I drugs were subdivided into potentiators and antagonists of warfarin effect (Table 3), although there was some evidence of a lower dose in the subgroup receiving "potentiating" drugs, the difference was not significant. Thrombotest values were, however, significantly lower in these patients thus demonstrating an increased anticoagulant effect. This study, using an epidemiological approach, has confirmed the known interaction of some drugs with warfarin and the approach used may therefore be of value in providing evidence of other previously unsuspected drug interactions.

The group aged over 70 spent significantly less time out of the 5 to 10% and 5 to 15% Thrombotest ranges than younger age groups (Fig. 2). At the same time, Thrombotest values of <5%, i.e., over-anticoagulation, were encountered predominantly in the elderly patients (Fig. 3). This is despite the fact that older patients were found to have received smaller doses of warfarin (Fig. 1). This study has therefore demonstrated quantitatively an increased susceptibility of the elderly to this drug. This may fit with the results of the general survey carried out by Hurwitz (7), which demonstrated the frequency of adverse drug reactions to be higher in a geriatric population. It is apparent from our study that the occurrence of Thrombotest values lower than 5% with their associated risk of anticoagulant-induced hemorrhage increased with patient age.

There are a number of possible explanations for this age-dependent difference in susceptibility to warfarin. With advancing years, changes may occur in lean body mass (8), in sensitivity to vitamin K or warfarin (9), in serum proteins, and in renal function. The most likely explanation however is that, as occurs with the metabolism of antipyrine and phenylbutazone (10), the rate of inactivation of warfarin is decreased in the elderly. Direct evidence of this would require measurement of steady-state plasma levels of warfarin in elderly patients and comparison with drug levels occurring in younger age groups.

Neither patient's sex nor the indication for anticoagulation had any great influence on anticoagulant control nor was there any significant difference in the warfarin dose given to male and female patients.

ACKNOWLEDGMENTS

This work was supported by grants from the Medical Research Council, the Scottish Home and Health Department, and the World Health Organization. We are grateful to Dr. A. J. Wood for identification of patients who had received warfarin.

REFERENCES

1. Loeliger, E. A., Hensen, A., Kroes, F., van Dyk, L. M., Fekkes, N., de Jonge, H., and Hemker, H. C. (1967): *Acta Med. Scand. 182,* 549.
2. Coull, D. C., Crooks, J., Dingwall-Fordyce, I., Scott, A. M., and Weir, R. D. (1970): *Europ. J. Clin. Pharmac. 3,* 51.
3. Hansten, P. D. (1971): *Drug Interactions.* Lea and Febiger, Philadelphia.
4. Owren, P. A. (1969): In: *Human Blood Coagulation* (ed. H. C. Hemker, E. A. Loeliger, and J. J. Velthamp), p. 300, Leiden University Press, Leiden.
5. Koch-Weser, J., and Sellers, E. M. (1971): *New Engl. J. Med. 285,* 487.
6. Koch-Weser, J., and Sellers, E. M. (1971): *New Engl. J. Med. 285,* 547.
7. Hurwitz, N. (1969): *Brit. Med. J. 1,* 536.
8. Forbes, G. B., and Reina, J. C. (1970): *Metabolism 19,* 653.
9. Hazel, K., and Baloch, K. H. (1970): *Geront. Clin. 12,* 10.
10. O'Malley, K., Crooks, J., Duke, E., and Stevenson, I. H. (1971): *Brit. Med. J. 3,* 607.

Drug Interactions, edited by P. L. Morselli,
S. Garattini, and S. N. Cohen. Raven Press,
New York © 1974

Methods Used for Evaluation of the Combined Effects of Alcohol and Drugs on Humans

M. Linnoila, I. Saario, T. Seppälä, J. Olkoniemi, and R. Liljeqvist

Departments of Pharmacology and Psychology, University of Helsinki, Helsinki, Finland

INTRODUCTION

In discussing methods used for the measurement of human psychomotor functions, we must first define this term. In this communication, I mean by it all the human functions needed in controlling technology, e.g., in driving or in occupational life. As a general concept psychomotor functions include sensory information processing and motor correction functions. In studying drug effects on human psychomotor skills, one has the urgent need of finding the point most vulnerable to drug effects in the chain of psychomotor functions. Indeed, we do have both convincing epidemiological and experimental evidence that this point is the human information processing system.

It has been demonstrated that sight has little correlation with individual road-traffic-accident records and that visually handicapped drivers drive more safely than normal drivers (5, 25). On the other hand, accident-prone drivers do have significantly poorer information processing capacity than normal ones (8), and alcohol, which is known to reduce information processing capacity, drastically increases accident risk and mortality in traffic as an exponential function of its blood concentration (3).

Epidemiological studies, which have revealed the above-mentioned increased traffic risks after alcohol, are useful tools to investigate drug effects on psychomotor functions. The type of epidemiological study used most frequently is a questionnaire filled in either by the subjects themselves or by the inquirer. Many such studies have proven unreliable because of either unskilled questions giving nonparametric distribution of answers, or because the subjects answered unreliably. When the answers concerning drug use in a drunk-driver population were monitored by serum analysis, the extent of drug use increased from 9 to 38% (18).

Another type of epidemiological study concerns serum or urine specimens taken from victims of traffic accidents brought to hospitals within a district during a certain time limit (18). Such studies have demonstrated that up to 40% of the participants in traffic accidents are under the influence of alcohol (9). The respective figures concerning drugs are lacking. This kind of study naturally excludes all minor accidents and the really severe ones, in other words those without human damage and those leading to immediate death.

Postmortem studies of the victims of traffic or occupational accidents give reliable results concerning drug levels because of the relative ease of obtaining specimens of blood, liver, bile, brain, or urine. Such studies have not shown any overrepresentation of drug users among the victims as compared to the number of drug users in the particular population (18).

Comparison of the accident records of known drug and/or alcohol users with those of matched controls gives us reliable information about the traffic risks of those persons if the observation time is long enough, from 2 to 4 years (7). The natural limit of this kind of study is the low number of road traffic accidents coming to the knowledge of police, estimated to be less than a half of the total in Scandinavia. The other important feature is that we can never determine the traffic risks caused by drugs directly from these figures because the drug users represent multiple social and psychological problems (18). The few critical studies of this kind have demonstrated the extra risks for traffic caused by use of LSD or amphetamine and its derivatives (23, 24). Marihuana on the other hand seemed not to increase accident risk in traffic (23, 24). The only epidemiological studies concerning occupational life have convinced us of the extra risks of alcohol (2).

The possibility of obtaining useful feedback in the future from epidemiological studies in this field encouraged us to approach the problem of drug effects on human psychomotor skills through investigation of psychomotor skills related to driving.

EXPERIMENTAL DESIGN

Choice of Subjects

The test performance varies slightly as a function of age, sex, educational level, and living district of the subject (7). Younger subjects generally react faster and more accurately than older ones, but the latter generally perform better in co-ordination tasks (7). Females show poorer psychomotor performance than males, and those subjects from urban areas with high educational level show better performance in acute test situations, after a short training period than rural ones with low educational level (7). This may be due to a better ability of adaptation to new situations among the urban population with high educational level. The above-mentioned subject-dependent factors should be taken into account when choosing subjects.

Old and even middle-aged subjects may be more sensitive to harmful drug effects than young ones. This holds particularly true with benzodiazepines (13). Females and males may differ in their sensitivity to drug effects as well (10). The testing of patients includes the general difficulties of clinical psychopharmacology.

Drugs Examined

The drugs examined may be chosen mainly in the interest of popularity or "pure pharmacology." In other words, they may be widely used or they may have interesting pharmacological effects without wide application for therapy. Generally, a program of a research center should include a suitable proportion of both kinds of drugs to be examined because the financial support can only be ensured by examining drugs having wide application.

Doses of Drug

The doses of the drugs examined should be therapeutic and dose-response curves should be produced (14). By repeating the tests, one can produce the time-response curve as well (10).

Duration of Treatment

The duration of treatment is a matter of crucial importance because of the strong adaptation capacity of the human brain. Acute studies should be conducted soon after the first dose of the drug. Our protocol contains three testing sessions at 30, 90, and 150 min after drug administration when testing psychotropic drugs, and six sessions at 2, 4, 6, 8, 10, and 24 hr when testing postanesthesia recovery periods. The subacute trials with healthy volunteers include tests 1 and 2 weeks after the beginning of treatment. With psychiatric outpatients we repeat the tests for up to 2 months.

Alcohol

The alcoholic drink should be pure alcohol mixed with a juice to avoid the effects of congeners, but then producing a placebo drink is difficult without extremes of taste that render the drinks impossible to be drunk quickly. So, one should compromise and a bitter substance with or without alcohol has proved a suitable combination (10). If the alcoholic drink is not many years old, the amount of congeners remains without major effect.

In acute experiments, up to 60% of the subjects can be misled by suitable drug-alcohol combinations (10), but in chronic experiments this is very difficult because the subjects mainly assess the nature of their treatment from its effects (14).

Trial Design

Trial design should not be too demanding and the tests not too difficult in order to maintain the motivation of subjects. This is more difficult in subjects who have extreme personality traits. The subjects should have enough time between the different tests for rest and concentration (10). In case the tests take only a few minutes, the subjects are able to pull themselves together and real drug effects may be hidden (10). Therefore, there is a correlation between the test duration and intensivity of effort, and a combination of tests differing in this respect gives the best and most reliable results (14). The subjects' motivation can be maintained better by short and intensive than prolonged tasks (12).

The drug administration must be double blind, but in acute experiments the cross-over design is not necessary, if the subjects are correctly matched according to the subject-dependent factors (10–12). In long-term studies with healthy subjects, the cross-over design is unavoidable but with patients some caution must be taken because of the large day-to-day variation in the symptomatology of mental disorders.

Psychomotor Test Pattern

The psychomotor test pattern should include at least three types of tests: choice reaction, co-ordination, and divided attention tasks. The *choice reaction tests* measure information retrieval from memory, from short- or long-term memory, respectively, as a function of the duration of training (6, 14). *Co-ordination tests* should measure eye-hand and multilimb coordination, because these functions have a satisfactory correlation with driving (6). *Attention tasks* should be designed to measure divided attention and information processing capacity (12) because of the sensitivity of these functions to drug effects (17).

Driving Simulators

Driving simulators should be as natural as possible and the less arbitrary the instructions are, the more reliable the results (15). Emergency situations are particularly effective in revealing drug effects (15).

Real driving tests do not yield very useful information because "skilled driving" between barrels with low speed tells us only of the ability to handle a car in a situation not common in traffic.

There are *clinical signs*, such as Romberg, positional nystagmus, or the finger-finger test, that have some correlation to blood-alcohol concentrations, but they are insufficient for interaction studies.

Sensory Tests

Sensory tests, such as flicker fusion and eye-movement studies, are sensitive tools for the examination of sedative and muscle-relaxing drugs providing us with the information sampling of the subject (20). Proprioception is seldom affected by drug doses generally used and reveals extra sensitivity to drug effects.

Motor and Psychological Tests

Pure motor measurements of power or speed are not of major importance in drug interaction studies.

Tests of anxiety, e.g., Taylor's manifest anxiety scale, and those measuring aggressiveness can explain some aspects of traffic behavior. The subjects may be psychologically examined before the tests and the results of those with extreme personality traits should be handled as a separate group.

Subjective Assessment

Subjective assessments of performance reveal possible disproportionalities between objective findings and these assessments. This may prove to be of real danger in traffic situations (10). The estimations of the nature of the treatment tell of the maintenance of the double-blind design during the experiment (10).

Statistical treatment of the data is generally according to the two-way analysis of variance, but some drug-alcohol interactions do not give results with normal distribution. Pearson's product-moment correlation coefficient is very useful for the estimation of psychomotor performance profiles (16).

There are some special problems with special drugs. With benzodiazepines, the drug-alcohol interaction and the effect on subjects of different ages are important (13). With antidepressants the nature of the drug-alcohol interaction may vary as a function of the treatment duration (19). The large interindividual variation of serum concentration of antidepressants is important but can be examined by tyramine pressor test. The neuroleptic drugs lead to deterioration of divided attention and information processing very strongly at the beginning of treatment (14). The eventual harmful psychomotor effects of hypnotics should be correlated with those caused by deprivation of sleep (13). Many drugs having active metabolites (1) may have delayed behavioral effects.

Drug-Alcohol Interactions

Drug-alcohol interactions do represent special problems if the agents are administered per os. Alcohol is known to delay the emptying of the stomach and alter the secretion of gastric acid; thus both delaying the absorption of the drug and possibly denaturing a part of it. On the other hand, alcohol may increase the solubility of some drugs, thus increasing their amount in the intestinal water phase. The metabolism of some drugs may also be altered by alcohol (21). Benzodiazepines may render the human brain very sensitive to the effect of increasing alcohol concentrations (10, 13), but they differ both qualitatively and quantitatively from each other in their interaction with alcohol (13, 14).

Drug-Drug Interactions

Drug-drug interactions also take place at the intestinal, blood, receptor, metabolism, and excretion level and two or more drugs interacting with alcohol may cause interactions that are highly difficult to anticipate (4).

SETTING UP A CENTER FOR STUDYING THE PSYCHOMOTOR DRUG-ALCOHOL INTERACTIONS

There are commercially available choice-reaction and coordination tests that are suitable for this kind of study. One should, however, be aware of exactly which psychomotor functions they measure. The attention tests and simulators should at present be constructed by the research team. Then one has to test several hundred subjects without any treatment in order to find out the significant subject-dependent factors and the correlation of the tests to traffic or occupational behavior, as well as their reliability and validity. Those tests requiring responses slightly but definitely different from the real ones should be excluded. In such tests, experienced drivers may react incorrectly because of extended repetition of their everyday functions.

Most important is to have a cooperative team of psychologists, sociologists, engineers, statisticians, and clinical pharmacologists for successful results to be achieved.

REFERENCES

1. Baird, E. S., and Hailey D. M. (1972): Delayed recovery from a sedative: Correlation of the plasma level of diazepam with clinical effects after oral and intravenous administration. *Brit. J. Anaest. 44*, 803–808.
2. Bierver, K. (1961): Alkoholproblem i industrin och trafiken. *Alkoholfrågan 55*, 159–162.
3. Borkenstein, R. F., Crowther, R. F., Shumate, R. P., Ziel, W. B., and Zylman, R. (1964): The role of drinking driver in traffic accidents. Dept. of Police Administration, Indiana Univ.
4. Bruener, H., Jovy, D., and Klein, K. (1961): Der Einfluss einiger verkehrsmedizinisch wichtiger Pharmaka auf die menschliche Leistungsbereitschaft. *Arzneim. Forsch. 11*, 995–1000.
5. Crancer, A., and McMurray, L. (1968): Accident and violation rates of Washington's medically restricted drivers. *J. Am. Med. Assoc. 205*, 74–78.
6. Dumas, J. (1973): Decision making in dynamic circumstances. Communication 730022, SAE meeting, Detroit.
7. Eklund, K. (1971): Selvitys ajokyvyn testausvaunun toiminnasta. *Taljan tutkimuksia 19*, 1–111.
8. Fergenson, P. E. (1971): The relationship between information processing, driving accident and violation record. *Human Factors 13*, 173–176.

9. Kielholz, P. (1973): International seminar. Research on alcohol, drugs and driving. *Pharm. Psychiatr. 6,* 65–66.
10. Linnoila, M., and Mattila, M. J. (1973): Drug interaction on psychomotor skills related to driving: Diazepam and alcohol. *Eur. J. Clin. Pharmacol. 5,* 186–194.
11. Linnoila, M. (1973): Effects of drugs on psychomotor skills related to driving: Antihistamines, chlormezanone and alcohol. *Eur. J. Clin. Pharmacol. 4,* 247–255.
12. Linnoila, M. (1973): Effects of drugs on psychomotor skills related to driving: Anticholinergics and alcohol. *Eur. J. Clin. Pharmacol. 6,* 107–113.
13. Linnoila, M. (1973): Effects of drugs on psychomotor skills related to driving: Hypnotics and alcohol. *Ann. Exp. Med. Biol. Fenn. 51,* 118–124.
14. Linnoila, M. (1973): Effects of drugs on psychomotor skills related to driving: Diazepam, chlordiazepoxide, thioridazine, haloperidole, flupenthixole and alcohol. *Ann. Exp. Med. Biol. Fenn. 51,* 125–132.
15. Linnoila, M., and Häkkinen, S. *(in press):* Effects of diazepam and codeine alone or in combination with alcohol on simulated driving. *J. Clin. Pharmacol. Ther.*
16. Linnoila, M., and Mäki, M. (1974): The effects of alcohol, diazepam, thioridazine, flupenthixole, and atropine on psychomotor performance profiles. *Arzneim. Forsch. 24,* 565–569.
17. Moskowitz, H., and DePry, D. (1968): The effects of alcohol upon auditory vigilance and divided attention tasks. *Q.J. Stud. Alc. 29,* 54–63.
18. Nichols, J. L. (1971): Drug use and highway safety, Review of the literature, DOT-HS-012-1-019, US Dept. of Transportation.
19. Patman, J., Landauer, A. A., and Milner, G. (1969): The combined effect of alcohol and amitriptyline on skills similar to motor car driving, *Med. J. Aust. 8,* 946–949.
20. Rockwell, T. H. (1971): Eye movement analyses of visual information acquisition in driving, North Carolina State University, Raleigh.
21. Rubin, E., and Lieber, C. S. (1971): Alcoholism, alcohol and drugs. *Science 172,* 1097.
22. Snapper, K., and Edwards, W. (1973): Effects of alcohol on psychomotor skills and decision making in a driving task. Ph.D. thesis, Department of Psychology, University of Michigan.
23. Waller, J. A., and Goo, J. T. (1969): Highway crash and citation patterns and chronic medical conditions. *J. Safety Res. 1,* 13–22.
24. Waller, J. A. (1965): Chronic medical conditions and traffic safety. *New Engl. J. Med. 273,* 1413–1420.
25. Ysander, L. (1966): The safety of physically disabled drivers. *Brit. J. Indust. Med. 23,* 173–180.

Drug Interactions, edited by P. L. Morselli,
S. Garattini, and S. N. Cohen. Raven Press,
New York © 1974

Some Principles of Combination
Chemotherapy of Animal Tumors*

John M. Venditti

*Drug Evaluation Branch, Division of Cancer Treatment, National Cancer Institute,
Bethesda, Maryland 20014*

There is abundant clinical evidence that a combination of drugs may provide more effective antitumor therapy than the individual drugs (Goldin et al., *in press*). It is the responsibility of the preclinical investigator not only to discover new and more effective combinations, but also to investigate the optimal conditions for their use and the underlying mechanisms leading to improved therapy.

Rationales for selecting drug combinations for experimental antitumor studies *in vivo* have included (a) the demonstrated antitumor activity of the individual drugs *in vivo*, (b) potentiating cytotoxicity to cells in culture, (c) less than additive toxicity to normal animals, (d) the observation that a tumor developed for resistance to drug A shows no change or an increase in its sensitivity to drug B, as well as (e) information relative to the effects of the individual drugs on host defense mechanisms, the stages of the cell life cycle, and specific biochemical sites of action (Goldin et al., *in press*).

In studying the combined actions of drugs, different investigators have used varying definitions of additivity, potentiation, and synergism (Venditti and Goldin, 1964). Often such definitions were appropriately derived from and applied to studies based on a single determinant or parameter of activity; e.g., cytotoxicity *in vitro* or tumor inhibition at specified doses *in vivo*. However, if one measures the value of antitumor therapy on the basis of cure or prolongation of life and if synergism indicates the cooperative action of agents to produce a therapeutic effect that cannot be achieved with either of the individual drugs, then one should feel free to define the improved therapy as therapeutic synergism (Venditti et al., 1956). This proposition follows from the realization that in the area of antitumor treatment, at least, the degree of therapeutic efficacy is the resultant of two responses to treatment,

---

* In recent years, the Division of Cancer Treatment (DCT), NCI, has placed increased emphasis on studies of combinations of therapeutic modalities. Most of the experimental data included in this presentation were developed in two of DCT's contract laboratories by Dr. F. M. Schabel, Jr., and his colleagues at the Southern Research Institute, Birmingham, Alabama, and Dr. I. Kline and his colleagues at Microbiological Associates, Inc., Bethesda, Maryland.

the destruction of tumor cells on the one hand, and the toxicity for the host on the other. For combinations of antitumor drugs, increased selective destruction of tumor cells leading to superior results may be attained when the sum of the individual drug effects against the tumor is greater than the sum of their effects against the host regardless of the degree of summation against the tumor cells alone or against the host cells alone, and regardless of the underlying mechanism leading to the improved therapy. Conceptually, one might expect therapeutic synergism when two antitumor drugs cooperate in a manner such that each retains its full effect against the tumor while their toxicities are less than completely additive or when one actually protects the host against the toxicity of the other. Therapeutic synergism might also be attained when an agent without antitumor action *per se* diminishes the host toxicity of an active antitumor drug without diminishing its capacity to destroy tumor cells. The data to be presented were selected to provide a few examples of such effects in the treatment of leukemia L1210 in mice.

The combination of cytosine arabinoside (Ara-C) and 6-thioguanine (6-TG) provides a striking example in which two antitumor agents cooperate to provide therapeutic synergism by virtue of the ability of one to protect against the host toxicity of the other with no apparent loss of either's ability to destroy tumor cells. LePage and Kaneko (1969) found that, under specific conditions, Ara-C blocked the incorporation of 6-TG into DNA, and they proposed treatment with the combination of Ara-C + 6-TG as an effective means of reducing toxicity without sacrificing antitumor efficacy. Gee et al. (1969) reported on the favorable response to this combination among patients with acute leukemia. Subsequently, Schmidt et al. (1970) demonstrated the antileukemic superiority of Ara-C + 6-TG over the individual drugs against L1210, also under very specific conditions of treatment scheduling, and also demonstrated the ability of Ara-C to protect against the toxicity of 6-TG.

The data summarized in Table 1 shows the protection by Ara-C against

TABLE 1. *Protection by cytosine arabinoside (Ara-C) against lethality of 6-thioguanine (6-TG) in normal mice*[a]

6-TG mg/kg/ injection[b]	Ara-C (mg/kg/injection)[b]						
	0	0.47	0.94	1.88	3.75	7.5	15
	Number of Survivors/Total						
0	39/40	10/10	10/10	10/10	10/10	10/10	10/10
0.45	7/7	10/10	10/10	10/10	9/9	10/10	9/10
0.90	0/10	9/10	9/10	10/10	10/10	10/10	10/10
1.35	1/10	1/10	9/10	9/9	10/10	8/10	9/10
1.80	0/10	0/10	0/10	3/10	3/10	4/10	0/10

[a] Data of L. H. Schmidt and F. M. Schabel, Jr. (see Schmidt et al., 1970).
[b] Treatment q3hr/24hr/days 1,5,9,13.

the lethal toxicity of 6-TG in normal mice. When given q3hr. on every 4th day, Ara-C alone was not lethal at doses up to and including 15 mg/kg/injection. This is close to the LD_{10} dose of Ara-C on this treatment schedule. The LD_{10} dose of 6-TG alone on this treatment schedule may be estimated at between 0.45 and 0.90 mg/kg/injection. It is clear that Ara-C, at less than LD_{10} doses, actually protected against the toxicity of 6-TG. That the combination of Ara-C and 6-TG is therapeutically synergistic against L1210 is shown by results of several experiments, pooled and summarized in Table 2. Inasmuch as Ara-C alone is generally curative when given on this intensive-intermittent treatment schedule to mice with 10^5 L1210 cells implanted i.p., the present study was designed to present a greater challenge to therapy, and 10^6 L1210 cells were injected i.v. on day 0. Under these conditions, untreated mice exhibited a median survival time of 5.0 days; 6-TG alone was only moderately effective, and Ara-C alone was substantially more effective, but neither of the individual drugs was curative. Examination of mortality among parallel groups of normal mice indicates that the optimal antileukemic dose of 6-TG alone (1.0 mg/kg/injection) was indeed lethal to the host. In contrast, when Ara-C (15 mg/kg) and 6-TG (1.0 mg/kg) were given in combination, 12 of 20 normal mice and nine of 18 leukemic mice survived.

Another example of therapeutic synergism arising from the ability of one antitumor drug to protect against the toxicity of a second is provided by

TABLE 2

EFFECTIVENESS OF DIVIDED-INTERMITTENT TREATMENT WITH CYTOSINE ARABINOSIDE (Ara-C) PLUS 6-THIOGUANINE (6-TG) AGAINST LEUKEMIA L1210[a]

IP Dose (Mg/Kg) q3hr/24hr. Days 1,5,9,13		Mice with Tumor			Normal Mice	
Ara-C	6-TG	ILS (%)	S/T	Pct. Surv.	S/T	Pct. Surv.
22	0	345	1/27	4	28/49	57
15	0	480	0/30	0	47/48	98
10	0	422	0/29	0	46/49	94
6.7	0	327	0/29	0	48/48	100
0	1.0	125	0/20	0	1/30	3
0	0.67	105	0/30	0	29/50	58
0	0.45	60	0/30	0	47/49	96
15	1.0	604	9/18	50	12/20	60
10	1.0	625	6/19	32	11/17	65
15	0.67	606	7/20	35	15/18	83
10	0.67	558	9/29	31	27/29	93
6.7	0.67	550	1/10	10	10/10	100

[a]Data of L.H. Schmidt and F.M. Schabel, Jr. (see Schmidt, et al. 1970). Tumor inoculum – 10^6 cells, IV.

the combination of ICRF-159 plus daunomycin. In attempting to elucidate the mechanisms of untoward cardiac effects attending the clinical use of daunomycin (Livingston and Carter, 1970); Herman et al. (1972) found that daunomycin-induced electrocardiographic abnormalities in the isolated dog heart could be partially reversed by preperfusion with the chelating agent Versene (EDTA) or ICRF-159 (Fig. 1). Woodman et al. (1972) showed that both EDTA or ICRF-159 protected mice against the lethal toxicity of daunomycin. Moreover, ICRF-159 was more effective than EDTA in this regard. Table 3 summarizes an experiment in which normal mice and leukemic (L1210) mice were given a single treatment with ICRF-159 and daunomycin, individually or combined. The optimal dose of ICRF-159 alone (400 mg/kg) produced a 67% ILS in leukemic mice, and was lethal to only one of six normal mice. The lowest dose of daunomycin alone (2.5 mg/kg) was not lethal to normal mice but was also not very effective in the leukemic mice. Higher doses of daunomycin alone (5.0 or 10 mg/kg) were lethal to the host. When the nonlethal dose of daunomycin was combined with ICRF-159, increasing dosages of the latter resulted in progressively increased antileukemic efficacy over that achieved with daunomycin alone; presumably this was due to the antitumor activity of ICRF-159. When ICRF-159 was combined with lethal doses of daunomycin, the former protected against the toxicity of the latter. Again, increasing ICRF-159 dosage resulted in an increase in antileukemic effectiveness. Maximum antileukemic activity (78% ILS) on this treatment schedule was achieved with the combination dosage of 400 mg/kg ICRF-

1,2-bis (3,5-dioxopiperazin-1-yl) propane

NSC 129,943   "ICRF 159"

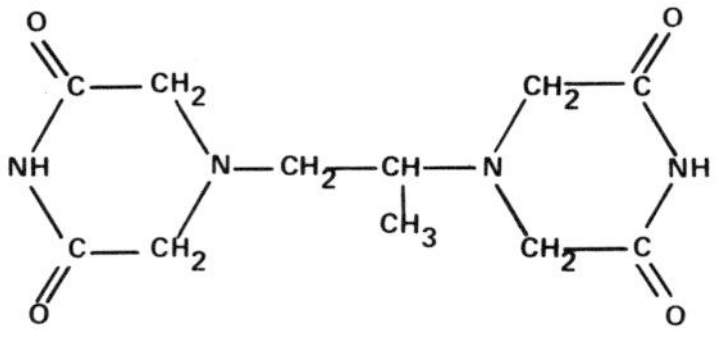

Ethylene diamine, tetracetic acid (VERSENE)

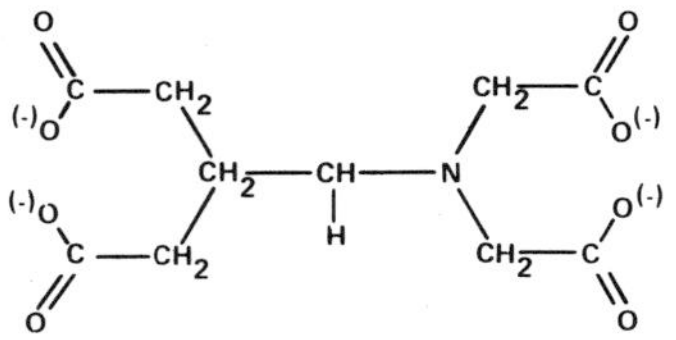

FIG. 1. Structure of ICRF-159 (NSC-129,943) and Versene (EDTA).

TABLE 3

INFLUENCE OF ICRF-159 ON DAUNOMYCIN ANTILEUKEMIC (L1210)* ACTIVITY
(ICRF-159 Given 10 Minutes Prior To Daunomycin — Day 1 Only)

(Mg/Kg-IP)		L1210 ILS (%)	Normal S/T Day 60	(Mg/Kg-IP)		L1210 ILS (%)	Normal S/T Day 60
ICRF-159	Daun.			ICRF-159	Daun.		
800	0	0	1/6	400	5.0	67	6/6
400	0	67	5/6	200	5.0	67	6/6
200	0	44	6/6	100	5.0	50	6/6
100	0	11	6/6	0	5.0	17	0/6
400	10	78	4/6	400	2.5	61	5/6
200	10	61	6/6	200	2.5	55	6/6
100	10	44	6/6	100	2.5	44	6/6
0	10	0	0/6	0	2.5	22	6/6

*IP tumor.

159 plus 10 mg/kg daunomycin but the efficacy of the combination was not substantially greater than that seen with optimal ICRF-159 alone treatment. However, when ICRF-159 and daunomycin were combined using intermittent or daily treatment, the therapeutically synergistic quality of the combination became evident and was most pronounced when treatment was given on every 4th day; 63% of the combination treated mice surviving for more than 60 days (Fig. 2). With the maximally effective q4d schedule the optimal combination dosage included ICRF-159 at its optimal dose when used alone plus daunomycin at a dose that was lethal for daunomycin alone treatment. In the experiments summarized in Table 3 and Fig. 2, both drugs were given i.p. to mice with ascites L1210. Lenaz and DiMarco (1972) reported that mice tolerated higher doses of either daunomycin or adriamycin when the agents were injected i.v. or s.c. than when they were injected i.p. More recent studies by Woodman et al. *(personal communication)* indicated that nonleukemic mice can tolerate 10 times the i.p. dose of daunomycin if the drug is given s.c. Further, the maximum tolerated s.c. dose of daunomycin could not be increased by concomitant ICRF-159 treatment. Nevertheless, s.c.-injected daunomycin showed therapeutic enhancement with i.p. injected ICRF-159 against early ascitic L1210 leukemia. In addition, preliminary studies have indicated ICRF-159 + adriamycin to be more effective against L1210 than either drug alone, but there was no suggestion that ICRF-159 protected normal animals against the lethal toxicity of adriamycin (Woodman et al., *personal communication).* However, this combination has been tested using only a limited number of treatment schedules.

The studies of the combinations of Ara-C + 6-TG and ICRF-159 + daunomycin provided clear-cut examples of therapeutic synergism arising

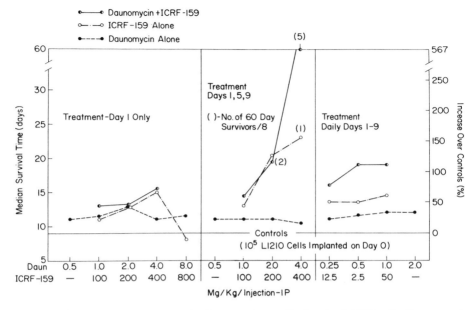

FIG. 2. Influence of treatment schedule on the antileukemic (L1210) effectiveness of combination chemotherapy with daunomycin (NSC-82151) and ICRF-159 (NSC-129,943).

from the ability of one antitumor drug to diminish the host toxicity of the other with no apparent diminution in antitumor effectiveness. The studies also emphasized the importance of the treatment schedule and route as factors influencing the efficacy of combination chemotherapy, and this adds to the complexities of experimental design in the evaluation of drug combinations.

The profound influence of the treatment schedule on the therapeutic efficacy of drug combinations is further illustrated by the studies of Schabel (1968 and *personal communication*) using Ara-C + 1-(2-chloroethyl)-3-cyclohexyl-1-nitrosourea (CCNU). This investigator had demonstrated the superiority of Ara-C + CCNU over either of the individual drugs in the treatment of L1210 when the drugs were combined concomitantly. In a subsequent study of the effects of sequential treatment with these drugs Ara-C followed by CCNU provided a marked enhancement in therapeutic efficacy whereas CCNU followed by Ara-C led to increased lethality for the mice (Table 4).

Therapeutic synergism may result from the ability of a therapeutically inactive agent to protect specifically the host from the toxicity of an antitumor drug. One procedure that has been used in an attempt to improve therapeutic efficacy is to treat with a combination of a metabolite plus a corresponding antimetabolite. For example, Goldin et al. (1955) reported

TABLE 4

SEQUENTIAL TREATMENT OF ADVANCED LEUKEMIA L1210*

IP Treatment	Schedule	Dose per Injection (Mg/Kg)	L1210		Normal
			MST (Days)	S/T D45	S/T D45
Controls	–	–	4.0	0/30	9/10
Ara-C alone	q3hr/24hr Days 2,6,10,14	15	20	0/10	8/10
CCNU alone	Once, day 2	50	15	0/10	4/10
		37.5	14	0/10	8/10
		25	9.5	0/10	10/10
Ara-C ↓ CCNU	q3hr/24hr/D2 ↓ Once, Day 5	15 ↓ 37.5	39	4/10	10/10
CCNU ↓ Ara-C	Once, Day 2 ↓ q3hr/24hr/D5	37.5 ↓ 15	10	0/10	0/10
CCNU ↓ Ara-C	Once, Day 2 ↓ q3hr/24hr/D5	25 ↓ 15	16	0/10	6/10

*10^7 cells implanted IV. Selected unpublished data of F. M. Schabel, Jr.

that simultaneous administration of citrovorum factor (CF) plus aminopterin or methotrexate (MTX) to mice with L1210 diminished the therapeutic efficacy of the folic-acid antagonists. However, when the CF was delayed for 12 or 24 hr following administration of either aminopterin or MTX, there was an increase in therapeutic efficacy. The advantages of the combinations were attributed to the ability of delayed CF to still protect the host against the toxicity of the antifols after the latter's actions against the tumor cells appeared to be complete.

In a more recent study (Goldin et al., *in press*), the combination of deoxycytidine plus Ara-C failed to provide a more effective antileukemic (L1210) therapy than treatment with Ara-C alone. In the experiment summarized in Table 5, Ara-C was given daily over a wide range of dosage levels and at varying time intervals following administration of deoxycytidine. The progressive increase in the optimal dose of Ara-C in the combination with decreasing time interval between the administration of metabolite and antimetabolite indicates that deoxycytidine was able to competitively protect the mice against the toxicity of Ara-C. However, under the conditions of this experiment, the combination did not result in increased therapeutic efficacy over that achieved with the optimal dose of Ara-C alone. A possible explanation for the apparent reduced effectiveness when deoxycytidine was given immediately prior to Ara-C (Table 5; "0" min) might be the failure to give the antimetabolite at a dosage level sufficiently high to compensate for the protective action of deoxycytidine against the tumor. In any case, from these data it was concluded that the combina-

TABLE 5

PROTECTION BY DEOXYCYTIDINE AGAINST TOXICITY AND ANTILEUKEMIC (L1210) EFFECTIVENESS OF CYTOSINE ARABINOSIDE (Ara-C)*

Ara-C Daily Dose	Ara-C Alone	Time (Minutes) of Administration of 320 Mg/Kg/Day Deoxycytidine Relative to Ara-C			
		− 120	− 60	0	+ 60
(Mg/Kg)	——— Median Day of Death (No. of 90-Day Survivors/8 Mice ———				
65	12.0 (0)	23.0 (0)	>97.0 (5)	29.0 (0)	18.0 (0)
39	41.0 (2)	>97.0 (5)	33.0 (0)	25.0 (0)	78.5 (2)
23	>97.0 (5)	80.0 (2)	29.0 (0)	23.5 (0)	>97.0 (6)
14	79.5 (3)	44.0 (0)	28.5 (0)	14.0 (0)	54.0 (2)
0	–	Deoxycytidine alone – 10.0 days (No survivors)			
0	–	Untreated controls – 11.0 days (No survivors)			

*SC treatment begun 3 days after SC tumor implantation and continued daily to death or day 70.

tion of deoxycytidine plus Ara-C resulted in a decrease in toxicity to the host that was offset by an essentially equivalent decrease in toxicity to the tumor.

The combination of N-acetylcysteine (NAC) plus isophosphamide (Isoph) does provide an additional example of therapeutic synergism resulting from the ability of an agent devoid of antitumor activity to protect the host but not the tumor against the toxicity of an active antitumor drug. Connors and Elson (1962) reported that thiol pretreatment of rats reduced the toxicity of the more chemically reactive nitrogen mustards, and Primack (1971) reported that irrigation of bladders of monkeys and dogs with acetylcysteine protected against cyclophosphamide-induced cystitis. Such findings prompted the investigation of the effects of NAC on the toxicity and antileukemic (L1210) effectiveness of cyclophosphamide and the related drug, Isoph (Kline et al., 1972). The experiment summarized in Fig. 3 shows the marked therapeutic advantage against L1210 of the combination of NAC plus Isoph over Isoph alone. The optimal dose of Isoph alone (300 mg/kg) produced three 90-day survivors among eight mice. At a higher dose of Isoph alone (500 mg/kg), one animal survived, but most succumbed to drug toxicity as evidenced by a median survival time of 3.5 days. NAC alone at 1,500 mg/kg was not toxic and had no antitumor activity. All of the mice that were given 1,500 mg/kg NAC + 500 mg/kg Isoph survived for more than 90 days. Whether bladder cystitis contributes to the lethal toxicity of Isoph in the mouse is not known. Clearly, however, NAC protected the mice from Isoph-induced lethality, an observation that has been repeatedly confirmed in nontumor-bearing animals. The resulting increase

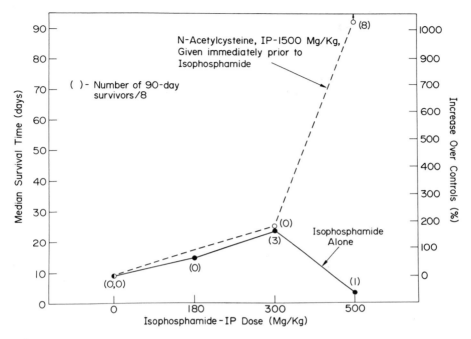

FIG. 3. Influence of N-acetylcysteine on isophosphamide activity against L1210 (Kline et al., 1972). Treatment was given once on the day following i.p. implantation of 10^5 L1210 cells.

in antileukemic specificity seen with the combination appeared to be due to the ability to safely give a higher dose of the active antitumor drug.

Skipper et al. (1970) in discussing cytokinetic, biochemical, toxicologic, and pharmacologic factors that influence antitumor efficacy emphasized the importance of the concentration (C) and duration of effect (T) of an active drug at the target site. In most cases, alterations in $C \times T$ leading to improved therapy have been brought about by modifications in treatment schedule. However, a growing number of investigators including Mellet et al. (1969) working with Skipper, and Donelli et al. (1972) in Garattini's laboratory, have studied alterations in $C \times T$ by modifying its rate of metabolic transformation to an active or inactive metabolite. Mellet et al. (1969) showed the ability of phenobarbital or SKF-525A to increase and retard, respectively, the conversion of Cy to its active metabolite. Recently, Field et al. (1972) studied the influence of phenobarbital or SKF-525A on the activity of Cy against L1210 leukemia. Leukemic mice, having been pretreated with phenobarbital or SKF-525A, were given Cy at various time intervals prior to tumor implantation. Chemical determinations of the alkylating metabolites of Cy in plasma showed that phenobarbital pretreatment accelerated both their production and depletion, whereas SKF-525A

TABLE 6

INFLUENCE OF PRETREATMENT WITH PHENOBARBITAL OR SKF-525A ON THE DURATION OF EFFECTIVE LEVELS OF CYCLOPHOSPHAMIDE ACTIVITY AGAINST LEUKEMIA L1210[a]

Cyclophosphamide IP-180 Mg/Kg	Cyclophosphamide Alone		Phenobarbital[b] + Cyclophosphamide		SKF-525A[c] + Cyclophosphamide	
Time Prior to Tumor Inoculation	Expt. 1	Expt. 2	Expt. 1	Expt. 2	Expt. 1	Expt. 2
(Minutes)	Mean Survival Time in Days (No. of 60-Day Survivors/Total)[d]					
0	29.4 (3/10)	27.5 (2/10)	41.3 (5/10)	53.4 (8/10)	50.2 (8/10)	37.2 (5/10)
20	43.4 (5/8)	32.5 (3/8)	22.1 (0/8)	18.4 (1/8)	43.3 (4/6)	42.9 (5/8)
40	11.6 (0/8)	11.9 (0/8)	8.6 (0/8)	10.1 (0/8)	40.5 (4/7)	32.1 (3/8)
60	8.7 (0/8)	10.4 (0/8)	8.4 (0/8)	8.7 (0/8)	25.0 (2/8)	26.5 (1/4)
90	–	–	–	–	–	13.4 (0/7)
180	–	–	–	–	–	11.5 (0/8)
Untreated Controls	9.1 (0/16)	8.9 (0/16)				
Phenobarbital Alone	9.2 (0/8)	8.3 (0/7)				
SKF-525A Alone	10.5 (0/8)	10.3 (0/8)				

[a] Field, et al. (1972). Tumor inoculum – 10^5 cells, IP.
[b] Phenobarbital (35 mg/kg) was given IP every 12 hrs. x 5; last injection 6 hr. prior to cyclophosphamide.
[c] SKF-525A (35 mg/kg) was given IP one hr. prior to cyclophosphamide.
[d] 60-Day survivors were assigned day 60 as the day of death for calculation of mean survival time.

retarded the activation of the drug. The survival times of the mice (Table 6) indicated that the duration of antileukemic activity was shortened by pheno-barbital and lengthened by SKF-525A. Whereas there seemed to be no profound effect on therapeutic efficacy, such studies do raise the question of the degree to which one drug might affect the activity or toxicity of a second drug by altering its rate of metabolic activation or inactivation either by specific effects on metabolizing enzyme systems or by nonspecific hepatotoxicity.

CONCLUSION

With an increasing number of drugs emerging as "active" from experi-mental screens, the possibilities for studies of two, three, or more drug combinations are abundant. Rationales for the selection of drug pairs for experimental combination studies have been based on a number of *in vitro, in vivo,* and biochemical approaches. A major rationale for selecting drugs for combination in clinical trials has been dissimilarity of qualitative toxicity of two or more known clinically active drugs. The few examples of thera-peutic synergism against mouse leukemia L1210 presented herein affirm the hypothesis that lack of additive toxicity is a reasonable basis for expect-ing a therapeutic advantage from the combination of antitumor drugs. However, it is also clear that reduction of an antitumor drug's toxicity for the host by administration of another agent, which may or may not have antitumor activity itself, need not be accompanied by an equivalent reduc-tion in toxicity for tumor cells. Finally, it is suggested that when drug com-binations are selected for clinical trial, the effect of treatment schedule on the therapeutic efficacy of the combination as well as the effect of one drug on the metabolism of the second drug should be thoroughly investigated at the preclinical level.

REFERENCES

Connors, T. A., and Elson, L. A. (1962): *Biochem. Pharmacol. 11,* 1221.

Donelli, M. G., Colombo, S., and Garattini, S. (1972): *Eur. J. Cancer 8,* 181.

Field, R. B., Gang, M., Kline, I., Venditti, J. M., and Waravdekar, V. S. (1972): *J. Pharmacol. Exp. Therap. 180,* 475.

Gee, T. S., Yu, K. P., Clarkson, B. D. (1969): *Cancer 23,* 1019.

Goldin, A., Venditti, J. M., Humphreys, S. R., Dennis, D., and Mantel, N. (1955): *Cancer Res. 15,* 742.

Goldin, A., Venditti, J. M., and Mantel, N. *(in press):* Combination chemotherapy: Basic considerations. In: *Handbook for Experimental Pharmacology.*

Herman, E. H., Mhatre, R. H., Lee, I. P., and Waravdekar, V. S. (1972): *Proc. Soc. Exp. Biol. Med. 140,* 234.

Kline, I., Woodman, R. J., and Venditti, J. M. (1972): *Proc. Amer. Assoc. Cancer Res. 13,* 29.

Lenaz, L., and DiMarco, A. (1972): *Cancer Chemother. Rep. 56,* 431.

LePage, G. A., and Kaneko, T.: Cancer Res. *29,* 2314, 1969.

Livingston, R. B., and Carter, S. K. (1970): *Single Agents in Cancer Chemotherapy,* p. 367, IFI/Plenum, New York.

Mellet, L. B., ElDareer, S. M., Luce, J. K., and Frei, E., III (1969): *Pharmacologist 11,* 273.

Primack, A. (1971): *J. Nat. Cancer Inst. 47,* 223.

Schabel, F. M., Jr. (1968): In: *The Proliferation and Spread of Neoplastic Cells* pp. 379–408, Williams and Wilkins, Baltimore.

Schmidt, L. H., Montgomery, J. A., Laster, W. R., Jr., and Schabel, F. M., Jr. (1970): *Proc. Amer. Assoc. Cancer Res. 11,* 70.

Skipper, H. E., Schabel, F. M., Jr., Mellet, L. B., Montgomery, J. A., Wilkoff, L. J., Lloyd, H. H., and Brockman, R. W. (1970): *Cancer Chemother. Rep. 54,* 431.

Venditti, J. M., and Goldin, A. (1964): Drug synergism in antineoplastic chemotherapy. In: *Advances in Chemotherapy,* Vol. 1, p. 397, Academic Press, New York.

Venditti, J. M., Humphreys, S. R., Mantel, N., and Goldin, A. (1956): *J. Nat. Cancer Inst. 17,* 631.

Woodman, R. J., Kline, I., Venditti, J. M. (1972): *Proc. Amer. Assoc. Cancer Res. 13,* 31.

Drug Interactions, edited by P. L. Morselli,
S. Garattini, and S. N. Cohen. Raven Press,
New York © 1974

A New Approach for the Quantitative Evaluation of the Respiratory Effect of Main Analgesic Combination in Man

György Rétsági,[1] J. Fischer,[2] and J. Knoll[3]

[1]*Third Medical Department, Semmelweis Medical University, Budapest, VIII. Mezö I. 17,*
[2]*Biomathematics Division, Institute of Computer Science, Hungarian Academy of Sciences, Budapest, Logodi 44/b, and* [3]*the Department of Pharmacology, Semmelweis Medical University, Budapest, VIII. Üllöi 26, Hungary*

INTRODUCTION

Up to the present, attempts to produce an analgesic drug suitable for relieving intractable pain without the risk of developing tolerance and dependence have been unsuccessful. Knoll (1) described two new substances, the combined application of which is supposed to approach the ideal analgesic. One of the two compounds, azidomorphine (6-deoxy-6-azido-dihydroizomorphine) (Am) is the most potent semisynthetic morphine derivative ever produced; the other, Rymazolium (1,6-dimethyl-3-carbethoxy-4-oxo-6,7,8, 9-tetrahydro-homopyrimidozol-methylsulphate) is a nonnarcotic analgesic having a new spectrum of activity that markedly potentiates the analgesic effect and reduces the respiratory depressant capacity of morphine derivatives.

The analgesic effect of AM in animal experiments is equal to that of fentanyl, and it is 300 times more potent than morphine. AM in gradually increasing analgesic doses over a period of 4 months proved to be significantly less toxic than morphine. The wide safety margin of the drug made it possible to treat rats and rhesus monkeys with constantly increasing doses.

The prolonged administration of morphine in an every second day increasing dosage resulted in the development of high-grade tolerance and physical dependence, and severe withdrawal symptoms were precipitated in rats by nalorphine and in monkeys on abrupt withdrawal of the drug. In parallel experiments with AM, the animals did not develop tolerance or physical dependence.

AM, in doses equivalent to morphine, suppressed withdrawal symptoms in morphine-addicted monkeys and did not abolish the abstinence syndrom (2, 3).

Rymazolium (R) is a new nonnarcotic analgesic, which in animal experiments highly potentiated the effect of AM (4–7). In man, it is a considerably more potent analgesic than novamidazophen, and it has very few side effects (8).

Our conclusions gained from over 8,000 applications can be summarized in the following:

(a) AM or AMR was found to be in man a 40 to 50 times more effective analgesic than morphine, thus about 0.2 mg of AM is equianalgesic to 10 mg of morphine.

(b) Euphoria could not be observed either by acute or by chronic application. No tolerance developed on chronic application. Examined by various methods, following prolonged administration of full doses, no signs of physical dependence were found.

(c) The side effects of AM or AMR as compared to morphine or pentazocine are negligible.

In the present study, the respiratory effects of AM and of the AMR combination are reported on the basis of our clinicopharmacological experiments.

MATERIAL AND METHODS

The investigations were carried out on 10 voluntary, healthy physicians aged 24 to 30. The applied substances were 0.2 mg of AM, 0.2 mg of AM and 150 mg of R, 10 mg of morphine, and 30 mg of pentazocine were used as referents. The administration occurred in all cases intravenously, at random, using a double-blind method.

The same staff performed all the examinations under uniform conditions. The participants were fasting, remained throughout the investigation in a sitting position, and stood up only for the examination of orthostasis.

In the present study the following of the obtained parameters are discussed in detail: ventilation/minute ($\dot{V}$), alveolar ventilation ($\dot{V}_A$), pH, and $PaCO_2$.

Respiratory function tests were performed by a water-sealed double-closed circulatory system (Pulmotest, Godart, Netherlands). Respiratory rate, ventilation volume, and ventilation/minute were measured; alveolar ventilation was estimated from the calculated value of anatomic dead space.

Blood gas analysis was carried out from capillary blood with the micromethod of Astrup (Astrup microanalyzer, Radiometer, Copenhagen). Ventilation volume, respiratory rate, $\dot{V}$ and $\dot{V}_A$, arterial blood pH, standard bicarbonate, $PaCO_2$ and BE were the parameters obtained. The $PaCO_2^{3.5}/\dot{V}_A$ ratio introduced on the basis of the computer discriminant analysis as a ninth parameter was found to have a valuable discriminatory power.

All parameters were measured four times in all cases, prior to and 10, 30, and 60 min following administration. Furthermore, the changes of pulse and blood pressure were registered continuously together with signs and symptoms concerning side effects. However, the conclusions suggested by these findings are beyond the scope of this report.

The methods of comparative drug action evaluation were based on a series of computer programs. In the authors' opinion, these are apt to evaluate quite a wide class of similar situations, too. The programs were run in the FORTRAN language of the CDC 3300 type computer of the Hungarian Academy of Sciences. Analyses were performed for three parallel metameters.

First were the basic data, i.e., parameter values in the original dimension of recording. These are very much subject to chance and serve primarily for comparison with alien results. Our second trial has been to relate values under drug effect to the respective initial ones. This kind of ratio, "normed data," proved to be more effective by eliminating most of the hazard in actual parameter levels. The most realistic image has been given by the third, namely the logarithmic metameter. This one was suggested by the property of the logarithm that it modifies, the shape of parameter frequency distributions toward symmetry enhancing effective statistical evaluation. Actually, when taking the logarithm of basic and normed data, numerically identical deviations from zero-minute values are gained; thus logarithmic analysis may be considered a joint refinement of both of these. It is worth mentioning that special programs produced a series of values within and between individual standard deviations of the parameters in order to see whether some normalization could be introduced for taking into account eventually different spreads. In our case, this normalization proved superfluous, but its necessity should be examined in similar situations.

Linear discriminant analyses were computed for all three metameter versions between the sets of before-and-after drug-administration data. The programs contain a number of evaluating statistics that establish an improved possibility of complex judgment. In fact, those complex analyses were also computed for sequentially selected subsets of the eight parameters. On the basis of the comparison of all these program results, the simple index $PaCO_2{}^{3.5}/\dot{V}_A$ lent itself as a rather characteristically discriminant ninth parameter. For this reason it has been introduced as such into all further calculations.

In the actual calculations, the value of the above index is divided by 10^4, which yields values of generally two integer digits. Since all preliminary calculations are based on deviations from initial values, it is quite natural that the changes rather than the absolute values of the index are characteristic of abnormal breathing function. From our cases, it can be stated that (within an hour) upward changes above 50% may be regarded as pathological rather than physiological and those above 100% can be considered abnormal with some certainty. Absolute values of the index are between 5 and 90; those above 60 can be regarded as pathological by themselves.

All that has been stated points to a very high sensitivity of the index just in the neighborhood of the physiological state.

Hence it is an adequate indicator of moderate dysfunction implementing the set of other parameters in this respect.

Another essential methodological innovation in statistical analysis is the following. The extreme mean, i.e., the arithmetic average of maximum and minimum after-administration values, is figured as "fifth observation time." This value has the advantage of expressing the range of changes independently of the time of their occurrence. Furthermore, it is a good basis for tests; under the assumption of symmetry in upward and downward deviations, it may be expected to fluctuate around the initial value.

Unfortunately it has been impossible to present completely even the main results of the whole evaluation. Thus we found it reasonable to give statistical tables for the five most informative parameters $\dot{V}$, $\dot{V}_A$, pH, $PaCO_2$, and $PaCO_2^{3.5}/\dot{V}_A$ with the most sensitive logarithmic metameter and the most characteristic "time," i.e., the extreme mean only. It has to be noticed that final biometric analysis with respect to differences of pre- and posttreatment values as representatives of "drug effect" has been based on results similar to those presented in Tables 1–4, taking into account the auxiliary information yielded by other parameters, metameters, and times as well.

These statistics are of the following types: drug-wise and between-drug difference averages are calculated together with the respective standard deviations and 95% confidence intervals constructed from the former. Significance levels to Student's t-values are computed one-sided toward depression for single drugs and two-sided between any two of them. The explanation of this fact is that depression can be assumed if there is any systematic change; yet it would be exaggerated to presume an exclusive direction also for differences between two drug effects. As to the latter, because of medium heterogenity in standard deviations, two-sample t-tests have been preferred against analyses of variance. Correlation coefficients are computed with their most exact normal confidence limits and Student's significance levels. All these are done between any two parameters for fixed drugs and conversely between any two drugs for fixed parameters.

Some rather important results and consequences that should be mentioned here are the following:

Table 1 shows the parameter-wise average, standard deviation and the Student's p values of extreme mean deviations for different drugs. (For sake of simplicity the words "parameter-wise" and "drug-wise" are to stand here for the expression "by parameters" and "by drugs.")

In the case of $\dot{V}$, $\dot{V}_A$, pH, and $PaCO_2$, morphine and pentazocine give generally significant (or almost significant) deviations from the initial values toward depression. It is natural that the index created for indicating slight deviations in the neighborhood of the physiological state does not work here anymore. From this point of view AM is a counterpart of the former: in

TABLE 1. Parameter-wise average, SD, and Student's p values of extreme mean deviations for different drugs

	AMR	Pe	Mo	AM
$\dot{V}$	−0.008	−0.126	−0.162	−0.069
	0.135	0.299	0.240	0.203
	0.426	0.108	0.031	0.155
$\dot{V}_A$	−0.013	−0.193	−0.226	−0.105
	0.170	0.427	0.311	0.260
	0.407	0.093	0.024	0.118
pH	−0.000	−0.003	−0.002	−0.000
	0.002	0.003	0.003	0.002
	0.201	0.004	0.045	0.673
$PaCO_2$	0.003	0.067	0.079	0.033
	0.052	0.086	0.107	0.045
	0.576	0.018	0.023	0.021
$PaCO_2^{3.5}/\dot{V}_A$	−0.113	0.039	0.057	0.113
	0.321	0.538	0.538	0.165
	0.853	0.411	0.373	0.029

$\dot{V}$, $\dot{V}_A$, and pH, the differences are smaller and not significant; the mean difference in the $PaCO_2$ is also smaller, and the $PaCO_2^{3.5}/\dot{V}_A$ shows the largest and significant deviations, pointing to the sensitivity domain of this index. As regards the combination AMR, the difference in the parameters $\dot{V}$, $\dot{V}_A$, and pH are less by an order of magnitude than under morphine and pentazocine (and naturally nonsignificant), whereas in the parameters

TABLE 2. Parameter-wise average, SD, and Student's p values of extreme mean deviations between pairs of drugs

	AMR-Pe	AMR-Mo	AMR-AM	Pe-Mo	Pe-AM	Mo-AM
$\dot{V}$	0.117	0.154	0.061	0.037	−0.056	−0.093
	0.281	0.233	0.119	0.407	0.320	0.232
	0.220	0.066	0.141	0.782	0.591	0.237
$\dot{V}_A$	0.180	0.213	0.092	0.033	−0.088	−0.121
	0.379	0.287	0.155	0.557	0.404	0.268
	0.168	0.044	0.094	0.856	0.509	0.188
pH	0.002	0.001	−0.001	−0.001	−0.003	−0.002
	0.003	0.003	0.003	0.003	0.003	0.004
	0.024	0.186	0.441	0.367	0.004	0.081
$PaCO_2$	−0.070	−0.082	−0.037	−0.012	0.033	0.045
	0.098	0.132	0.067	0.097	0.107	0.112
	0.049	0.082	0.116	0.709	0.348	0.233
$PaCO_2^{3.5}/\dot{V}_A$	−0.153	−0.170	−0.227	−0.018	−0.074	−0.056
	0.430	0.658	0.274	0.754	0.521	0.566
	0.291	0.435	0.028	0.943	0.664	0.760

TABLE 3a. *Drug-wise estimate, confidence limits, and Student's p values of correlation coefficients between pairs of parameters*

	AMR	Pe	Mo	AM
$\dot{V}$-$\dot{V}_A$	0.986	0.980	0.970	0.992
	0.951	0.928	0.893	0.971
	0.998	0.994	0.994	0.998
	0.000	0.000	0.000	0.000
$\dot{V}$-pH	0.489	−0.092	−0.628	−0.396
	−0.199	−0.693	−0.904	−0.828
	0.861	0.580	−0.018	0.313
	0.151	0.800	0.052	0.257
$\dot{V}$-$PaCO_2$	−0.545	−0.025	0.146	0.113
	−0.881	−0.654	−0.543	−0.566
	0.119	0.625	0.721	0.705
	0.104	0.946	0.687	0.755
$\dot{V}$-$PaCO_2^{3.5}/V_A$	0.489	0.831	0.643	0.831
	−0.199	0.461	0.043	0.461
	0.861	0.959	0.910	0.959
	0.151	0.003	0.045	0.003
$\dot{V}_A$-pH	0.572	−0.050	−0.585	−0.430
	−0.078	−0.670	−0.893	−0.842
	0.889	0.609	0.057	0.273
	0.084	0.891	0.076	0.215

TABLE 3b.

	AMR	Pe	Mo	AM
$\dot{V}_A$-$PaCO_2$	−0.506	−0.042	0.089	0.134
	−0.867	−0.666	−0.584	−0.551
	0.174	0.615	0.691	0.715
	0.135	0.909	0.807	0.712
$\dot{V}_A$-$PaCO_2^{3.5}/\dot{V}_A$	0.539	0.841	0.630	0.853
	−0.129	0.488	0.020	0.523
	0.877	0.963	0.906	0.967
	0.108	0.002	0.051	0.002
pH-$PaCO_2$	−0.278	−0.893	−0.685	−0.571
	−0.781	−0.975	−0.922	−0.889
	0.434	−0.639	−0.123	0.080
	0.436	0.001	0.029	0.085
pH-$PaCO_2^{3.5}/\dot{V}_A$	0.215	−0.523	−0.849	−0.638
	−0.488	−0.873	−0.967	−0.908
	0.754	0.152	−0.512	−0.035
	0.550	0.121	0.002	0.047
$PaCO_2$-$PaCO_2^{3.5}/\dot{V}_A$	0.427	0.502	0.817	0.619
	0.277	−0.180	0.426	0.002
	0.840	0.865	0.959	0.904
	0.219	0.139	0.004	0.056

$PaCO_2$, $PaCO_2^{3.5}/\dot{V}_A$ the direction of the average deviations is even the opposite of depression.

Table 2 shows the parameter-wise average, standard deviation and Student's p values of extreme mean deviations between pairs of drugs.

No significant deviation could be found between morphine and pentazocine. Although AM shows essential deviations from the two former drugs concerning pH only, the AMR combination shows such deviations of almost this order in $\dot{V}$, $\dot{V}_A$, and $PaCO_2$, too. When confronting the AMR combination with AM, we can see that the differences in favor of the combination in the $\dot{V}$, $\dot{V}_A$, and $PaCO_2$ are not far from significance, the difference in pH is very slight and that in the index is significant, as expected.

Table 3a,b shows the drug-wise estimate, confidence limits, and Student's p values of correlation coefficients between pairs of parameters.

Here we find worth mentioning that parameters $\dot{V}$ and $\dot{V}_A$ offer almost the same information concerning our problem; all the correlations are very highly significant. As the correlations between $\dot{V}_A$ and the index are generally higher than those between $PaCO_2$ and $PaCO_2^{3.5}/\dot{V}_A$, this fact proves the important role of the $\dot{V}_A$ in the index. It is seen from the row regarding $\dot{V}_A - PaCO_2$ (and naturally $\dot{V} - PaCO_2$) that these are the lines of lowest correlations, which shows that we succeeded in combining the most independent relevant information in our index.

Table 4 shows the parameter-wise estimate, confidence limits, and Student's p values of correlation coefficients between pairs of drugs.

The connection between the reaction to morphine and pentazocine is the most explicit of all and is significant for all parameters examined. Not one significant correlation was found between any of the parameter reactions to the two former drugs and those to the drugs containing AM. The correlations between the latter drugs are highly significant for the spirometric parameters and nonsignificant for others. This fact is a hint that Rymazolium has a less immediate effect on respiration than on blood gas parameters.

Considering the biological aspect of the reported mathematical data, we are justified in stating that the respiratory-depressant capacity of AM or of the AMR combination is significantly lower than that of equianalgesic doses of morphine or pentazocine. AM, which is about 40 times more potent an analgesic in man than morphine and has a safety margin about five- to sixfold to that of morphine in animal experiments, shows even in itself a considerably less respiratory depressant effect than morphine or pentazocine. The AMR combination does not reveal a respiratory depressant capacity even using the index suggested by us, with a high sensitivity in the border of physiological values.

Finally bearing in mind the most important fact, that neither AM nor the AMR combination led to the development of tolerance or physical dependence, we may hope with reasonable assurance that the introduction of these drugs might actually serve as an approach to the ideal analgesic.

TABLE 4. *Parameter-wise estimate, confidence limits, and Student's p values of correlation coefficients between pairs of drugs*

	AMR-Pe	AMR-Mo	AMR-AM	Pe-Mo	Pe-AM	Mo-AM
$\dot{V}$	0.377	0.332	0.826	0.858	0.391	0.461
	−0.291	−0.340	0.482	0.566	−0.275	−0.190
	0.805	0.787	0.955	0.963	0.811	0.838
	0.279	0.345	0.003	0.001	0.260	0.175
$\dot{V}_A$	0.521	0.411	0.820	0.859	0.527	0.572
	−0.107	−0.252	0.467	0.568	−0.098	−0.031
	0.861	0.818	0.955	0.963	0.861	0.877
	0.118	0.235	0.003	0.001	0.113	0.080
pH	0.148	0.237	−0.214	0.865	0.186	0.162
	−0.506	−0.432	−0.732	0.586	−0.475	−0.494
	0.697	0.742	0.451	0.967	0.717	0.705
	0.683	0.508	0.551	0.001	0.605	0.653
$PaCO_2$	−0.302	−0.288	0.065	0.799	0.020	0.104
	−0.771	−0.768	−0.566	0.414	−0.598	−0.539
	0.369	0.383	0.650	0.947	0.623	0.674
	0.393	0.417	0.857	0.005	0.957	0.774
$PaCO_2^{3.5}/\dot{V}_A$	−0.057	−0.117	0.521	0.773	0.165	−0.019
	−0.647	−0.682	−0.107	0.354	−0.492	−0.623
	0.572	0.529	0.861	0.940	0.705	0.600
	0.876	0.746	0.118	0.007	0.648	0.959

SUMMARY

Several authors have examined the respiratory effect of a newly synthetized major analgesic, azidomorphine (AM), a morphine derivative in itself and in its combination with Rymazolium (R). R is a new nonnarcotic analgesic increasing considerably the analgesic effect of AM in animal experiments. Spirometrical and blood gas analytical investigations were carried out on 10 normal voluntary participants in a double-blind trial and 10 mg of morphine and 30 mg of pentazocine were applied as reference substances. The about 4,000 data gained by measurements before and 10, 30, and 60 min after the intravenous administration of the drugs, including ventilation volume, respiratory rate, $\dot{V}$ and $\dot{V}_A$, arterial blood pH, standard bicarbonate, $PaCO_2$ and BE changes were analyzed. The $PaCO_2^{3.5}/\dot{V}_A$ ratio introduced on the basis of the computer discriminant analysis as a fifth parameter was found to have a valuable discriminatory power. Based upon preliminary data, three ways of relating were estimated simultaneously: differences, relative values, and logarithmic differences. The average of the maximal and minimal drug values were considered as a fifth time. The relevant versions of Student's *t*-test were employed to evaluate the mean values, correlations, and the between-drug differences. The depressive effect exercised by morphine and pentazocine upon the respiration could be proved by the usual statistical methods at various times concerning different parameters; on the other hand such alterations referring to AM or AMR combination could be demonstrated only by our newly introduced method. The latter rendered statistical proof that the combined preparation exercises the least depressant effect upon respiration.

ACKNOWLEDGMENT

Our most sincere thanks for their important contributions are expressed to Mrs. Eva Baumgarten concerning the mathematical activities as well as to Dr. Eva Schwarczmann and Dr. Ottó Székely regarding the medical activities in the present work.

REFERENCES

1. Knoll, J. (1973): *Pharm. Res. Comm. 5*, 175.
2. Knoll, J., Fürst, Z., and Kelemen, K. (1971): *Orvostudomány 22*, 265.
3. Knoll, J. (1973): *J. Pharm. and Pharmacol. 25*, 929.
4. Knoll, J., Mészáros, Z., Szentmiklósi, P., and Fürst, Z. (1971): *Arzneim. Forsch. 21*, 717.
5. Knoll, J., Fürst, Z., and Mészáros, Z. (1971): *Arzneim. Forsch. 21*, 719.
6. Knoll, J., Fürst, Z., and Mészáros, Z. (1971): *Arzneim. Forsch. 21*, 727.
7. Knoll, J., Magyar, K., and Bánfi, D. (1971): *Arzneim. Forsch. 21*, 733.
8. Graber, H. (1972): *Int. J. Clin. Pharmacol. 64*, 354.

Drug Interactions, edited by P. L. Morselli,
S. Garattini, and S. N. Cohen. Raven Press,
New York © 1974

The Isobolographic Method
Applied to Drug Interactions

Peter K. Gessner

*Department of Pharmacology, School of Medicine, State University of New York at Buffalo,
Buffalo, New York 14214*

The study of drug interactions always poses the problem of how to best characterize the effects observed when two agents are administered together. Secondly, it raises the question of whether the effects observed following administration of the combination, deviate significantly from what could have been predicted from the individual action of the two agents. Both of these questions can best be dealt with by the use of isobolographic analysis. I shall attempt to illustrate this with examples of its application in our work on drug interactions.

The isobolographic method was first introduced in 1926 by Loewe (Loewe and Muischnek, 1926); it had, however, associated with it a complex and exotic terminology. Moreover, its introduction preceded the development of rigorous mathematical methods for the calculation of ED_{50}'s and their 95% confidence limits (Finney, 1952). Consequently, the method as initially introduced was not a truly quantitative one. For these and other reasons Loewe's later writings on the subject (Loewe, 1928, 1953, 1957, 1958, 1959, 1961) failed to make the method widely accepted.

Nonetheless, isobolographic analysis is an essentially simple yet powerful technique for the study of drug interactions. It employs rectangular coordinates to represent drug combinations, defining thereby both the dose and the proportion of the two agents in the combination. This allows one to plot doses exhibiting equal effectiveness as points on the graph. Normally, the parameter of effectiveness employed is the occurrence of the effect in question in 50% of the animals tested and the points plotted are accordingly the ED_{50} doses. The locus of all such experimentally observed points, obtained using binary mixtures of the two drugs, is the isobol for that effect and the resulting plot is termed an isobologram.

The advantages derived from using this approach are best discussed in the context of Fig. 1. This represents the results of a study of the interaction of hexobarbital and phenobarbital with respect to their anesthetic effects in mice. In this experiment the loss of righting reflex was selected as an appropriate effect end point. Mice were administered various doses of hexobarbital i.p. in saline and from the incidence of righting reflex loss at

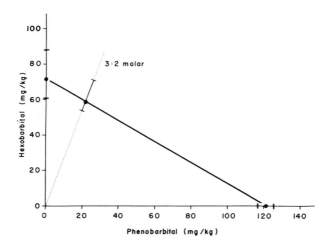

FIG. 1. Isobologram for the interaction of hexobarbital and phenobarbital with respect to righting-reflex loss in mice following their intraperitoneal administration. The ED_{50} points are plotted with their 95% confidence limits. The expected location of ED_{50} points, given the occurrence of a simple additive synergism, is given by the solid diagonal. The dotted diagonal going through the origin gives the loci of mixtures of hexobarbital and phenobarbital in a 3:2 molar ratio.

these doses the ED_{50} for hexobarbital and the 95% confidence limits of this ED_{50} were computed and marked on the abscissa. The procedure was repeated for phenobarbital; its ED_{50} point and 95% confidence limits were plotted on the ordinate. The procedure was repeated again using various doses of hexobarbital and phenobarbital combined in a 3 to 2 molar ratio. The ED_{50} for this mixture and its 95% confidence limits were computed and plotted on a line passing through the origin and representing the locus of all possible combinations of hexobarbital and phenobarbital in a 3 to 2 molar ratio.

The next question that arises is whether the effect experimentally observed with the drug combination is smaller or larger than would have been simple predicted on the basis of the individual pharmacological properties of the two agents. The arguments regarding this can be very complex, yet there is a very simple way of resolving them. For the sake of argument then let's consider what the isobologram would be like if hexobarbital and phenobarbital were different forms of the same compound, possibly in one case diluted down with an inert substance. The ED_{50} dose of either form would represent the same amount of active compound. Accordingly, a mixture of $\frac{1}{2}$ of the ED_{50} dose of one form plus $\frac{1}{4}$ of the ED_{50} dose of the other (or $\frac{1}{4}$ of one plus $\frac{3}{4}$ of the other, etc.) would contain an amount of active compound equal to the ED_{50} of either form and if administered would yield a 50% response. The location of all such points would be the diagonal joining the ED_{50} points of the two preparations. It can be seen from Fig. 1 that the ED_{50} point for hexobarbital and phenobarbital combined in a 3 to 2 molar ratio is not significantly displaced from this line. Accordingly, it can be said that for this combination of the two agents there was an interaction but that it was one of a simple additive nature. If the ED_{50} had fallen below the diagonal, this would have meant that a 50% response had been obtained with a dose smaller than expected, i.e., that the mixture had proved more potent than expected. This would have allowed one to state that potentiation had occurred, or, alternatively, that supra-additivity had been observed.

An alternative manner in which ED_{50}'s of combinations can be determined is to keep the dose of one agent constant and vary the dose of the other. If ED_{50}'s are determined in this manner, however, their computation requires special handling (Gessner and Cabana, 1970). An example of an isobologram where ED_{50}'s were determined in this way is that for the interaction between ethanol and trichloroethanol with respect to righting-reflex loss in mice (Fig. 2). This isobologram presents a further instance of

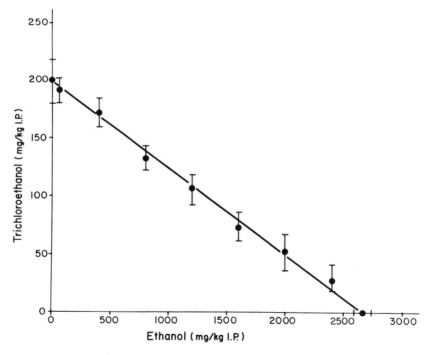

FIG. 2. Isobologram for the interaction of trichloroethanol and ethanol with respect to righting reflex loss in mice following their intraperitoneal administration. ED_{50} points are plotted with their 95% confidence limits. The expected location of the ED_{50} points, given the occurrence of a simple additive synergism, is given by the solid diagonal. Reprinted from Gessner and Cabana (1970).

an interaction of a simple additive nature with no deviations from expectation. Additionally, it might be noted that, although not all possible combinations of ethanol and trichloroethanol were employed, enough were so that it becomes possible to claim that the interaction between these two agents in mice follows simple additivity throughout.

A departure from simple additivity was observed, on the other hand, for the interaction between chloral hydrate and ethanol with respect to righting-reflex loss in mice. From the isobologram (Fig. 3) it is evident at a glance that the deviation from simple additivity is a significant one, but that it is seen only with some chloral hydrate–ethanol combinations. The degree of potentiation can be expressed quantitatively by a potentiation coefficient (Gessner and Cabana, 1970). Calculation of the coefficient for the chloral hydrate–ethanol interaction revealed that the potentiation was maximal when chloral hydrate and ethanol were combined in an equimolar ratio.

It would appear rational to suppose that investigation of the mechanisms

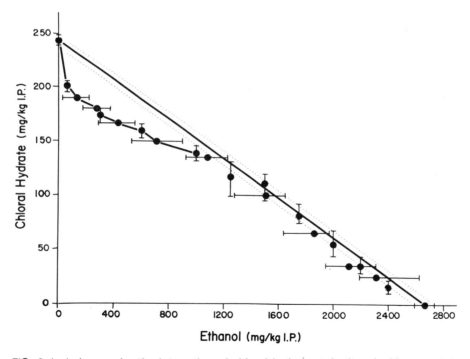

FIG. 3. Isobologram for the interaction of chloral hydrate and ethanol with respect to righting-reflex loss in mice following their intraperitoneal administration. ED_{50} points are plotted with their 95% confidence limits. The expected location of the ED_{50} points, given the occurrence of a simple additive synergism, is given together with the 95% confidence limits by the solid and dotted straight line diagonals, respectively. In the area of significant potentiation, the ED_{50} isobol has been generated by connecting adjacent ED_{50} points. Reprinted from Gessner and Cabana (1970).

of the interaction would be most likely to be successful if such an investigation would employ the two drugs in their maximally potentiating ratio. Accordingly, the opportunity afforded by the isobolographic method to identify this ratio adds to its power as a method for the investigation of drug interactions. It also provides a powerful test of any hypothesis advanced as explaining the mechanism of the interaction since such a hypothesis should be able to account for the potentiation being maximal when the two agents are combined in that particular ratio.

In the study of the chloral hydrate–ethanol interaction, as of the ones previously discussed, the two agents were administered simultaneously. Once a potentiation is observed, however, the question arises whether a further potentiation would be observed if the two agents were not administered simultaneously. We undertook to explore the optimal timing of the administration of the two agents relative to each other and found the potentiation to be greater when ethanol was administered 2 min before chloral hydrate (Gessner and Cabana, 1970). Any proposed mechanism should also be capable of explaining this type of finding.

To elucidate the mechanism of the interaction, we undertook a study in mice of the pharmacokinetics of chloral hydrate and ethanol metabolism when administered (a) singly and (b) jointly in an equimolar ratio to each other. We found that chloral hydrate, which has hypnotic properties of its own, was rapidly metabolized (*in vivo* half-life = 12 min), 56% being reduced to trichloroethanol, which is a slightly more potent hypnotic than chloral hydrate and possesses a much longer half-life (211 min). When coadministered with an equimolar amount of ethanol, chloral hydrate disappeared faster, and more of it (74%) was reduced to trichloroethanol (Cabana and Gessner, 1970). Ethanol on the other hand when it was coadministered with an equimolar amount of chloral hydrate disappeared less rapidly than when administered alone (Gessner, 1973a). The contribution made by ethanol to the hypnotic effects of the mixture and the contribution made to the interaction by the decreased rate of ethanol disappearance were, however, both minor because, given its relative lack of potency, the amount of ethanol in the mixture was small. Accordingly, the major reason for the observed potentiation was the formation of larger than normal amounts of trichloroethanol (Gessner, 1973*a*). As to the mechanism responsible for these biochemical events, these appeared to be due to the fact that the reduction of chloral hydrate to trichloroethanol is mediated by alcohol dehydrogenase, that is, by the same enzyme that is responsible for the oxidation of ethanol. Thus, it would appear that the two reactions become coupled. The higher than normal levels of alcohol dehydrogenase–NADH complex being available for reaction with chloral hydrate lead to an increase in the rate of its reduction. Since the product of the reduction, trichloroethanol, is an inhibitor of alcohol dehydrogenase, ethanol oxidation is significantly inhibited. However, the normal rate of ethanol oxidation in mice is some six times faster than the normal rate of chloral hydrate reduction. Accordingly, although under the conditions of the interaction the rate of ethanol oxidation is decreased and that of chloral hydrate reduction increased, the resultant absolute rates of the two reactions are virtually the same (Gessner, 1973a).

We investigated whether the potentiation between chloral hydrate and ethanol extended to the toxic properties of these agents (Gessner and Cabana, 1970). To this end, LD_{50}'s of chloral hydrate, ethanol, and combinations of the two agents in mice were determined and plotted on a multiple isobologram (Fig. 4), that is, an isobologram on which isobols for more than one parameter of effectiveness are plotted. In this instance, the isobols plotted were that for the ED_{50}'s for loss of righting reflex and the LD_{50} isobol. The former of these isobols is in effect reproduced from Fig. 3. Consideration of Fig. 4 reveals that some supra-additivity of the lethal effects of chloral hydrate and ethanol did occur when the drugs were coadministered in an equimolar ratio. On the other hand, when combinations of the drugs containing a higher proportion of ethanol were administered, LD_{50} points significantly above the line of simple additivity were obtained. Thus,

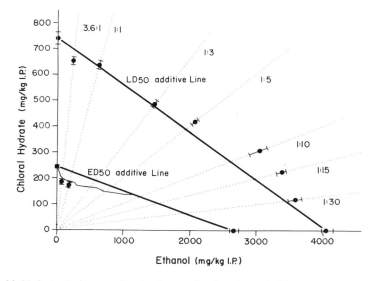

FIG. 4. Multiple isobologram for the interaction in mice of chloral hydrate and ethanol with respect to righting-reflex loss and mortality, respectively. All administrations were intraperitoneal. LD_{50} and ED_{50} points are plotted with their 95% confidence limits. The expected location of LD_{50} points, given the occurrence of simple additive synergism, is given by the upper solid diagonal. Similarly the expected location of ED_{50} points is given by the lower solid diagonal. The location of the line joining the points of significant potentiation in Fig. 3 is also given. The dotted diagonals passing through the origin give the loci of mixture points of chloral hydrate and ethanol in the stated ratios. Reprinted from Gessner and Cabana (1970).

more of the mixture was required to obtain an LD_{50} with such combinations than would have been predicted on the basis of simple dose additivity. It might be said that with these combinations significant infra-additivity was observed.

The multiple isobologram of Fig. 4 illustrates an additional point, namely that the kind of interaction that is observed depends not only on the proportion of the two agents in the combination but also on what parameter of effectiveness is employed. Thus, it might be noted that, when chloral hydrate and ethanol were coadministered in a 1:5 ratio, infra-additivity was observed with respect to mortality and supra-additivity with respect to righting-reflex loss.

The combination of chloral hydrate with alcoholic beverages has long been held to give rise to a potent mixture variously known as "Mickey Finn" or "knockout drops" (Gessner and Cabana, 1967). It is, therefore, not surprising that contemporaneously with our studies three other groups undertook to investigate the mechanism of this interaction (Craeven and Roach, 1969; Kaplan et al., 1969; Sellers et al., 1972a, b). In all instances differences in dosages, dosage ratios, and, in one instance, species, preclude direct comparison of their work with our results. None of these groups, however, employed the isobolographic method and none sought to investigate what the optimal interval between administration of the two agents might be. Of the two groups working with mice, one administered the two agents in a ratio that Gessner and Cabana (1970) had found not to lead to supra-additivity; the other administered the chloral hydrate 30 min prior to ethanol. Since chloral hydrate has a short half-life, there would have been very little of it left to interact with the ethanol administered 30 min later. Interestingly, both groups reported finding significant biochemical effects although it is not immediately clear with what pharmacological phenomenology these correlate.

The isobolographic method can also be applied to interactions where, for maximal potentiation, the two agents have to be administered several hours apart. An example of this is the tranylcypromine-meperidine interaction in mice with respect to their LD_{50}'s (Gessner and Soble, 1973). Preliminary experiments revealed that a 4-hr interval between the administration of the two drugs was optimal for a maximal potentiation. Other experiments showed that those animals that did die after the administration of tranylcypromine and meperidine 4 hr apart died within 4 hr of the meperidine administration. Therefore, in determining LD_{50}'s for the combination of tranylcypromine and meperidine the tranylcypromine was administered 4 hr before the meperidine administration and mortalities were noted 4 hr after meperidine administration. Accordingly, we proceeded to construct an isobologram for this interaction (Fig. 5) by plotting on one axis the 8-hr mortality of tranylcypromine and on the other the 4-hr mortality of meperidine. The resultant isobologram clearly shows supra-additivity, both with

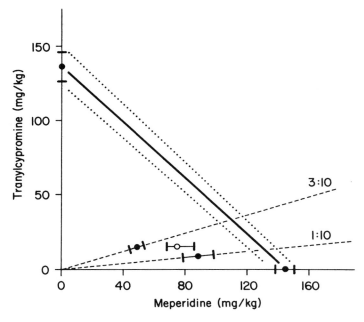

FIG. 5. Isobologram for the interaction of the toxic effects of tranylcypromine and meperidine administered 4 hr apart. LD_{50}'s were determined 4 hr after meperidine and 8 hr after tranylcypromine administration; they are plotted together with their 95% confidence limits. The expected location of LD_{50} points of combinations, given the occurrence of simple additive synergism, is given together with the 95% confidence limits by the solid and dotted diagonals, respectively. The dotted lines passing through the origin give the loci of tranylcypromine and meperidine doses in 3:10 and 1:10 ratios, respectively. The experimentally observed LD_{50} of these combinations is plotted together with its 95% confidence limits as solid points. The open point represents the position and 95% confidence limits of the LD_{50} reported for a combination of tranylcypromine and meperidine by Rogers and Thornton (1969). Reprinted from Gessner and Soble (1973).

respect to our data (black dots) and that of Rogers and Thornton (1969) who employed identical conditions and whose LD_{50}'s for tranylcypromine and meperidine were very similar to ours. Eade and Renton (1970), who were also interested in this interaction, explored whether its mechanism might involve inhibition of meperidine metabolism by the tranylcypromine pretreatment. They were able to show that tranylcypromine pretreatment did result in an inhibition of meperidine metabolism but also showed that under the conditions of dose, etc., employed by them this pretreatment did not potentiate meperidine toxicity. The ratio of tranylcypromine to meperidine in the LD_{50} dose reported by Eade and Renton was 1:30. Since the dose ratios employed by us and Rogers and Thornton (1969) were significantly higher than this, there is no conflict between the two sets of findings. It is, however, another instance of a biochemical observation that has no pharmacological phenomenology clearly associated with it. Our results (Gessner and Soble, 1973) support the hypothesis of Rogers and Thornton (1969) that 5-hydroxytryptamine, accumulated as a result of the inhibition of monoamine oxidase by tranylcypromine, is released onto its receptors by meperidine.

The tranylcypromine-meperidine interaction is one of considerable clinical interest. This is evidenced by interaction of tranylcypromine, as well as several other monoamine oxidase inhibitors, with meperidine all having been first observed clinically (see Gessner and Soble, 1973 for references). To study the mechanism of this interaction in an animal model we felt it essential to demonstrate the appropriateness of the model. To achieve this we turned to the isobolographic method. Such a demonstration of the appropriateness of the animal model would appear to be a logical prerequisite to the laboratory investigation of a clinically observed interaction. Yet, presumably because the isobolographic method is not well known, it is not used as widely as it might be. A case in point is the interaction between disulfiram and ethanol. It is well known that humans pretreated with disulfiram experience marked toxic effects when they ingest ethanol. There is continuing interest in trying to elucidate the mechanism of this interaction. The question arises as to what constitutes an appropriate animal model for the study of the interaction. Figure 6 is the isobologram for the lethal interaction of disulfiram and ethanol in the rat. It was constructed from the data reported by Child et al. (1952). Clearly the data show no supra-additivity, and therefore, one must conclude that either the species or the parameter of toxicity is inappropriate. Yet I know of no data clearly identifying an animal model as one in which supra-additivity between disulfiram and ethanol does occur.

Up to this point we have discussed dose addition. As stressed in the initial discussion, this is the type of addition that would necessarily occur with two forms of the same compound. Any two compounds producing effects by similar mechanisms would be expected to behave likewise. In the terminology of Bliss (1939) this corresponds to similar joint action. It has been argued on logical grounds, however, that for two compounds producing the same effect by entirely different mechanisms, effect addition rather than dose addition would occur (Bliss, 1939; Zipf and Hamacher, 1966). Bliss (1939) and later Finney (1952) term this independent joint action. Because of the S shape of the dose response curve, and because the effect observed over a wide range of low doses is virtually zero after which the dose response curve rises steeply with dose, the line of simple effect addition is radically different from that of simple dose addition. This theoretical effect addition line can be constructed by supposing (Finney, 1952) that, if the administration of the two agents used separately results in the effect being seen in fraction P_1 and P_2, respectively, then following their joint administration a fraction P_2 of the animals not showing the effect due to the first agent

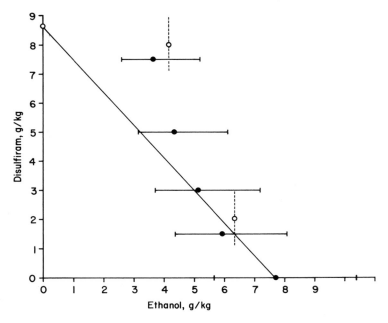

FIG. 6. Isobologram for the interaction of ethanol and disulfiram with respect to their lethal effects in rats constructed from the data of Child et al. (1952). Where Child et al. reported mortality data, the LD_{50}'s (●) and their 95% confidence limits were calculated by use of the ISOBOL program (Gessner and Cabana, 1970); in other instances the LD_{50}'s (○) are given as reported by Child et al. (1952) and are without 95% confidence limits. The dashed lines represent the manner in which mixture composition was varied in these latter cases. Reprinted from Gessner (1973b).

will show it due to the action of the second one. Accordingly, P, the total fraction showing an effect, is given by

$$P = P_1 + P_2(1 - P_1). \tag{1}$$

Since the question of effect addition had not been explored experimentally we looked for two drugs that would bring about the loss of righting reflex by mechanisms as dissimilar as possible. We selected ethanol and d-tubocurarine and we determined the ED_{50}'s for righting-reflex loss following administration of these agents i.v. to mice both singly and in combination. These were plotted on an isobologram (Fig. 7) as were the expected isobols for simple dose addition (straight-line diagonal) and simple effect addition of the two agents. It can be seen that in terms of simple dose addition all three d-tubocurarine–ethanol combinations showed infra-additivity. The effect addition isobol as constructed from the dose response curves of the two agents, using Eq. (1) above, had a very rectangular shape. Two of the combinations of d-tubocurarine and ethanol behaved as predicted by the

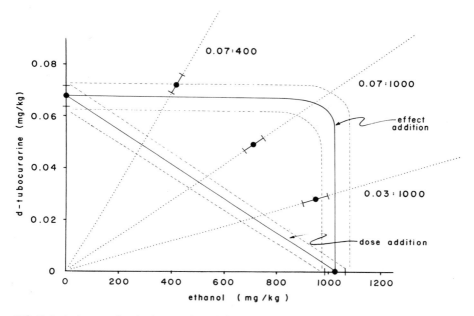

FIG. 7. Isobologram for the interaction of *d*-tubocurarine and ethanol in mice with respect to righting-reflex loss following their intravenous administration. ED_{50} points are plotted with their 95% confidence limits. The expected location of the ED_{50} points given simple dose addition is given together with the 95% confidence limits by the solid and dotted straight line diagonals, respectively. The expected location of the ED_{50} points given simple effect addition is given together with its 95% confidence limits by the solid and dotted quasi rectangular lines connecting the ED_{50}'s of *d*-tubocurarine and ethanol, respectively. The dotted diagonals passing through the origin give the loci of mixture points of *d*-tubocurarine and ethanol in the stated ratios.

effect addition isobol and showed no significant synergism. Thus the ED_{50} dose for *d*-tubocurarine and ethanol combined in a ratio of 0.07 to 400 by weight did not contain significantly less *d*-tubocurarine than that contained in the ED_{50} dose of *d*-tubocurarine when administered by itself. Similarly the ED_{50} for these two agents when combined in a ratio of 0.03 to 1000 by weight did not contain significantly less ethanol than found in the ED_{50} dose of this compound when administered by itself. When the two agents were combined, however, in a ratio similar to that of their ED_{50}'s, significant synergism was observed. The term synergism is used to indicate that the ED_{50} dose of the combination contained less than the ED_{50} dose of either compound. Additionally, this *d*-tubocurarine–ethanol combination had greater potency than would have predicted on the basis of simple effect additions. Whether simple effect addition might govern the interaction of some other pair of drugs is a moot point; however, logic would appear to argue against it. Given the high degree of integration of a living organism

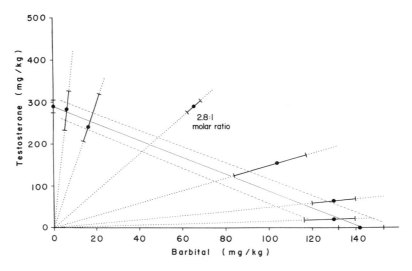

FIG. 8. Isobologram of the interaction of testosterone and barbital in mice relative to righting-reflex loss following their intraperitoneal administration. ED_{50} points are plotted with their 95% confidence limits. The expected location of the ED_{50} points, given the occurrence of simple dose addition, is given, together with its 95% confidence limits, by the solid and dotted straight line diagonals, respectively. The dotted diagonals passing through the origin give the loci of mixture points of testosterone and barbital for the various ratios employed. Reprinted from Gessner and Gessner (1973).

it seems doubtful whether an action on one target organ or system can be envisaged that in no way would alter the responsiveness of other organs or systems. Thus the effect addition isobol, while useful conceptually, cannot at this time be considered to have significant predictive power.

Isobolograms with experimentally observed ED_{50} falling in the area between the dose addition and effect addition isobols present problems of interpretation. In such instances, the question arises whether the apparent infra-additivity is due to the agents acting by different mechanisms or whether other explanations should be sought. This type of question arose in the study of the interaction of barbital and testosterone (Fig. 8) with respect to their hypnotic effect in mice (Gessner and Gessner, 1973). In a very large dose, testosterone is a hypnotic, but its interaction with barbital shows infra-additivity. Is this so because testosterone acts by a different mechanism? We thought there might be a simpler explanation for we noticed onset times for the effects of testosterone were much more rapid than those for barbital. On further investigation, it became apparent that when doses of equivalent potency were compared, the onset times for testosterone and barbital combined in a 2.8:1 molar ratio and were very much like those of testosterone and much shorter than those of barbital. Thus, it would appear that the effects observed with this combination represent, in the main, an action of testosterone.

ACKNOWLEDGMENT

The technical assistance of Mr. Michael I. Madeja is gratefully acknowledged. This investigation was supported in part by U.S. Public Health Service Grants 5T1 FM 107 and R01 MH 12542.

REFERENCES

Bliss, C. I. (1939): The toxicity of poisons applied jointly. *Ann. Appl. Biol. 26,* 585–615.
Cabana, B. E., and Gessner, P. K. (1970): The kinetics of chloral hydrate metabolism in mice and the effect thereon of ethanol. *J. Pharmacol. Exp. Therap. 174,* 260–275.
Child, G. P., Crump, M., and Leonard, P. (1952): Studies on the disulfiram-ethanol reaction. *Quart. J. Studies Alc. 13,* 571–582.
Creaven, P. J., and Roach, M. K. (1969): The effect of chloral hydrate on the metabolism of ethanol in mice. *J. Pharm. Pharmacol. 21,* 332–333.
Eade, N. R., and Renton, K. W. (1970): The effect of phenelzine and tranylcypromine on the degradation of meperidine. *J. Pharmacol. Exp. Ther. 173,* 31–36.
Fingl, E., and Woodbury, D. M. (1970): General principles. In: *The Pharmacological Basis of Therapeutics* (ed., L. S. Goodman and A. Gilman), 4th Ed., p. 25, Macmillan, New York.
Finney, D. J. (1952): *Probit Analysis,* 2nd Ed., Cambridge Univ. Press, Cambridge.
Gessner, P. K. (1973a): Effect of trichloroethanol and chloral hydrate on the *in vivo* rate of disappearance of ethanol in mice. *Arch. Int. Pharmacodyn. 202,* 392–401.
Gessner, P. K. (1973b): *In vivo* ethanol metabolism: kinetics of inhibition. *Proceeding of First Annual Alcoholism Conference of the National Institute of Alcohol Abuse and Alcoholism,* pp. 79–99, U.S. Government Printing Office, Washington, D.C.
Gessner, P. K., and Cabana, B. E. (1967): Chloral alcoholate: reevaluation of its role in the interaction between the hypnotic effects of chloral hydrate and ethanol. *J. Pharmacol. Exp. Therap. 156,* 602–605.
Gessner, P. K., and Cabana, B. E. (1970): A study of the interaction of the hypnotic effects and of the toxic effects of chloral hydrate and ethanol. *J. Pharmacol. Exp. Therap. 174,* 247–259.
Gessner, P. K., and Soble, A. G. (1973): A study of the tranylcypromine-meperidine interaction: effects of *p*-chlorophenylalanine and 5-hydroxytryptophan. *J. Pharmacol. Exp. Therap. 186,* 276–287.
Gessner, P. K., and Gessner, T. (1973): The interaction of barbital and testosterone relative to their hypnotic effects. *Arch. Int. Pharmacodyn. 201,* 55–58.
Kaplan, H. L., Jain, N. C., Forney, R. B., and Richards, A. B. (1969): Chloral hydrate-ethanol interaction in the mouse and dog. *Toxicol. Appl. Pharmacol. 14,* 127–137.
Loewe, S., and Muischnek, H. (1926): Über Kombinatsionswirkungen. I. Mitteilung: Hilfsmittel der Fragstellung. *Naun. Schmied. Arch. Exp. Path. Pharmak. 114,* 313–326.
Loewe, S. (1928): Die quantitativen Probleme der Pharmacologie. *Ergenbn. Physiol. 27,* 47–187.
Loewe, S. (1953): The problem of synergism and antagonism of combined drugs. *Arzeim. Forsch. 3,* 285–290.
Loewe, S. (1957): Antagonism and antagonists. *Pharmacol. Rev. 9,* 237–242.
Loewe, S. (1959): Randbemerkungen zur quantitativen Pharmakologie der Kombinationen. *Arzeim. Forsch. 9,* 449–456.
Loewe, S. (1961): Fragen zur Praxis der quantitativen Leistungs prüfung von Wirkstoffkombinationen. *Arzneim. Forsch. 11,* 899–902.
Rogers, K. J., and Thornton, J. A. (1969): The interaction between monoamino oxidase inhibitors and narcotic analgesics in mice. *Brit. J. Pharmacol. 36,* 470–480.

Sellers, E. M., Lang, M., Koch-Weser, J., LeBlanc, E., and Kalant, H. (1972a): Interaction of chloral hydrate and ethanol in man. I. Metabolism. *Clin. Pharmacol. Therap. 13*, 49.

Sellers, E. M., Carr, G., Bernstein, J. G., Sellers, S., and Koch-Weser, J. (1972b): Interaction of chloral hydrate and ethanol in man. II. Hemodynamics and performance. *Clin. Pharmacol. Therap. 13*, 58.

Zipf, H. F., and Hamacher, J. (1966): Kombinatsionseffekte. 2. Mitteilung: Experimentalle Erfassung und Darstellung von Kombinationseffekten. *Arzneim. Forsch. 16*, 329–339.

Drug Interactions, edited by P. L. Morselli,
S. Garattini, and S. N. Cohen. Raven Press,
New York © 1974

A Computer-Based System for the Study and Control of Drug Interactions in Hospitalized Patients

Stanley N. Cohen, Marsha F. Armstrong, Russell L. Briggs, Laurie S. Feinberg, John F. Hannigan, Philip D. Hansten, Gilbert S. Hunn, Terrence N. Moore, Tadashi G. Nishimura, Michael D. Podlone, Edward H. Shortliffe, Laurel A. Smith, and Linda Yosten

Division of Clinical Pharmacology, Stanford University School of Medicine, Stanford, California 94305

INTRODUCTION

Data presented elsewhere in this volume provide convincing evidence that drug interactions can be a significant factor in determining human response to drug therapy. Unlike genetic or pathophysiological factors, which may also influence clinical response to medications, drug interactions are usually the direct result of the physician's therapeutic decisions, and their clinical consequences are potentially preventable. Whereas certain examples of enhancement of toxicity or negation of beneficial therapeutic effects resulting from the use of specific drug combinations are widely recognized by physicians, the substantial number of potential drug interactions and the pharmacological complexities involved in many of these interactions have made it impractical for most physicians to have adequate drug interaction information on hand when therapy is prescribed. Moreover, the widespread circulation of information that is inaccurate, poorly documented, or clinically irrelevant has impeded general acceptance of the medical significance of such interactions (1). Whereas the pharmacological community requires better methods for carrying out prospective studies of drug interactions in a clinical setting and more rigorous assessment of the incidence and clinical relevance of specific interactions, the needs of practicing physicians require a mechanism for accumulation and maintenance of an accurate data base of information about drug interactions that *already* have been well documented, and a technology for disseminating this information in a clinically useful way.

This report describes a computer-based system, the MEDIPHOR System (i.e., Monitoring and Evaluation of Drug Interactions by a Pharmacy-Oriented Reporting System) developed at the Stanford University Medical

Center for the control and study of drug interactions in hospitalized patients. In designing this system, our goals have included the following:

(a) The establishment of procedures for collecting drug interaction information from the medical and scientific literature, and for critically assessing its scientific validity and clinical relevance.

(b) The creation and implementation of computer technology capable of prospective detection and prevention of clinically significant drug interactions.

(c) The development of procedures that utilize the capabilities of the MEDIPHOR System to identify patients receiving specific drug combinations in order to carry out prospective studies of the incidence and clinical consequences of specific drug interactions.

(d) Evaluation of the effects of the MEDIPHOR System on medication use and physician prescribing practices, on specific adverse consequences of drug interactions, and on general parameters of health care.

The MEDIPHOR System employs a large well-documented computer data base of drug interaction information accumulated by the Division of Clinical Pharmacology at Stanford during the past 4 yr, and a series of interactive computer programs to provide rapid and automatic notification to pharmacists, nursing staff, and physicians when potentially interacting drug combinations are prescribed. The system utilizes information entered at a central in-patient pharmacy to monitor drug use, create patient medication profiles, and generate drug interaction reports. It carries out the additional tasks of automatically producing prescription labels for the hospital pharmacy and has the capability for printing out or displaying patient medication profiles. The system enables rapid retrieval of specific items of drug interaction information contained in its data base and is useful as a teaching instrument for physicians and pharmacists. Finally, it provides the framework for prospective clinical investigation of the consequences of administering putative interacting-drug combinations by enabling identification of patients who are about to receive any individual drug or drug combination specified by the investigator.

The general concept of operation for the MEDIPHOR System, which has been operational in its present form at the Stanford University Medical Center since early 1973, is shown in Fig. 1 (2). Each prescription for a hospitalized patient is entered at a cathode-ray-tube (CRT) terminal in the hospital pharmacy, and a computer-stored drug record is created and maintained for each patient. This record is updated by entries of relevant information about all medication changes, and newly prescribed drugs are checked for potential interactions against drugs already listed in the patient drug profile. When an interaction is found by the search programs, the computer generates a report, which is printed at a terminal located in the hospital pharmacy and is sent to the nursing unit along with the medication.

MEDIPHOR SYSTEM CONFIGURATION (SEPTEMBER, 1973)

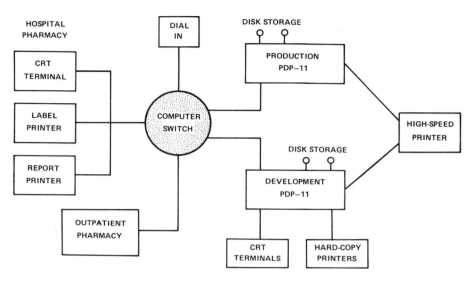

FIG. 1. General operational scheme for MEDIPHOR System. Prescription information entered at a pharmacy terminal is stored in a patient drug profile. Newly prescribed drugs are checked for potential interaction with medications the patient is already receiving, using the drug interaction table and master drug-list files.

Although conceptually simple, the actual development of a drug-interaction monitoring and reporting system capable of meeting the practical needs of an acute-care hospital and able to function within the framework of pre-existing hospital operations has proved to be surprisingly complex. Thus, it appears useful to describe the design and function of the system in some detail.

ACCUMULATION OF DATA BASE

Whereas the problem of drug interactions has attracted considerable attention in the medical and pharmaceutical literature in recent years, the scarcity of primary references documenting the interactions listed in most published compilations has been a continuing problem. The literature contains many examples of purported interactions that are included in tabulations on no more strength than an unreferenced statement in a drug package insert, or on the basis of a single case report. Such citations have been cross-quoted by authors of other articles, leading to accumulation of lists of publication references, which are cited as so-called "supporting documentation" for still later tabulations. Moreover, whereas the stated intent of most drug interaction tabulations has been to assist the physician and pharmacist in dealing with drug interactions in clinical practice, the regular extrapolation of animal or *in vitro* data to humans has led to inclusion of interactions of very doubtful clinical significance. Finally, even when primary literature references have been provided as documentation for a particular interaction, little attention has usually been given by the author of the tabulation to assessing the validity of experimental design of such studies, to evaluating the data obtained, or to determining their clinical relevance. Because no suitable drug-interaction data base was available at the time this project was started in early 1970, the Division of Clinical Pharmacology at Stanford undertook to establish literature search and evaluation procedures for accumulating its own data base.

In collecting and evaluating drug interaction information, the validity of design of experimental studies and the quality and clinical relevance of the data presented have been considerations of primary importance. Standard bibliographic search methods have been used to locate primary clinical and pharmacologic reports of possible drug interactions, and these reports have been reviewed and evaluated by the staff of the division. Information that has been compiled, interpreted, and documented with primary references is then coded in a predetermined format for entry into the computer. Each entry includes information about (a) the *pharmacological effects* of the interaction, (b) its *mechanisms*, (c) *clinical findings* that might result in administration of the interacting drug combination, (d) the *clinical significance* of the interaction (e.g. "effects are dosage dependent," "probably significant but needs more study," etc.), (e) a *report class* designation that presently reflects both the clinical relevance of the interaction and the immediacy of its potential consequences.

The report class designation, which is largely a matter of medical and pharmacological judgment, provides guidelines that the physician may use in dealing with the interaction in a practical way. Although drug interactions are often thought of in absolute terms, they represent only one of many factors capable of influencing clinical response to drugs; moreover, most interacting drug combinations *can* be given concurrently if the interactive potential is kept in mind by the physician and appropriate adjustments in dosage or route of administration are made. In part, the report class provides this information. In addition, the report class designation provides guidelines for the nursing staff to use in responding to drug-interaction reports produced by the computer.

In general, class 1 contains interactions having effects of demonstrated clinical significance that would be expected to occur relatively quickly after administering the drug combination. In this case, the patient's physician is informed about the potential interaction before the first dose of the interacting drug is administered. For example, the interaction between mono-amine oxidase inhibitors and certain sympathomimetic amines is included in this class. Class 2 interactions have consequences that may be somewhat less immediate, but nonetheless serious; in this case, the first dose of the interacting drug may be administered, but the physician is contacted before the drug combination is continued as prescribed. The interference with the hypertensive effects of guanethidine when a tricyclic antidepressant is given concurrently is an example of a class 2 interaction. Class 3 is assigned to interactions that have well-documented clinical significance but do not ordinarily lead to clinically apparent consequences until the interacting drug combination has been administered for at least several doses. Information about such an interaction is placed in a conspicuous location in the patient's chart, but the drugs are administered as prescribed unless the physician changes his order. The interaction between phenobarbital and coumarin anticoagulants is included in this class. In every instance, the physician retains the prerogative of making all decisions about administration of the interacting drug combination; the MEDIPHOR System has been designed to be a method for dissemination of clinically relevant drug-interaction information, rather than an attempt to control the physician's practice of medicine. The drug-interaction report is viewed simply as an item of information about a factor that may influence the patient's response to a therapeutically administered drug and must be considered in the context of other clinical information available to the physician.

Class 4 contains interactions that, we believe, are not sufficiently well documented to warrant distributing reports to physicians; class 4 reports, which concern interactions for which the clinical relevance has not been adequately demonstrated, are used for investigational purposes only. This class of interactions provides a mechanism for identifying patients that are about to receive a specific drug combination which was selected for study, and thus establishes a framework for prospective clinical evaluation of the consequences of administering therapeutic agents which are suspected of interacting.

The entries also include (f) *duration information*. In certain instances, the potential for a drug interaction may exist for up to 2 weeks after one of the interacting drugs has been discontinued. Thus, once monoamine oxidase (MAO) has been irreversibly inactivated by an MAO inhibitor, certain interacting drugs may have the potential of causing adverse effects until the new enzyme is synthesized. This information is included in the duration field of the data base and is used by the computer in determining whether an interaction report is to be generated.

(g) *Clinical management suggestions* that may be useful to the medical staff in responding to the interaction report are included in the data base (e.g. "monitor prothrombin time closely and adjust anticoagulant dosage accordingly," or "reduction of anticoagulant dosage may be required following cessation of phenobarbital therapy").

(h) *Primary literature references* document the information presented in the report.

The last inclusion in each entry is a section for (i) *comments*. This section includes brief textual statements that may be useful in interpreting the information contained in the report or in assessing the likelihood of adverse consequences of the interaction in a particular patient.

All drug interaction information collected by the staff of the Division of Clinical Pharmacology is reviewed by a senior clinical pharmacologist and its accuracy and validity are appraised and verified—or it is modified— before it is entered into the computer. Once entered, information can be retrieved by programs that search for specific journal articles either by the author's name or by "key words" contained in the title of the articles or in the accompanying brief summary of subject matter. In addition, updating and/or modification of the data base can be carried out interactively at computer terminals.

Therapeutic agents are grouped into "interaction classes" to facilitate the computer's search for interacting drug combinations. An interaction class is defined functionally as a group of drugs capable of interacting with another interaction class in a specific and homogeneous way. Interaction classes may contain a single member or many drugs and are often identical with more commonly used pharmacological or chemical groupings such as tricyclic antidepressants, barbiturates, etc. However, some drugs may differ from other members of their pharmacological group in their ability to participate in a particular interaction, and in certain instances a drug may belong to more than one interaction class. In situations where it does not seem appropriate to split pharmacologic groupings into separate drug interaction classes, the system allows a list of excluded drugs to be specifically flagged as differing from other members of the pharmacologic group with regard to involvement in a particular interaction.

The MEDIPHOR System drug file currently contains a total of more than 4,000 pharmaceutical preparations: in the case of multicomponent medications, entries identify each generic component of the preparation and specify the interaction class for the component. Thus, the computer can search for interactions of drugs included in various "brand-name" compounds and in other multicomponent preparations. Drug entries also include information that enables the computer to determine whether the occurrence of the specific interaction is dependent upon a particular route of administration. For example, the interaction between tetracyclines and the divalent cations of certain antacid preparations occurs at the level of drug absorption and thus is observed only when the tetracycline is administered orally. This type of information is included in the master drug file and is utilized by the computer in its search for possible interactions.

The hardware configuration for the MEDIPHOR System is shown in Fig. 2. Although an earlier version of the system was developed using the

GENERAL OPERATIONAL SCHEME FOR MEDIPHOR SYSTEM

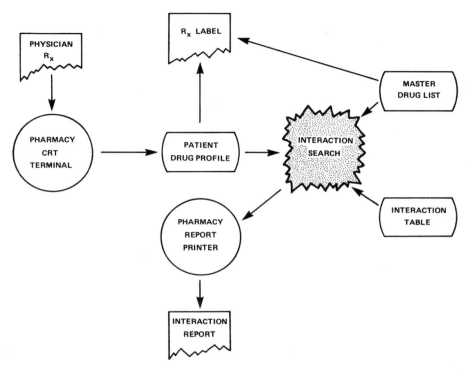

FIG. 2. MEDIPHOR System configuration (September, 1973). A pharmacy station consists of CRT terminal(s), label printer(s), and a drug-interaction report printer. Remote access to information in the MEDIPHOR System data base is available through dial-in capacity. A version of the MEDIPHOR System capable of meeting the special needs of out-patient pharmacies and ambulatory patients is currently under development.

ACME time-sharing computer system at Stanford (2), pharmacy operations are currently managed by a Digital Equipment Corporation PDP-11 computer in MUMPS[1] (3), using cathode-ray-tube terminals for data entry and hard-copy printers to produce medication labels and interaction reports. Since the processing of prescriptions at Stanford is now dependent upon operation of the computer, a second PDP-11 machine is employed to provide reserve capacity during rare periods of failure of the primary hardware. The second computer is also used for program development, data base and bibliography entry and retrieval, and for processing the statistical programs used in analyzing and evaluating the system.

---

[1] MUMPS is an acronym for Massachusetts General Hospital Utility Multi-Programming System.

OPERATION OF THE SYSTEM

In operation of the system, patient identification information and medication data are entered by the pharmacist or pharmacy clerk using CRT terminals placed in the hospital pharmacy. In entering data, pharmacists respond to a series of prompts on the screen; to simplify and accelerate prescription entry, a series of three or four letter codes have been devised for approximately 200 commonly used drugs, and abbreviations are employed for instructions relating to the administration of medications. In the most frequently used mode of operation, which is shown in the hard-copy print out in Fig. 3, the pharmacist enters the patient's identification number followed by a three letter code for a prepackaged drug. The patient's name, the nursing unit location, and full name of the drug are retrieved from the data file and are displayed on the video screen along with the necessary label information such as drug strength and prepackaged quantity. The pharmacist then enters the dosage regimen prescribed for that particular patient, verifies other information retrieved by the computer, and modifies the entry as required. Upon his approval, the information is stored in a patient drug profile, which may be retrieved for review by the pharmacist at any time, and relevant prescription data are printed on a gummed label (Fig. 4), which is then affixed to the medication container being sent to the nursing unit. When an interaction between the newly entered drug and a previously prescribed medication is found by the computer, an interaction report (Fig. 5) is automatically produced on a printer located in the pharmacy.

```
ID NUMBER?  189680, DC, DC65

  ** ID# DOES NOT VERIFY.  ID NUMBER?  189690, DC, DC65

     NAME:  BOND, JAMES

     WARD:  E1A

     ACTUAL DRUG NAME:  DARVON COMPOUND: PO: - 65 CAPSUL

     QUANTITY:  12

     SIG?  PO1CAFDPN

     INSTRUCTIONS?  N

     SPECIAL INSTRUCTIONS?  N

     DOCTOR?  DR. NO

     OK?  Y

     STORING REQUEST
```

FIG. 3. Print-out of format used by pharmacy personnel entering prescriptions at CRT terminals. Information entered by pharmacy clerk is underlined. All other information is retrieved by computer.

<u>LABEL</u>

E1A   RX 212776 9/11/73

BOND JAMES

DARVON COMPOUND - 65

CAPSULES #12

TAKE 1 CAPSULE(S) 4 TIMES A DAY

FOR PAIN AS NEEDED

DOCTOR NO

FIG. 4. Print-out of medication label produced by computer from information shown in Fig. 3.

STANFORD UNIVERSITY MEDICAL CENTER • DIVISION OF CLINICAL PHARMACOLOGY • DRUG INTERACTION REPORT

JAMES BOND   007 E1A
PATIENT NAME   ACCOUNT NO.   MED. REC. NO.
09/1/73   ALERT CLASS 2. GIVE FIRST DOSE ONLY.
REPORT DATE   CONTACT PHYSICIAN AND FILE REPORT IN PROGRESS NOTES.

AMITRIPTYLINE (ELAVIL) AND GUANETHIDINE (ISMELIN)

OLD DRUG : GUANETHIDINE (ISMELIN)
    MEMBER OF CLASS : GUANETHIDINE
    DRUG STARTED ON : 8/1/73

NEW DRUG : AMITRIPTYLINE (ELAVIL)
    MEMBER OF CLASS : TRICYCLIC ANTIDEPRESSANTS

INTERACTIONS :

    PHARMACOLOGICAL EFFECTS :
        PHARMACOLOGICAL EFFECTS OF GUANETHIDINE ANTAGONIZED

    MECHANISMS :
        INTERFERENCE WITH NEURONAL UPTAKE OF GUANETHIDINE BY AMITRIPTYLINE

    EXPECTED CLINICAL FINDINGS :
        EXACERBATION OF PROBLEM BEING TREATED BY GUANETHIDINE. HYPERTENSION.

    CLINICAL SIGNIFICANCE :
        CLINICAL SIGNIFICANCE DEMONSTRATED IN HUMANS.

    CLINICAL MANAGEMENT SUGGESTIONS :
        AVOID AMITRIPTYLINE. HIGHER DOSE OF GUANETHIDINE WILL USUALLY BE REQUIRED
        DURING AND FOLLOWING ADMINISTRATION OF AMITRIPTYLINE.

REFERENCES :
    STONE, C.A. ET AL. (1969) J. PHARMACOL. EXP. THER. 144: 196.
    MITCHELL, J.R. ET AL. (1970) J. CLIN. INVEST. 49: 1596.
    MITCHELL, J.R. ET AL. (1967) J.A.M.A. 202: 973.
    MEYER, J.F. ET AL. (1970) J.A.M.A. 213: 1487.
    LEISHMAN, A.W.D. ET AL. (1963) LANCET 1: 112.
    FANN, W.E. ET AL. (1971) PSYCHOPHARMACOLOGIA 22: 111.

COMMENTS :
    THE VARIOUS TRICYCLIC ANTIDEPRESSANTS ALL APPEAR TO BE CAPABLE OF REVERSING THE
    ANTIHYPERTENSIVE EFFECTS OF GUANETHIDINE AND ITS ANALOGUES BY INHIBITING UPTAKE
    INTO ADRENERGIC NEURONS.

FIG. 5. Sample drug interaction report produced on pharmacy report printer.

A variety of programs enable rapid entry and computer storage of various kinds of medication orders, such as renewal prescriptions (which do not result in the generation of a second drug-interaction report), drug discontinuations, or prescriptions dispensed directly from the nursing unit floor stock of drugs. Since the system maintains a computer record of *all* patient medications, information about drugs dispensed directly from nursing units is sent to the pharmacy and is entered there by pharmacists or pharmacy clerks.

The interaction search, which occurs following entry of a new prescription to the patient's medication record, sometimes requires a substantial amount of computing time (occasionally, as long as 1 to 2 min) when a patient is receiving a large amount of drugs concurrently. Certain patients in our records have received more than 40 medications concurrently, and many of these have been multicomponent preparations. As noted earlier, every new prescription is checked for possible interactions with the components of *each* of these medications. In order to satisfy the operational needs of the pharmacy to process prescriptions rapidly, a series of control programs has been developed to handle the various functions of the MEDIPHOR System on a predetermined priority basis. Thus, the need of the pharmacists and pharmacy clerks entering data at the CRT terminals to have the computer accept information rapidly is given the highest priority. Production of prescription labels is given a slightly lower priority, and the interaction search, which need not be instantaneous, a still lower priority in the computer-data queue. This arrangement enables the rapid processing of prescriptions, but also ensures that drug interaction reports are available by the time a medication is ready to leave the pharmacy.

EVALUATION

Our evaluation of the effects of the MEDIPHOR System on drug use and on the incidence and clinical consequences of drug interactions is still in progress. A major aspect of this evaluation has involved utilization of baseline data accumulated during a period when drug interaction frequency and consequences were being monitored, but before the MEDIPHOR System was capable of generating drug interaction reports. Although only very preliminary data are presently available, it may nevertheless be useful to review briefly some of the information obtained thus far in order to illustrate the types of questions we have been attempting to answer.

(a) During a recent 3-month period of study, 50,101 prescriptions dispensed to patients hospitalized at the Stanford University Medical Center resulted in the generation of 647 valid drug-interaction reports (i.e., instances where a patient actually received a drug combination involving a Class 1, 2, or 3 interaction) or frequency about 1.2%. Approximately 10 to 12 reports were generated each day, or approximately one report for every

50 patients hospitalized at Stanford. This observed incidence of drug interactions is substantially lower than the frequency reported in most earlier investigations (4–8); we believe that this low frequency results from our use of stringent criteria for defining drug interactions that are clinically relevant and for inclusion of specific interactions in our data base. In part, it may also reflect a relatively high level of prior awareness about drug interactions by physicians practicing at Stanford.

(b) the MEDIPHOR System has proved to be extremely sensitive in reflecting errors in the medication administration by the hospital staff; reports that have been produced incorrectly because of such errors have been a cause of continuing concern. Conversely, the production of such reports provides a useful method for detecting and recording medication errors for the purposes of peer review and quality assurance.

(c) Among the potentially interacting drug combinations prescribed most frequently during the period studied are (i) barbiturates and coumarin anticoagulants, (ii) aluminum-containing adsorbents and oral phenothiazines, (iii) polyvalent cations and oral tetracyclines, (iv) potassium preparations and spironolactone or triampterine, (v) coumarin anticoagulants and salycilates, and (vi) coumarin anticoagulants and quinine derivatives. In addition, the concurrent use of multiple central nervous system (CNS) depressant drugs in a single patient is a common occurrence.

(d) In agreement with the results published by others (9, 10), clinicians at Stanford usually utilized laboratory determinations of prothrombin levels to adjust oral anticoagulant dosage appropriately in patients who were experiencing the effects of anticoagulant drug interactions during a "control" period. In most instances, there was no indication in the medical record that physicians were aware that they were compensating for the clinical effects of drug interactions. Interactions causing both excessive and inadequate lowering of prothrombin level potentially attributable to drug interactions were also observed during the control period.

(e) Most physicians receiving drug interaction reports reacted promptly to the information provided by the report when it was clinically relevant in the context of overall patient care. In most instances, the appropriate medical response to an interaction report did not involve discontinuation of one or both the interacting drugs, but instead required modification of the drug dose or route of administration.

(f) A preliminary survey of physician attitudes about the MEDIPHOR System indicates that the majority of physicians served by the system found the information provided to be clinically useful and/or informative, and that they favor continuation and extension of the system.

(g) The MEDIPHOR System has proved to be an effective tool for rapidly identifying patients who are about to receive or who have received a particular drug combination for the purposes of clinical studies of drug interactions in hospitalized patients.

Although the long-term clinical value and cost effectiveness of the MEDIPHOR System have yet to be determined, it presently appears that an on-line computer-based drug interaction monitoring and reporting system of this type is capable of modifying the use of potentially interacting drug combinations by physicians and consequently of preventing certain adverse clinical consequences of drug interactions. In addition, such a system may also be useful for clinical and pharmacological studies of drug interactions in hospitalized patients.

ACKNOWLEDGMENTS

These investigations were supported by grant HS00739 from the U.S. National Center for Health Services Research and Development and by an award from the Burroughs Wellcome Fund. S.N.C. is the recipient of a Research Career Development Award from the U.S. Public Health Service.

REFERENCES

1. Puckett, W. H., Jr., and Visconti, J. A. (1971): *Am. J. Hosp. Pharm. 28*, 247.
2. Cohen, S. N., Armstrong, M. F., Crouse, L., and Hunn, G. S. (1972): *Drug Inf. J. 72*, 81.
3. Greenes, R. A., Pappalardo, A. N., Marble, C. W., and Barnett, G. O. (1969): *Comput. Biomed. Res. 2*, 469.
4. Borda, L. T., Slone, D., and Jick, H. (1968): *J. Am. Med. Assoc. 205*, 645.
5. Ogilvie, R. I., and Ruedy, J. (1967): *Can. Med. Assoc. J. 97*, 1445.
6. Seidl, L. G., Thronton, G. F., Smith, J. W., and Cluff, L. E. (1966): *Bull. Johns Hopkins Hosp. 119*, 299.
7. Laventurier, M. F., and Talley, R. B. (1972): *Calif. Pharm. 20*, 18.
8. Stewart, R. B., and Cluff, L. E. (1971): *Johns Hopkins Med. J. 129*, 319.
9. Sellers, E. M., and Koch-Weser, J. (1970): *New Engl. J. Med. 283*, 827.
10. Boston Collaborative Drug Surveillance Program (1972): *New Eng. J. Med. 286*, 53.

Drug Interactions, edited by P. L. Morselli,
S. Garattini, and S. N. Cohen. Raven Press,
New York © 1974

Identification of Drug Interactions from Clinical Epidemiological Data

Dennis Slone and Samuel Shapiro

Boston Collaborative Drug Surveillance Program, Boston University Medical Center, 400 Totten Pond Road, Waltham, Massachusetts 02154

The manner in which drugs ultimately come to be employed in a clinical setting may differ substantially from the relatively structured and carefully controlled conditions under which they were first evaluated. Possible interactions between drugs, environmental and genetic factors, and diseases, in addition to variable dose regimens, might influence the toxicity or effectiveness of any given drug and do so in unforeseen ways.

There are thus several major concerns in the epidemiologic evaluation of drugs after they come into widespread use. One is to provide reliable, quantitative estimates of the frequencies of known adverse effects of individual drugs, or classes of drugs, and to identify those populations that are particularly susceptible. Another is to provide for the discovery of previously unsuspected adverse drug effects. The identification of such effects may be confined to a single drug, or may be the result of a drug interaction. Attempts to obtain these types of information in human populations have involved a number of approaches, including direct clinical observation and retrospective or prospective studies.

The availability of modern computers has made it possible to organize a system of comprehensive drug monitoring. Such a system has been used by the Boston Collaborative Drug Surveillance Program since its inception in 1966 (1–4). The objectives of this program are as follows: to detect and evaluate previously unknown effects of drugs, including drug interactions; to quantitate and evaluate known adverse effects of drugs; to evaluate the role of factors that influence toxicity and efficacy; to describe drug utilization patterns; and, ultimately, to establish a clinical data base as a resource for the evaluation of a variety of pharmacologic, clinical, and epidemiologic problems. This chapter is concerned with the organization, methods of data collection, computer handling, and principles of analysis and interpretation employed by the Boston Collaborative Drug Surveillance Program.

The Boston Collaborative Drug Surveillance Program consists of the systematic, standardized recording of a wide variety of well-specified items of information in a setting of routine medical or psychiatric wards (Fig. 1). The primary data recording is performed by specially trained nurses who

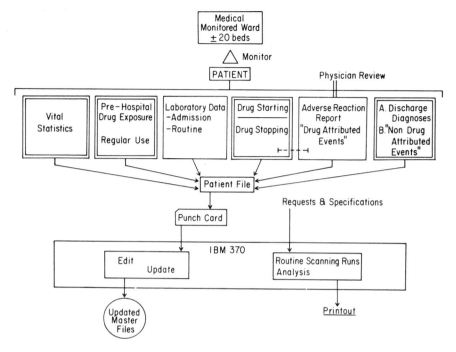

FIG. 1. The modular organization of data acquisition in the BCDSP is illustrated. Modules, consisting of medical wards with about 20 beds, are each monitored by one nurse monitor who is responsible for obtaining data on all patients admitted to the ward. The data items contained in double boxes are obtained on all patients: the remaining data are obtained when available or when appropriate.

are stationed in selected general medical wards in a number of hospitals both within the United States and other countries. Each monitored ward unit consists of approximately 20 beds. Biased selection of patients entering the system is largely avoided by a strictly enforced set of rules governing the conditions under which a new patient may be entered into the study.

The overall program is designed as a modular system, and additional monitoring units or wards can be added or deleted at will. The central facility provides for the management of the program and for quality control of data derived from the various participating units (Fig. 2). This includes appropriate coding, filing, and storage of data. A staff of clinical pharmacologists, epidemiologists, and biostatisticians is involved in the analysis and interpretation of the data, and the central facility maintains a group of computer scientists having close access to major computing facilities. The nurse monitors, while full-time employees of the surveillance program, are nonetheless an integral part of the staff of the monitored ward. The monitors, following a common protocol and using standard sets of self-coding forms,

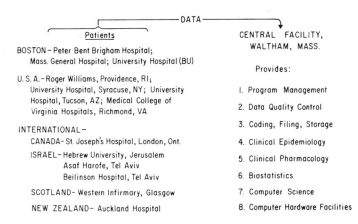

THE BOSTON COLLABORATIVE DRUG SURVEILLANCE PROGRAM
BOSTON UNIVERSITY MEDICAL CENTER

MEDICAL IN-PATIENT PROGRAM

DATA

Patients

BOSTON - Peter Bent Brigham Hospital;
Mass. General Hospital; University Hospital (BU)

U. S. A.- Roger Williams, Providence, RI;
University Hospital, Syracuse, NY; University
Hospital, Tucson, AZ; Medical College of
Virginia Hospitals, Richmond, VA

INTERNATIONAL -
CANADA- St. Joseph's Hospital, London, Ont.

ISRAEL-Hebrew University, Jerusalem
Asaf Harofe, Tel Aviv
Beilinson Hospital, Tel Aviv

SCOTLAND- Western Infirmary, Glasgow

NEW ZEALAND- Auckland Hospital

CENTRAL FACILITY,
WALTHAM, MASS.

Provides:

1. Program Management

2. Data Quality Control

3. Coding, Filing, Storage

4. Clinical Epidemiology

5. Clinical Pharmacology

6. Biostatistics

7. Computer Science

8. Computer Hardware Facilities

FIG. 2. Overall program.

obtain the data by interviewing the attending physicians, and where appropriate, patients and by examining the medical records.

The data collected on each patient fall into five broad categories of information: (a) drug utilization prior to entry into hospital (Table 1,A), (b) patient characteristics (Table 2), (c) treatment regimens administered during hospitalization (Table 1,B), (d) recorded measures of drug efficacy (Table 3,A), and finally, (e) drug-attributed or routinely observed clinical events occurring during hospitalization (Table 3,B).

Under the heading of patient characteristics, information such as age, sex, race, and occupation is collected. In addition, certain routine laboratory tests performed within 48 hr of admission, such as the blood urea nitrogen level, white cell count, hematocrit, total serum protein, and urinalysis are

TABLE 1. *Drug exposure data*

A. Drug utilization prior to entry into hospital
  1. Obtained on admission
  2. Derived from a standard set of 27 questions, e.g., drugs for pain,
     blood pressure, seizures, diabetes, etc.

B. Drug exposure during hospitalization

Aspect	Particulars and examples	Source
Treatment ID	Drugs, fluids, blood, ±1,500 items	Order sheet
Indication	Insomnia, pain, etc.; ±100	Doctor interview
Specifics	Form, dose, route, frequency	Order sheet
Timing	Starting and stopping dates	Order sheet

TABLE 2. *Routinely monitored admission and discharge characteristics*

Demographic
age, sex, race, parity, etc.
Social habits
tobacco, alcohol, coffee, etc.
Cause of admission
drug induced or related
Medical history
selected items, i.e., allergy, radiotherapy
Routine admission laboratory data
hematocrit, BUN, WBC, etc.
Diagnoses
first four discharge diagnoses
Type of discharge
home, transfer, death

recorded; at the time of discharge, subsequent to the completion of the diagnostic procedures performed in hospital, up to four discharge diagnoses are recorded and coded according to the International Classification of Diseases.

All drug orders are recorded, as written by the attending physician, on the routine ward drug order sheet. The name of the drug, date started, dosage, frequency, and instructions are all noted. In addition, the nurse monitor interviews the attending physician to determine the indication. Subsequently, she interviews the physician each time a drug is stopped to de-

TABLE 3. *Drug efficacy ratings and clinical events recorded during hospitalization*

A. Drug efficacy

Type of information	Source
Discontinuation of drug because ineffective	Doctor interview
Rating as "satisfactory," "unsatisfactory," or "don't know"	Doctor interview, Patient interview, where feasible and/or relevant

B. Clinical events during hospitalization

Adverse reactions (AR) or events
Drug attributed
1. Drug discontinued due to AR
2. Drug continued but AR recorded
Not drug attributed
Routine recording of a set of clinical events occurring during hospitalization

termine the reason for discontinuation. At the same time she asks the physician to rate the efficacy of the drug in terms of the choices, "satisfactory," "unsatisfactory," and "don't know." She also asks whether any suspected adverse reactions occurred. All adverse reactions are reviewed by a team from the Boston Collaborative Drug Surveillance Program and relevant supplementary information is obtained and recorded. Finally, at the time of discharge the nurse monitor determines whether any of a number of specified serious events, irrespective of whether or not they were drug-attributed, occurred during hospitalization.

After a patient is discharged, all data sheets are edited for completeness by the nurse monitor and then coded and re-edited by specially trained personnel at the central facility. An additional computer editing procedure checks the data for completeness, plausibility, and internal consistency. Documents that are in some way inconsistent are then referred back to either the nurse monitor or the special central facility personnel for correction. Periodically, the new data are updated on the master tape files, which contain virtually all of the collected information on each patient. In addition, the original patient records are stored on microfilm and are available for scrutiny when necessary. It then becomes possible to run a series of routine computer analyses and, when indicated, especially designed *ad hoc* analyses to provide a wide range of information.

It is clear that the data allow for the description of drug utilization patterns, quantitation of known and suspected drug effects, and the evaluation of a variety of nonpharmacologic clinical problems. However, the focus and main challenge in the data analysis is concerned with (a) the discovery and evaluation of previously unknown drug effects and (b) the discovery and evaluation of effect-modifying factors, whether they be patient characteristics or interacting drugs.

The first stage in the discovery-oriented process is to comprehensively scan the data base for associations. With reference to the identification of drug interactions, it is frequently useful to perform a screening comparison between those experiencing and those not experiencing a given adverse reaction. All drugs received by the two comparison groups are tallied to determine which of them have been received significantly more often by the reactors. If patients experiencing drug rashes, for example (ignoring the particular drug incriminated in each case), are compared with those who did not develop rashes, the use of ampicillin is significantly higher in those with drug rashes. The potential for signaling previously unsuspected relationships in this type of screening procedure is obvious. In the ampicillin example we were able to show that the concomitant receipt of allopurinol further increased the risk of ampicillin rashes (5). Further elaborations of this finding, as well as others, are presented by Jick in this volume (8).

In addition to the above general analysis, we also screen directly for possible drug interactions. In this procedure all patients who receive a given drug are divided into those who had an adverse reaction attributed to it and those who did not. The object of the screen is then to tally all other drugs given to the two comparison groups and to determine whether any particular drug received by the patients was administered with a greater than expected frequency to the "reactors."

The above-mentioned screens are designed to alert the investigator to the existence of an association. However, its mere existence does not necessarily imply cause and effect. A strong statistical association between the receipt of neomycin and gastrointestinal bleeding, for example, does not imply that neomycin causes bleeding: it simply indicates that patients with cirrhosis of the liver are both at high risk for gastrointestinal bleeding and are treated with neomycin. Similarly, an association between drug rashes due to ampicillin and receipt of diphenhydramine does not indicate that the two drugs interact to produce rashes: it merely indicates that diphenhydramine is used to treat ampicillin rashes.

It is obvious that the screening procedures are designed only to provide tentative clues at best (Fig. 3). In fact, they invariably present the investigator with a multitude of associations, most of them being noncausal. The selection of any particular association for further evaluation depends on a complex set of scientific and clinical judgments. It involves considerations of the strength and statistical significance of the observed association, the clinical importance of the phenomenon at issue, and the advance intrinsic credibility of a causal explanation for the association in the light of available medical knowledge.

After such considerations, any decision to further evaluate an association requires precise definition of the hypothesis at issue, and the removal of the effects of various confounding factors defined specifically for the problem under investigation. This is achieved by a combination of the following procedures: (a) restriction of the types of subjects to be included within the analysis, (b) analysis with stratification of the subjects according to confounding factors, and (c), in more complex situations, the use of multi-

BOSTON COLLABORATIVE DRUG SURVEILLANCE PROGRAM

ROUTINE SCANNING ─────────────────────→ ASSOCIATIONS
  between   *reflecting*

  Drug usage and clinical events   *Known clinical facts*
  Drug usage and patient modifying factors *Possibly spurious associations* }─→ FURTHER ANALYSIS
  Diagnoses and patient modifying factors   *Potential discoveries*   *involving*

                                                        Restriction of subjects
                                                        Stratification by confounding
                                                          factors
                                                        Multivariate analyses
                                                        Temporal relationships
                                                        Dose response
                                                        Analogous associations
                                                        Analysis of other data banks

FIG. 3. Schema for data analysis.

variate analysis. In deciding how to proceed, the investigator is influenced by the nature of the problem and its tractability to the various analytical options available.

In the event that an association being studied remains after control of confounding, the analytical process continues in terms of the search for collateral evidence within the data base to help evaluate whether a causal interpretation can be entertained. In the absence of a controlled trial, the classical means of gaining further confidence in a causal explanation is that of checking the veracity of a variety of predications under the causal hypothesis. For example, in the case of an association between a drug and an adverse event, there would tend to be a characteristic time sequence between an antecedent drug exposure and the adverse event. Similarly, a dependence on dose or route of administration or both may often be expected if the association is causal. Yet another type of supporting evidence for causal interpretation is the existence of associations between the drug at issue and events analogous to the one under study. Thus, a causal explanation of an association between a drug and gastrointestinal bleeding gains credence if the drug is also associated with other types of bleeding.

Even after elaborate analysis, there are occasions when a causal explanation may still appear to be tenuous. Under such circumstances, it may be necessary to design further *ad hoc* studies.

Any judgment concerning the credibility of a causal explanation for an association is an extremely complex matter. In addition to its statistical significance, this judgment involves a consideration of the following: the success of the attempted control of known confounders, the extent of totally uncontrolled (mainly unknown) confounding, the magnitude of selection bias, the extent of bias from the lack of comparability of the observations and finally, the magnitude of the total bias from all possible sources in relation to the magnitude of the association under study in the data.

As attested to by this volume, a large and bewildering array of drug interactions has been identified in recent years. For the most part, these have been identified experimentally, and the question of their clinical importance often remains unanswered, particularly in the context of the everyday practice of clinical medicine. An epidemiological approach using comprehensive drug monitoring and the types of screening analyses described in this chapter should be capable of identifying clinically important drug interactions.

Finally, the accumulated data base can be used to check hypotheses suggested by other workers. For example, clinical evidence (6) confirming experimental findings of Sellers and Koch-Weser (7) that an interaction exists between chloral hydrate and warfarin was found in this way.

To date, the BCDSP has monitored some 16,500 consecutive medical patients. The utility of this body of data in both the identification of interactions and testing for postulated interactions has been demonstrated (8). As more data are accumulated, the utility should increase.

ACKNOWLEDGMENTS

Hospitals currently participating in the Boston Collaborative Drug Surveillance Program are: Boston, Massachusetts — Peter Bent Brigham Hospital, Massachusetts General Hospital, and University Hospital; Providence, Rhode Island — Roger Williams General Hospital; Syracuse, New York — State University Hospital of the Upstate Medical Center; Tucson, Arizona — University Hospital; Richmond, Virginia — Medical College of Virginia Hospitals; Canada — St. Joseph's Hospital, London, Ontario; New Zealand — Auckland, Hospital; Israel — Hadassah-Hebrew University Hospital, Jerusalem, Beilinson Hospital, Tel-Aviv, and Asaf-Harofe Hospital, Tel-Aviv; Scotland — Western Infirmary, Glasgow.

The Boston Collaborative Drug Surveillance Program is supported by Public Health Service Contract No. NIH-72-2010 from the National Institute of General Medical Sciences (NIGMS); and *in part* by grants from the United States Food and Drug Administration; the Canadian Food and Drug Directorate; the Israeli Ministry of Health; the Kupat-Holim; Auckland Hospital, Auckland, New Zealand; the Roger Williams General Hospital (Brown University NIGMS grant No. GM 165–38–02); and Hoffmann LaRoche, Inc.

REFERENCES

1. Slone, D., Jick, H., Borda, I., Chalmers, T. C., Feinleib, M., Muench, H., Lipworth, L., Bellotti, C., and Gilman, B. (1966): *Lancet 2*, 901.
2. Slone, D., Gaetano, L. F., Lipworth, L., Shapiro, S., Lewis, G. P., and Jick, H. (1969): *Public Health Rep. 84*, 39.
3. Jick, H., Miettinen, O. S., Shapiro, S., Lewis, G. P., Siskind, V., and Slone, D. (1970): *JAMA 213*, 1455.
4. Miller, R. (1973): *Am. J. Hosp. Pharm. 30*, 584.
5. Boston Collaborative Drug Surveillance Program (1972): *N. Engl. J. Med. 286*, 505.
6. Boston Collaborative Drug Surveillance Program (1972): *N. Engl. J. Med. 286*, 53.
7. Sellers, E. M., and Koch-Weser, J. (1970): *N. Engl. J. Med. 283*, 827.
8. Jick, H. (1974): This volume.

Drug Interactions, edited by P. L. Morselli,
S. Garattini, and S. N. Cohen. Raven Press,
New York © 1974

Drug Interactions Evaluated from Drug Surveillance

Hershel Jick

Boston Collaborative Drug Surveillance Program, Boston University Medical Center,
400 Totten Pond Road, Waltham, Massachusetts 02154

The standardized recording of data on drug exposures and various medical "events" has been carried out on medical patients in many hospitals in four countries for some years by the Boston Collaborative Drug Surveillance Program (1). Details of dosage and route of administration of all drugs is obtained as well as date information on when the drugs are started and stopped and when events occur.

With the aid of computers, the relationship of a drug or combinations of drugs to medical events can be explored by appropriate programming of the computer.

Since the study began, we have routinely evaluated possible drug interactions for all drugs used in the monitored hospitals by the use of certain routine scanning programs. These are designed to tabulate the frequency of drug exposures for all other drugs in patients who have developed an alleged adverse reaction to one particular drug. In addition, unsuspected relationships between all drugs and certain events are searched. When these associations arise, the possible interaction relationships with other drugs are then evaluated.

Finally, when certain hypotheses have been raised by other investigators relating to alleged drug interactions, we sometimes have sufficient data to carry out specific analyses to evaluate the clinical significance of these proposed drug interactions.

Sometime ago we noted, on routine screening of the data, a strong association between the drug allopurinol and drug-attributed rashes. Such rashes were recorded in 300 patients, and the drug most commonly implicated by the attending medical staff as causing them was ampicillin (109 patients). The remaining rashes were attributed to a large variety of drugs, including allopurinol, which was itself implicated in only six of 347 patients receiving this drug. A detailed evaluation of each case of rash revealed that allopurinol was received by an unusually large number of patients whose rashes were attributed to ampicillin. On the other hand, the frequency of allopurinol use *per se* was not related to the use of ampicillin.

These observations raised the possibility that allopurinol may potentiate the allergenicity of ampicillin and prompted a more detailed evaluation of this hypothesis.

A preliminary analysis was confined to patients who *did not receive ampicillin*. The rash frequencies were compared between recipients and nonrecipients of allopurinol. There were 283 patients who received allopurinol (but not ampicillin) and rashes occurred in six (2.1%), whereas the corresponding frequency for nonrecipients was 185 out of 8,759 (2.1%). Thus, in nonrecipients of ampicillin the rash frequency with allopurinol was no different from the remainder of the monitored population.

The final analyses were confined to *patients receiving ampicillin*. The frequencies of rashes were compared between (a) "allopurinol recipients" who received both allopurinol and ampicillin together for one or more days and (b) "nonrecipients" comprising the remaining patients. The following rashes were not included: (1) those occurring within 24 hr of transfusion of blood or its derivatives and attributed to these agents and (b) those appearing either before administration of the two drugs in combination or more than 21 days after the initiation of ampicillin treatment.

The final study material consisted of 1,325 patients who received ampicillin. Of these, 67 were allopurinol recipients and 1,257 were nonrecipients (Table 1).

The sex ratios in the two treatment groups were similar. The frequency of malignant diseases was higher among allopurinol recipients, but overall rash frequencies were similar for patients with malignant diseases and for patients with other diseases. While the rash frequency was high in the case of gout, this was not controlled because of small numbers (seven patients, four rashes).

The frequencies of rashes among allopurinol recipients and nonrecipients were 22.4 and 7.5%, respectively ($p < 0.00005$) (Table 1). Apart from allopurinol, there were no other drugs significantly associated with ampicillin rashes.

The data thus suggest that the allergenicity of ampicillin is enhanced by

TABLE 1. *Frequencies of rashes in relation to use of allopurinol among patients receiving ampicillin by sex*

	Allopurinol recipients			Allopurinol nonrecipients			Total		
	No. of rashes	No. of patients	Percent rashes	No. of rashes	No. of patients	Percent rashes	No. of rashes	No. of patients	Percent rashes
Males	5	38	13.2	36	681	5.3	41	719	5.7
Females	10	29	34.5	58	576	10.1	68	605	11.2
Total	15	67	22.4	94	1,257	7.5	109	1,324	8.2

All recipients versus all nonrecipients: X^2 (1 d.f.) $= 16.80$; $p < 0.00005$.
Point estimate of relative risk: 2.99; 95% confidence limits, 1.76–4.62.

allopurinol, or alternatively, by hyperuricemia. This relationship cannot be explained without invoking interaction because the frequency of drug-attributed rashes among recipients of allopurinol who did not receive ampicillin was only 2.1%, a rate similar to that observed among ampicillin nonusers in general.

The data do not permit an evaluation as to whether the potentiation should be ascribed to allopurinol or to its indication, hyperuricemia, since in the surveillance program, there is no routine assessment of uric acid levels. Moreover, whereas gout could be taken as an indirect indicator of hyperuricemia, there was only one patient with this diagnosis who received ampicillin without allopurinol.

Finally, the data could be interpreted to indicate that ampicillin potentiates allopurinol eruptions, rather than the reverse. However, ampicillin is clearly the more allergenic of the two drugs when given alone. For this reason, it seems likely that it is ampicillin rashes that occur in excess when allopurinol is administered concomitantly.

Another finding resulting from our study related an association noted between tetracycline administration and drug-attributed rises in BUN. This association, first seen on a routine scan, was not entirely unexpected since numerous case reports have appeared in the literature that suggest that tetracyclines may induce a clinically significant rise in BUN. The current data base allowed us to evaluate this problem to a considerable degree in terms of verifying this potential undesired effect, providing some quantitation of the effect, if it exists, and evaluating patient factors and the concomitant administration of other drugs that may contribute to the effect.

The data revealed that, whereas 25 of the 147 patients in whom a rise in BUN was reported received tetracycline, the drug itself was implicated by the attending physician in only seven instances.

In the detailed investigation of this finding, the study material was restricted by excluding patients who received known nephrotoxic antibiotics (amphotericin, polymixin B, colistin, kanamycin, gentamycin, and neomycin) and patients who did not receive diuretics. The latter restriction was applied because the vast majority of the patients (not receiving nephrotoxic drugs) with reported rise in BUN had received diuretics (82/89 = 92%).

The remaining patients were divided into three comparison groups: Group T — patients receiving tetracycline; Group A — patients receiving any antibiotic other than tetracycline; and Group N — patients receiving no antibiotics. The homogeneity of Group A was verified: all antibiotics in this group had closely similar frequencies of drug-attributed rise in BUN.

Factors explored as possibly providing an explanation for the observed association between tetracycline and rise in BUN included age, sex, hospital, BUN level of admission, survival, and first discharge diagnosis.

Stratification and discriminant function analysis were employed in this evaluation.

VALIDITY OF COMPARISONS

The numbers of patients in Groups T, A, and N were 204, 596, and 1,137, respectively. The distributions of these groups by age and sex were similar, and therefore, these factors were not controlled in further analysis. In addition, the distribution of patients with rise in BUN and those without were similar with respect to hospital, survival and discharge diagnosis, and so the latter factors also were not controlled. However, there were differences between the comparison groups with regard to admission BUN, and this factor was taken into account in evaluating the relationship between tetracycline-diuretic receipt and recorded rise in BUN.

TETRACYCLINE AND RISE IN BUN (TABLE 2)

The observed, unadjusted frequency of drug-attributed rise in BUN among diuretic recipients was 9.8% for Group T, 3.5% for Group A, and 3.4% for Group N. When the subjects were stratified by admission BUN, there was a higher frequency of recorded rise in BUN in the tetracycline group in each stratum. By the Mantel-Haenszel test (2) the differences between Groups T and A, and separately, between Groups T and N, were significant at p values of less than 0.001 and 0.0005, respectively. The discriminant function analysis gave no evidence of confounding in this relationship.

The mean rise in those with a recorded rise in BUN was 28.3 mg/100 ml (range, 6 to 77 mg/100 ml). The mean rise was similar in the three groups. In five of the 20 patients in Group T, serial creatinine levels were available, and of these, four had a rise in creatinine reported at the time of the rise in BUN.

TABLE 2. *Frequency of recorded rise in BUN among recipients of diuretics in relation to admission BUN levels[a]*

Admission BUN level (mg/100 ml)	Group T	Group A	Group N
≤25	8/112 = 7.1%	5/333 = 1.5%	20/790 = 2.5%
>25	12/92 = 13.0%	16/263 = 6.1%	19/367 = 5.2%
All levels	20/204 = 9.8%	21/596 = 3.5%	39/1157 = 3.4%

Group T = tetracycline recipients.
Group A = recipients of other antibiotics.
Group N = recipients of other drugs.
[a] These data are to be read in a comparative rather than a quantitative sense, because only a fraction of BUN rises are detected.

DOSE, ROUTE, AND TIME RELATIONSHIP

There were no differences in the mean daily dose and route of administration of tetracycline between patients with reported rises in BUN and those without.

In 18 out of 20 cases of rise in BUN in association with tetracycline-diuretic exposure, tetracycline was administered within 1 week prior to the reported rise. In the remaining two instances, one patient received tetracycline 8 weeks before, and the other 3 weeks after, the detected rise in BUN.

This study of a large series of hospitalized medical patients is the first systematic evaluation of the existence of a relationship between tetracycline treatment and a clinically important rise in BUN level. It showed that, when this drug was given together with diuretics, the recorded frequency of this event was threefold, relative to patients receiving diuretics without tetracycline. The statistical significance ($p < 0.001$) of the difference between tetracycline recipients and those in the comparison groups was high, and the association remained strong and highly significant, even when taking into account various patient characteristics, whether by stratification, or by discriminant function analysis.

Whereas there was no apparent relationship between the rise in BUN and dose or route of administration of tetracycline, the time relationship between tetracycline exposure and rise in BUN was striking, in that 18 out of 20 patients received tetracycline within the week immediately preceding the rise in BUN.

We were also able to demonstrate that patients in the tetracycline-diuretic group who developed a rise in BUN had admission BUN levels which were higher than those who did not, suggesting that those with pre-existing renal impairment are more prone to develop this complication.

Little information is available from the surveillance program on the tendency of tetracycline to produce uremia in the absence of diuretics, because a search for this event is generally prompted by diuretic treatment. In addition, the data from this study do not allow for speculation as to the etiology of the tetracycline-associated rise in BUN, particularly as the finding relates to patients who received other drugs (i.e., diuretics) that act on the kidney. However, the finding of a coincidental rise in creatinine levels in four out of five cases in the tetracycline group where this information was available suggests that, at least in those cases, deterioration in renal function was a factor in the observed rise.

These data, derived from an intensive drug surveillance program, provide evidence that tetracycline therapy in patients receiving diuretics is associated with an increased risk of developing clinically significant uremia, particularly in those with an initially elevated BUN level.

Finally, I would like to present data that were obtained following a detailed analysis of our entire data base designed to evaluate a hypothesis of a drug interaction recently reported in the literature.

Sellers and Koch-Weser demonstrated that trichloracetic acid, a major metabolite of chloral hydrate, displaces warfarin from its binding sites on plasma albumin (3). This action temporarily raises plasma levels of unbound warfarin, and this increases the pharmacologic effect per unit dose. In their studies, Sellers and Koch-Weser also demonstrated that increased plasma levels of unbound warfarin are associated with a decrease in the plasma half-life of the drug.

Griner et al. (4) and Udall (5) studied the potential interaction of warfarin and chloral hydrate in a clinical setting and failed to show an increased prothrombin time in patients given warfarin and chloral hydrate together. However, these authors studied patients for periods of months, and specific detailed data on a possible early effect were not presented.

For the present study, all patients who received warfarin were identified. Details of warfarin therapy were examined, and a record was made of other relevant drugs administered to each patient. In particular, all patients who received chloral hydrate were identified, and the potential influence of this drug on warfarin therapy was explored.

Since the primary purpose of this study was to evaluate the influence of chloral hydrate on early stages of anticoagulation, patients who entered the hospital on continuous long-term warfarin therapy were excluded from subsequent analyses. Thus, only those anticoagulated in the hospital were included. These patients were divided into three treatment groups: Group N–patients who did not receive chloral hydrate; Group CH–patients who received chloral hydrate daily during the first 4 days of warfarin therapy; and Group O–patients who received at least one but less than four doses of chloral hydrate during the first 4 days of warfarin therapy.

For each treatment group, the following data were tabulated: loading dose of warfarin (1st day), total dose of warfarin given on the following 3 days (2nd to 4th days), and mean daily maintenance dose for the remainder of the warfarin therapy.

Unless an adverse reaction occurred, no information was available on the prothrombin levels in these patients, since these data were not routinely collected by the nurse monitors.

PATIENT CHARACTERISTICS AND VALIDITY OF COMPARISON

Of the 10,447 patients monitored, 408 received warfarin (4%). Of these, 134 were anticoagulated in the hospital (33%). The mean age of the latter patients was 57 years; 55% were male and the mean weight was 75 kg. The number of patients in Groups N, CH, and O were 67, 32, and 35, respec· tively. Age, sex, weight, and duration of stay in hospital were similar in the three groups. The frequency of barbiturate administration among patients in Groups N, CH, and O was also similar (27%, 31%, and 34%, respectively).

LOADING DOSE OF WARFARIN (TABLE 3)

The mean loading dose of warfarin was similar in the three treatment groups – 23.1 mg in Group N, 24.5 mg in Group CH, and 23.9 mg in Group O (*p* greater than 0.4).

EARLY WAFARIN DOSE (2ND TO 4TH DAYS)

The mean (±SEM) total dose of warfarin given during the 3 days after the loading dose was highest among patients in Group N (22.3 ± 1.8 mg), and lowest among patients in Group CH (15.4 ± 2.2 mg). The difference was statistically significant (*p* less than 0.01). The mean dose (±SEM) in Group O was intermediate between the other groups (18.6 ± 2.1 mg), but was not significantly different from either.

MAINTENANCE DOSE OF WARFARIN

The mean daily dose of warfarin given after the 4th day was similar in the three treatment groups – 6.3 mg in Group N, 6.8 mg in Group CH, and 6.6 mg in Group O (*p* greater than 0.5).

Reported adverse reactions related to hypoprothrombinemia were infrequent in the comparison groups (four of 67 in Group N, one of 32 in Group CH, and one of 35 in Group O).

This study demonstrates that, in the routine clinical setting, patients given continuous chloral hydrate therapy receive less warfarin during the induc-

TABLE 3. *Influence of chloral hydrate on warfarin dosage*

Group	Warfarin therapy		
	Loading dose (mg ± SE)[a]	Total dose (days 2–4) (mg ± SE)	Daily maintenance dose (mg ± SE)
N	23.1 ± 1.0 (67)	22.3 ± 1.8 (67)	6.3 ± 0.5 (67)
CH	24.5 ± 1.7 (32)	15.4 ± 2.2 (32)	6.8 ± 0.9 (32)
O	23.9 ± 1.6 (35)	18.6 ± 2.1 (35)	6.6 ± 0.8 (35)

[a] SE = Standard Error
Figures in parentheses give number of patients in each group.
Group N = No chloral hydrate.
Group CH = Daily chloral hydrate for first 4 days of warfarin therapy.
Group O = Occasional chloral hydrate for first 4 days of warfarin therapy.

tion phase of anticoagulation. The magnitude of the decrease during the 2nd to 4th days is approximately one-third, averaging 22.3 mg in those who received no chloral hydrate, as compared with 15.4 mg in those who received continuous chloral hydrate during this period. In addition, similar maintenance doses of warfarin were given to newly anticoagulated patients when those who did and those who did not receive chloral hydrate were compared.

Although the prothrombin levels attained in these patients were not routinely measured by nurse monitors, it is unlikely that physicians would accept a lower level of anticoagulation in patients receiving chloral hydrate than in those not receiving this hypnotic. Moreover, if such a level were accepted, it would have to be assumed that the policy operated only during the induction phase of anticoagulation – an assumption that seems highly unlikely. It is therefore concluded that patients receiving continuous chloral hydrate therapy require less warfarin during the induction phase of anticoagulant therapy.

The data are fully consistent with the finding of Sellers and Koch-Weser that a transient rise in prothrombin time follows the displacement of warfarin from plasma albumin by chloral hydrate metabolites. This rise is due to an increase in the level of unbound (active) drug, which subsequently falls owing to increased metabolic inactivation leading to a reduction in the half-life of the drug in the plasma.

Finally, we now have data to suggest an interaction between allopurinol and antitumor agents, leading to increased clinically detrimental bone marrow depression. Our series included 160 patients with neoplastic disease (other than leukemia) who were treated with cytotoxic drugs. Drug-attributed, undesired bone marrow depression was more common in 65 patients who also received allopurinol, as compared with 95 patients who did not ($p < 0.005$). Among 58 recipients of cyclophosphamide, the frequencies of bone marrow depression in allopurinol recipients and nonrecipients were 58 and 19%, respectively. In 102 patients who received other cytotoxic drugs bone marrow depression occurred in 18% of patients who also received allopurinol, as compared to 10% of those who did not. An interaction between allopurinol and cytotoxic drugs is a possible explanation of these findings.

In summary, I have presented a number of findings relating to possible drug interactions which have resulted from a comprehensive drug monitoring study. It is our impression that this study can be of substantial value in uncovering and evaluating such interactions in the clinical setting.

ACKNOWLEDGMENTS

Hospitals currently participating in the Boston Collaborative Drug Surveillance Program are: Boston, Massachusetts – Peter Bent Brigham

Hospital, Massachusetts General Hospital, and University Hospital; Providence, Rhode Island — Roger Williams General Hospital; Canada — St. Joseph's Hospital, London, Ontario; New Zealand — Auckland Hospital; Israel — Hadassah-Hebrew University Hospital.

The Boston Collaborative Drug Surveillance Program is supported by Public Health Service Contract No. NIH-72–2010 from the National Institute of General Medical Sciences (NIGMS), and *in part* by grants from the Veterans Administration, the Canadian Food and Drug Directorate, the Israeli Ministry of Health, Auckland Hospital, Auckland, New Zealand, the Roger Williams General Hospital (Brown University NIGMS grant No. GM 165–38–02), and Hoffmann LaRoche, Inc.

REFERENCES

1. Jick, H., Miettinen, O. S., Shapiro, S., Lewis, G. P., Siskind, V., and Slone, D. (1970): *JAMA 213*, 1455.
2. Mantel, M., and Haenszel, W. (1959): *J. Nat. Cancer Inst. 22*, 719.
3. Sellers, E. M., and Koch-Weser, J. (1970): *N. Engl. J. Med. 283*, 827.
4. Griner, P. F., Raisz, L. G., Rickles, F. R., et al. (1971): *Ann. Intern. Med., 75*, 540.
5. Udall, J. A. (1971): *Ann. Intern. Med. 75*, 141.

Drug Interactions, edited by P. L. Morselli,
S. Garattini, and S. N. Cohen. Raven Press,
New York © 1974

Automatic Monitoring of Drug–Laboratory Test Interactions

D. S. Young,* R. B. Friedman,† and L. C. Pestaner*

Clinical Pathology Department, Clinical Center, National Institutes of Health, Bethesda, Maryland 20014 and †Department of Medicine, University of Wisconsin, Madison, Wisconsin 53706

INTRODUCTION

With the advances that have been made in analytical instrumentation and methodology for clinical laboratory tests, it is possible to observe that the physiological regulation of the concentration of many blood constituents is very precise. When specimens are obtained and analyzed under reproducible conditions biological variability becomes the major source of day-to-day differences in laboratory data for healthy individuals. In a hospital patient, considerable changes in laboratory data may occur over a period of time. Although much of this is probably due to alteration of the disease processes, we have become concerned about the role of drug therapy in modifying test values.

The major influences on laboratory data in healthy individuals are summarized in Table 1. Therapeutic drugs may affect laboratory data through three of the mechanisms listed. In the normal individual various physiological processes may be altered and in the sick person the underlying disease process may also be modified. Blood collected shortly after the administration of a drug is likely to show the maximum effect of the drug as well as the highest concentration of the drug. In a clinical laboratory when nonspecific analytical procedures are used, certain drugs may be measured as the major analyte or interfere with the method, so that incorrect results are reported to the patient-care physician.

It is now quite common for as many as 10 drugs to be prescribed at one time for a patient and more than 20 laboratory tests may be ordered on a single sample of blood. It is impossible for a physician to know all the physiological influences of drugs that he commonly prescribes and he is likely to be even less certain about those drugs that he uses occasionally. Few patient-care physicians are aware of the possible effects of drugs on chemical methods, and most are ignorant of the analytical procedures used to derive the data on which they depend for making their diagnoses and determining treatment.

TABLE 1. *Factors influencing laboratory data*

Genetic (interindividual) influences
Physiological (intraindividual) factors
Sampling related physiological influences
Specimen-collection procedures
Specimen-handling procedures
Analytical factors in the laboratory

To reduce misinterpretations, we have developed a computer-based system whereby the drugs prescribed for a patient may be matched with the laboratory tests ordered on specimens from the same patient. The central computer file contains a listing of the effects of drugs on laboratory tests. By use of the system, it is possible to produce reports indicating the possible modification of test values by the drugs administered to a patient. The system permits the clinical laboratory staff to obtain information that is essential for proper interpretation of laboratory data without placing any additional burden on patient-care physicians or the pharmacy staff (Fig. 1).

STRUCTURE OF THE DATA FILE

The file has been organized so that it may be used in response to typed-in queries or on-line when the identity of a patient and the administered drugs are entered. The file that has been used for the initial evaluation of the on-line mode of operation contains approximately 8,000 entries, although the number currently available is almost double this.

The file is so structured that, if the proprietary name of a drug is entered into the computer, it will respond with the generic name. If the name of a mixture is entered, the computer will list all the components. Searches are

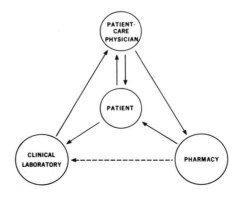

FIG. 1. Information flow required for optimal utilization of laboratory data. The dotted line indicates the critical step necessary for the automatic monitoring program.

MORPHINE	B	PCO2 INC	V	DIMINISHES VENTILATION, CAUSES HYPERCAPNIA	R0026
MORPHINE	O	BMR DEC	V	METABOLIC EFFECT OF DRUG	R0596
MORPHINE	O	GASTRIC JUICE HCL DEC	V	SLIGHT DEC IN SECRETION OF ACID	R0384
MORPHINE	P	AMMONIA INC	V	IMPAIRS ABILITY OF LIVER TO METABOLIZE NH3 IN DOGS	R0931
MORPHINE	P	EPINEPHRINE INC	V	MECHANISM OBSCURE ALSO INVOLVED IN GLUCOSE RELEASE	R0496
MORPHINE	P	HISTAMINE INC	V	OBSERVED WITH INJECT ASSOC WITH ANESTHESIA	R2828
MORPHINE	P	NOREPINEPHRINE DEC	V	MECHANISM OBSCURE	R0496
MORPHINE	P	17 KETOSTEROIDS DEC	V	INHIBITS ACTH AND PIT GONADOTROPIN RELEASE	R0384
MORPHINE	P	17 OH CORTICOSTEROIDS DEC	V	INHIBITS ACTH AND PIT GONADOTROPIN RELEASE	R0384
MORPHINE	S	ALKALINE PHOSPHATASE INC	V	ASSOCIATED WITH ABNORMAL LIVER FUNCTION	R0620
MORPHINE	S	AMYLASE INC	V	CAUSES SPASM OF SPHINCTER OF ODDI FOR 48 HOURS	R0907
MORPHINE	S	BARBITURATE Z	N	NO INTERFERENCE WITH UV ABSORPTION METHODS	R0779
MORPHINE	S	BILIRUBIN INC	V	ASSOCIATED WITH ABNORMAL LIVER FUNCTION	R0620
MORPHINE	S	BSP RETENTION INC	V	ABNORMAL LIVER FUNCTION TESTS REPORTED	R1001
MORPHINE	S	CPK INC	V	RESPONSE TO FREQUENT I.M. INJECTIONS	R0080
MORPHINE	S	CPK Z	V	NO CHANGE, ALTHOUGH OTHER ENZYMES INC	R0657
MORPHINE	S	GLUCOSE INC	V	MINOR, CLINICALLY INSIGNIFICANT INCREASE	R0384
MORPHINE	S	HBD INC	V	PROB DUE TO SPASM OF SPHINCTER OF ODDI	R0657
MORPHINE	S	INDOCYANINE GREEN DEC	V	OBSERVED IN SMALL SERIES, NORMAL LFT	R5007
MORPHINE	S	LACTIC DEHYDROGENASE INC	V	MAY CAUSE RISE IN INTRABILIARY PRESSURE	R0907

FIG. 2. Partial print-out from the file of the effects of morphine on laboratory tests.

then made on the basis of each component. Searches may also be made by class of compound, e.g., diuretics or as a member of a subclass, e.g., thiazide diuretics. Each drug-test effect comprises a single line entry as illustrated in Fig. 2. The drug name is followed by a single letter abbreviation to indicate the body fluid involved in the interaction. This is followed by the name of the test and a statement indicating whether the result is decreased, increased, or unaffected by the drug. A single letter is used to indicate whether the reported effect is of physiological (*in vivo*) origin or whether it is due to interference with an analytical method in use in the laboratory. For automatic interpretation, only those methods actually in use in the laboratory of the hospital involved in the study are considered.

For the physiological effects included in the latest version of the file, we have attempted to indicate the probability of an effect occurring by the use of subscripts. Thus, 0 indicates an isolated case report, whereas 3 indicates that it occurs in more than 20% of all instances in which the drug is used. In each entry, we include a brief English-language description of the effect and where possible indicate the dose of drug or its concentration in serum at which the effect has been observed. The entry also contains a reference number, and in a separate file we list the authors, title of article, and journal citation of an appropriate reference to this effect. The entry in the main file is completed by our three-digit laboratory test number which, with the number we have assigned each drug, is essential for matching of drugs and tests in the on-line mode.

Approximately 75% of the entries in the file are physiological effects, whereas the remainder are methodological. The information used for the file is obtained from the clinical, pharmacological, and chemical literature for the most part, but we also make use of our personal experience and information supplied by pharmaceutical manufacturers.

USE OF THE SYSTEM

The data base is used as a system to warn physicians or laboratory scientists of potential effects of drugs on laboratory tests. We stress that the information contained in it can not be used to provide a literal explanation for unusual laboratory results when a patient is receiving the drugs included in the file. The file information is accessible in three forms: (a) published version, (b) written or telephone query, and (c) on-line operation.

At appropriate intervals, the file will be published in a scientific journal with widespread distribution throughout clinical laboratories so that individuals who require the information have it available for interpretation of results. We envisage a microfiche version so that it may be scanned readily in a central location such as a hospital library or ward. Publication at intervals does not permit all the information in the file to be made available to potential users, so that we are providing additional information in response to enquiries. These have come from patient-care physicians and laboratory scientists at the National Institutes of Health, and elsewhere, who have been unable to explain abnormal results on a patient's medical condition alone, and also from manufacturers of pharmaceuticals seeking information required for new drug applications to the Food and Drug Administration and other purposes.

Whereas, in theory, it is possible for any individual with a telephone communication terminal to interrogate the file in the National Institutes of Health time-shared computer system, we have not yet made the file freely accessible so that all requests for information must be processed by one of the laboratory staff. This enables us to determine the purpose for which the information is used and the clinical usefulness of the system.

On several occasions, it has been possible to provide information that has led to new diagnoses. In one case, the large doses of ascorbic acid that a patient was ingesting caused falsely negative tests for occult blood in spite of gastrointestinal bleeding to which her anemia could be attributed. In another patient, chlorpromazine was determined to be the cause of a falsely positive immunological pregnancy test. On these occasions search of the file also was able to provide possible explanations rapidly for the unanticipated results.

Although the system was not developed initially for on-line interpretation of laboratory data, this appeared to be a logical application in view of the number of queries the laboratory received concerning the effects of drugs on laboratory tests. Fortunately, the file was so structured that it could be used equally well in an automatic mode with correlation of the drugs administered to patients and the tests ordered on many patients at the same time, as in the look-up made in response to individual queries.

On-line use of the system was initially evaluated in one ward at the Clinical Center of the National Institutes of Health, but because of the need to study a greater variety of diseases and therapeutic regimes than available at the National Institutes of Health the trial evaluation was continued in two wards in the University of Wisconsin Hospital. Some minor modifications were made to the system to allow for different analytical methods, etc., in use in the clinical laboratories there.

ON-LINE INTERPRETATION OF DATA

The data base for the trial at the University of Wisconsin consisted of approximately 8,000 drug-laboratory test combinations. It has been used in two wards. Ward A is nominally a general medical ward but with almost half the patients having a gynecological malignancy and subjected to radiation therapy and radium implants. Ward B is an acute medical ward and the patients typically have a myocardial infarct, pneumonia, diabetes, or similar acute disorder. From January to July over 5,500 patient-days have been followed. Most of the patients studied have been in Ward A.

The drugs in use in the University of Wisconsin are assigned a numerical code. Each component of a mixture is assigned the appropriate code. Information on the drugs used in the hospital is obtained from the pharmacy and incorporated into a matrix in the computer file in which the drugs and the laboratory tests are correlated. The matrix is stored on magnetic tape and loaded into the computer each day. Rather than matching all test values with the drugs ordered, the computer is programmed to produce a report only when abnormal values are obtained or when marked trends develop for data within the normal range over 3-day intervals. The decision-making process that is used is illustrated in Fig. 3. A report is only generated when a specific match of drug and test is made and thus is linked to the physician requisitioning of laboratory tests. The system is concerned with chemistry and hematology laboratory tests only at the present time; although if interactions between drugs and other laboratory tests existed, it would be possible to incorporate this information into the program. A summary of the findings to the present time is illustrated in Table 2.

During the preliminary evaluation period approximately 4,000 drug–laboratory test interactions were printed. Listing occurred when abnormal laboratory test values were identified. The normal range of values used within the University of Wisconsin Hospital was used to determine the threshold values. On one occasion only, a report was initiated by a 3-day trend developing within the normal range. We observed that when a trend did develop values on the 3rd day were abnormal, which provided the main mechanism for the listing of an interaction. Physicians rarely ordered the

DECISION-MAKING PROCESS — WHICH PATIENTS WILL BE PROCESSED?

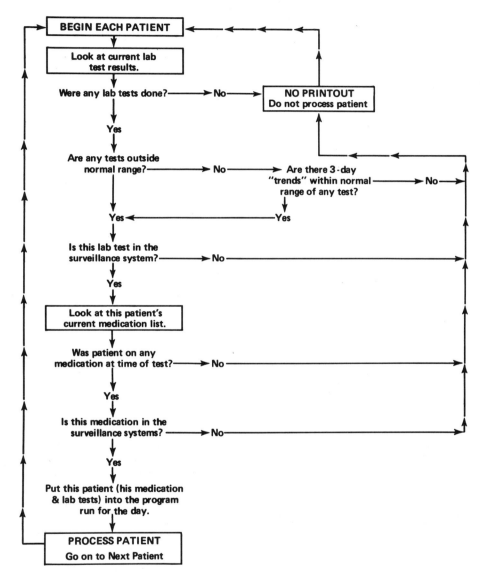

FIG. 3. Logic used to determine which patients are processed for the automatic interpretation of laboratory data.

TABLE 2. *Summary of observations*

	Ward A	Ward B
Days in use	246	45
Average daily census (patients)	24.1	23.4
Patients meeting criteria for processing (P.P.[a]) per day	4.0	3.9
Average no. of drugs received per P.P. per day	9.0	6.3
Drugs with interactions per P.P. per day	3.3	2.0
Abnormal tests per P.P. per day	3.7	3.8
Tests with interactions per P.P. per day	2.7	2.0
Total no. of interactions/day/ward	20.7	13.1
Interactions per P.P. per ward	5.2	3.4
Interactions per patient (processed and unprocessed) per day	0.9	0.6

[a] P.P. indicates a patient meeting the criteria for processing in Fig. 3.

same laboratory test with sufficient frequency, when test values were within the normal range, to obtain enough data over successive days for the trend program to be initiated.

The drug–laboratory test interaction reports were evaluated by the interns and resident physicians in charge of the patients. Subsequently, 150 of the patient charts — mainly from the general medical ward — were evaluated by one of us (R.B.F.). The evaluations yielded similar information. Eight percent of the interactions implicated toxic doses of drugs and 40% cited toxic effects of drugs. None of these was likely to be the correct explanation in a hospital population under well-controlled therapeutic regimes. Of the remaining 52% the effect listed provided a possible explanation for the change in laboratory data. However, for 31% an alternative explanation was provided by alteration of the patients' medical condition. In almost 21% of the drug–test interactions the file provided the most probable explanation for alteration of the laboratory data, although the effect had already been recognized by the patient-care physicians without the assistance of the file. Many of these effects were related to the influence of diuretic drugs and dietary supplements.

Of the 4,000 interactions reported to the patient-care physicians, there were four admitted instances in which therapy was changed as a result of the alerting of the physician to a potential problem by the drug interaction report. We suspect that there were more cases, but, as admission of change by a physician in response to the print-out could be interpreted as a reflection on his knowledge, we believe that the incidence is underestimated. One case involved the possible action of allopurinol and colchicine on liver function and a liver biopsy was postponed when it was noted that changes of liver function coincided with administration of the drugs. In the second case in a patient receiving warfarin, prothrombin activity was modified markedly when reserpine was administered and the dose of the anticoagulant was modified in response to the combined action of the drugs.

In the third case, an intensive work-up of a low serum phosphate was postponed in a patient with a peptic ulcer when it was noted that an aluminum salt administered as an antacid could cause binding of phosphate ions in the gastrointestinal tract and inhibit their absorption. In the fourth case, the initial diagnosis of pheochromocytoma in a patient was excluded when it was noted that α-methyl-DOPA which had been used to treat the patient's hypertension also reacted chemically as if it were vanillylmandelic acid in the quantitative test to measure the compound.

COST OF THE SYSTEM

In the computer in use for the trial at the University of Wisconsin, the file is stored on magnetic tape and is loaded into the computer each day from the tape. The cost of loading the tape is $0.40 per day included in the total cost of using the system of approximately $2.50 per day. At present, approximately 48 patients are monitored daily so that the overall cost averages $0.05 per patient per day. If the number of patients was to be increased, the cost per patient would be decreased slightly.

PHYSICIAN ACCEPTANCE

Initially the reports were not as well received by physicians as we had anticipated until we learned that repetitive listing every day of the same effect caused by the same drug irritated the patient-care staff. When the program was modified to list the same drug-test combination twice only, the medical staff was more enthusiastic. In general, specialists in internal medicine were much more receptive to the program than gynecologists. We will assess the responsiveness of surgeons in the next phase of the study. On questioning the interns, residents, and attending physicians who actually reviewed the reports, more than 90% expressed their enthusiasm for the scheme, citing in particular its educational benefits, and 85% advocated its expansion to include the entire hospital.

STRENGTHS AND WEAKNESSES OF THE SYSTEM

The file was not initially developed for use in interpreting laboratory results automatically. We did not include probabilities of an effect occurring. For this purpose, it is unnecessary to include those effects which are, in effect, the intent of the administration of the drug. Again in hospital practice, there is little need to include drug overdoses or toxicity effects as these are rare except in a toxicological center. It would be desirable to correlate the cumulative dose, or serum concentration of drugs that had been required to produce some of the rare effects that had been reported, especially with reference to depression of the bone marrow. It would be desirable to include changes in laboratory data that might arise through the interaction of two drugs that did not occur when each was administered separately. It would be helpful to indicate the possible magnitude of response that could be anticipated with a particular regime.

When tests are ordered on an intermittent basis, it is impossible to follow in detail the development of trends in laboratory data, yet our own experience has indicated that trends within the normal range may precede overt abnormalities by many days. It is difficult to observe the effects of one drug in isolation because rarely is only one drug administered to a patient. It is difficult to gain the background data required to build the information needed in the detail that is required for the system to be fully effective.

FUTURE PLANS

As far as possible, we intend to eliminate the major weaknesses that are outlined above. The improved system, which will also be enlarged, will be evaluated in a community hospital to determine the response of less academically orientated physicians. Again we will study the medical benefits to the hospital patients from use of the program. In another hospital, we intend to study the cost-benefits to patients arising solely from not performing certain laboratory tests when the patient was exposed to certain medications. In both of these situations, we anticipate that the system will lead to an overall improvement in health care. Further, we intend to continue the use of the expanded system (now approaching 16,000 entries) for interpretation of abnormal data both within our laboratories, and in response to written or telephone queries.

INDEX